Infection Prevention and Control

Infection Prevention and Control

Theory and Clinical Practice for Healthcare Professionals

DEBBIE WESTON
Infection Control Advisor, East Kent Hospital

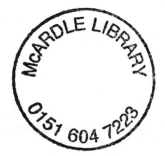

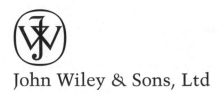

John Wiley & Sons, Ltd

Other Wiley Editorial Offices

John Wiley & Sons Inc., 111 River Street, Hoboken, NJ 07030, USA

Jossey-Bass, 989 Market Street, San Francisco, CA 94103-1741, USA

Wiley-VCH Verlag GmbH, Boschstr. 12, D-69469 Weinheim, Germany

John Wiley & Sons Australia Ltd, 42 McDougall Street, Milton, Queensland 4064, Australia

John Wiley & Sons (Asia) Pte Ltd, 2 Clementi Loop #02-01, Jin Xing Distripark, Singapore 129809

John Wiley & Sons Canada Ltd, 6045 Freemont Blvd, Mississauga, ONT, L5R 4J3, Canada

Wiley also publishes its books in a variety of electronic formats. Some content that appears in print
may not be available in electronic books.

Library of Congress Cataloging-in-Publication Data

Weston, Debbie.
    Infection prevention and control : theory and clinical practice for healthcare
    professionals / Debbie Weston.
        p.   cm.
    Includes bibliographical references and index.
    ISBN 978-0-470-05907-4 (alk. paper)
    1. Infection—Prevention.   2. Nosocomial infections—Prevention.   I. Title.
    [DNLM: 1. Cross Infection—prevention & control.   2. Hospitals.   3. Infection
    Control—methods. WX 167 W534i 2007]
    RA761.W38 2007
    362.196′9—dc22

                                                                           2007027379

British Library Cataloguing in Publication Data

A catalogue record for this book is available from the British Library

ISBN-13: 978-0-470-05907-4 (P/B)

Typeset in 10/12pt Times by Integra Software Services Pvt. Ltd, Pondicherry, India
Printed and bound in Great Britain by TJ International, Cornwall, UK.

Contents

Foreword

During the past two decades, healthcare-associated infections have become a significant risk to patient safety and acquiring a new infection during episodes of healthcare is a worldwide hazard for both patients and healthcare providers. Prevalence surveys in Europe, Australasia and North America suggest that approximately 5–10 per cent of all inpatients will have acquired a healthcare-associated infection during periods of hospital care. Many of these infections are serious and sometimes fatal. Many are resistant to the antimicrobial drugs usually used to treat them and all of them are distressing and expensive. The financial and personal costs of healthcare-associated infections, in terms of the economic consequences to the National Health Service in the United Kingdom, and the physical, social and psychological costs to patients and their relatives, are severe. The perceived threat of becoming infected during care is undermining the public's confidence in our ability to safely and competently care for them and to protect them from adverse consequences of care.

Although not all of these infections are avoidable, research suggests that at least 20 per cent are potentially preventable. Clinically effective care, i.e. infection prevention and control practices based on reliable evidence of efficacy, is a core component of an effective strategy designed to protect patients from infection. Today's healthcare practitioners need a complex repertoire of knowledge and skills in order to develop and implement evidence-based care that consistently and effectively minimise infection risks to patients and others.

Ready access to current and reliable best evidence for practice is a central feature for ensuring practitioners have the necessary knowledge to plan and deliver safe and clinically effective care. This new text by one of today's most respected senior infection control and prevention specialists is an ideal resource for ensuring access to pertinent and reliable evidence and associated practice information. It is written in an engaging and easily understandable style, and throughout the text the underpinning evidence for best practice recommendations is made crystal clear and applicable. The description of critical learning outcomes at the beginning of each chapter will be appreciated by students and practitioners, as will the comprehensive bibliography of current policy and evidence that is the foundation for best practice.

Debbie Weston has focused on the essential body of infection prevention and control knowledge that all healthcare practitioners need to acquire, understand and then translate into everyday clinical practice. This is a remarkable and totally relevant resource that can support practitioners in continuing to develop more effective evidence-based approaches to protecting patients from infection. For many, it will be the seminal basis for their enhanced understanding of one of the key issues in healthcare that practitioners are confronting.

Protecting patients from harm is at the heart of everything we do. Understanding the background science, evidence and infection prevention and control practices described in this text can positively influence our potential to do just that and ensure that patients are safe during care.

Robert J. Pratt CBE FRCN RN
Professor of Nursing
Director, Richard Wells Research Centre
Thames Valley University

Preface

The prevention and control of infection is everybody's business since it is a fundamental and integral part of healthcare provision. Historically, infection prevention and control has been a speciality with a relatively low profile compared to other areas of health service development, and it has been viewed very much as a 'Cinderella' service, but now the tide is turning and it has become one of the most talked about subjects in both the healthcare and public arena. The high media profile given over to topics such as MRSA, dirty hospitals and poor compliance with hand hygiene, old infectious diseases and the emergence of new ones, together with the changing face of healthcare and new guidance, initiatives and drives to reduce infection rates, should make infection control a priority for everyone involved in patient care. It is, however, a complex and challenging speciality. Unlike most other specialist areas, infection control encompasses not only clinical practice issues in relation to patient care, but also the infection control aspects of the environment, together with the health and safety of members of the public and healthcare workers. It is therefore essential that healthcare professionals have a firm grasp of both the principles of infection control which they can relate to clinical practice, and the current issues. The aim of this book is to provide the reader with a valuable resource that will not only enhance their knowledge and understanding of infection control but also encourage them to look at their own clinical practice, and that of others, and develop a real interest in, and enthusiasm for, the subject so that they can make a difference to patient care.

Acknowledgements

I would like to acknowledge the invaluable support and assistance given to me by the following individuals:

Dr James Nash, Consultant Microbiologist/Deputy Director Infection Prevention and Control, East Kent Hospitals NHS Trust, for reading the chapter drafts and providing me with so many useful and much appreciated constructive comments.

Dr Graeme Calver, Consultant Microbiologist, East Kent Hospitals NHS Trust, for his assistance with, and contributions to, some of the earlier chapter drafts.

My infection prevention and control nursing team colleagues at East Kent Hospitals NHS Trust – Sue Roberts, Alison Burgess and Sandra Tomlin – for reading the chapter drafts and for their support and encouragement while I was writing this book.

Emma Hatfield, Nicky Skinner, Laura Ferrier and the rest of the team at Wiley.

Edwina Rowling – Editor

Jim McCarthy – Commissioning Editor

Professor Robert Pratt for writing the Foreword

James Murray – Director of Communications, East Kent Hospitals NHS Trust

East Kent Hospitals NHS Trust for permission to reproduce the Trust guidelines (with thanks to Ann Broadhead in the Practice Development Team), and infection control '10 point plans'.

My family and friends.

Finally, I would like to acknowledge Celia Carson, who sadly died in March 2007. Celia provided me with much support and made many valuable comments on the manuscript.

List of Figures

List of Tables

Introduction

This book is written with the intention of providing all healthcare professionals with a valuable and comprehensive text that will equip them with the necessary knowledge base so they can apply the principles and practice of infection prevention and control in their day-to-day work. It is also envisaged that this book will be a useful resource for nurses undertaking undergraduate and postgraduate education and infection control nurses who are new in post. Although it is primarily written for those working in an acute hospital setting, it is hoped that healthcare professionals working in the community also find this book a helpful and useful resource.

The book is in two parts. Part One consists of chapters 1–8. Chapters 1–2 provide the reader with an overview of the history of infectious diseases and infection control, and introduce the reader to the structure and function of bacteria and viruses. Chapters 3–4 aim to enable the reader to gain an insight into the importance of obtaining good quality clinical specimens and the workings of the clinical microbiology laboratory, so that they will understand some of the processes that occur in order to arrive at identifying the cause of the patient's infection, which in turn influences the patient's treatment. Chapter 5 describes the basic components of the immune system and how an immune response is generated in patients with an infection, giving rise to systemic signs and symptoms of illness. Chapter 6 discusses the basic principles that should be applied in everyday clinical practice to prevent cross-infection occurring, and Chapter 7 looks at four of the commonest types of healthcare-associated infections and measures to prevent them from occurring in the first instance. Part One concludes with Chapter 8 which examines the problem of antimicrobial resistance, and the challenges that this presents for patient care and public health. In Part Two, specific organisms, associated infections and preventative measures are discussed. Chapters 9, 10, and 11 examine three infections that are rarely out of the media spotlight – MRSA, tuberculosis and *Clostridium difficile* – with reference in Chapter 11 to the *Clostridium difficile* outbreak at Buckinghamshire NHS Trust in 2003–2005. In Chapters 12 and 13, two particularly virulent organisms which can have devastating consequences for patients, invasive group A streptococcal disease and meningococcal meningitis, are discussed in detail. Chapter 14 looks at norovirus, a viral infection that causes widespread disruption during winter months and generates media interest in the event of ward/hospital closures. The most common bacterial causes of food poisoning are discussed in Chapter 15, along with the Stanley Royd Hospital Salmonella outbreak which occurred in 1984. The public health implications of infections with blood-borne viruses are examined in Chapter 16. Chapters 17 and 18 are given over to SARS and Pandemic Influenza which have huge implications for global health. As the threat of an influenza pandemic is becoming an increasingly likely event at some point in the future, it is important that healthcare workers understand the implications and are aware of pandemic preparedness planning. The BSE crisis and the emergence of variant CJD and implications for public health and clinical practice are discussed in Chapter 19. Finally, Chapter 20 looks at the specific problems associated with Legionella and the potential risks that this organism poses to healthcare premises.

The book can be read as a whole from cover to cover, or dipped in and out of, as each individual chapter stands alone. Chapters are introduced with clear learning outcomes that can be used as self assessment tools, and a general account of the subject matter. Where specific infections are discussed, information relating to the organism and the nature of the resulting infection is given. Throughout the book, national and international guidance, and Department of Health policies, drives and initiatives are discussed. Infection control management and recommendations for clinical practice are highlighted and are evidence based. The glossary at the back of the book explains terms used (in **bold italic**) in the book.

Part I

1 Infection Prevention and Control: Past, Present and Future

INTRODUCTION

Starting with the appointment of the first infection control nurse in 1959, this introductory chapter sets the scene, looking at the profile of the prevention and control of healthcare-associated infection today in conjunction with the challenges facing infection prevention and control teams and the National Health Service as an organisation.

Disease threats old and new are discussed, along with the rising media profile of organisms such as meticillin-resistant *Staphylococcus aureus* and *Clostridium difficile*. The background to the latest Department of Health drives, guidance and initiatives is also discussed, emphasising the root and branch shift towards making the prevention and control of healthcare-associated infection a priority for the NHS and everyone involved in patient care.

THE DEVELOPMENT OF INFECTION PREVENTION AND CONTROL AS A SPECIALITY IN HOSPITALS

In 1941, the British Medical Council recommended that control of infection officers were appointed in hospitals to oversee the control of infection. This was followed in 1944 by the setting up of control of infection committees consisting of clinical and laboratory staff, nurses and administrators. The first infection control nurse, however wasn't appointed in the UK until 1959.[1] The appointment of Miss EM Cottrell, formerly an operating theatre superintendent, as infection control sister at Torbay Hospital, Devon, was in response to a large outbreak of staphylococcal infections, affecting both patients and staff. Staphylococci had been causing problems in hospitals in the UK since 1955, and staphylococcal *surveillance* revealed that the carriage rate amongst nursing staff on two of the major hospital wards was 100%, with high staff absentee levels due to staphylococcal skin sepsis, and evidence of post-operative wound infections and skin sepsis amongst the patients.[1] Miss Cottrell was appointed for an experimental period to assist in the collection of surveillance data and advise on the prevention of cross-infection through rigorous adherence to the principles of *asepsis*. In 1961, a report on the development of the post of an infection control sister was submitted by Dr Brendan Moore, Director of the Public Laboratory in Exeter, to the Joint Advisory Committee on Research of the South West Region Hospital Board. Although the appointment of a nurse as a full-time member of the infection control team was nationally opposed by consultants, infection control sisters were subsequently appointed in many other hospitals.

During the 1960s, an increase in infections caused by Gram-negative bacteria such as *Escherichia, Klebsiella, Pseudomonas* and *Proteus* started to overtake *S. aureus* as agents of cross infection.[2] *Pseudomonas* in particular established itself as a major **opportunistic** hospital **pathogen** in those with underlying illness. The discovery of penicillin by Alexander Fleming in 1928, and its further development and subsequent use in clinical practice in the 1940s, completely transformed the management of infections and infectious diseases. Penicillin was seen as the 'golden bullet' (see Chapter 8 The Problem of Antimicrobial Resistance) and there was enormous expectation that the development of antibiotics would rid the world of infectious diseases. However, during the 1960s and 1970s antibiotic resistance was recognised as an increasing problem and lurking just around the corner were major resistance problems with staphylococci against meticillin, which gave rise to meticillin-resistant *Staphylococcus aureus*. MRSA really started to be become problematic in the 1970s, and exploded during the 1980s (see Chapter 9 Meticillin-resistant *Staphylococcus aureus*). Since then, antibiotic resistance has become increasingly common with most strains of bacteria now resistant to one or more antibiotics, thus representing a major threat to public health.

DISEASE THREATS, OLD AND NEW

It is difficult to predict when a new disease with the potential to wreak havoc and destruction on the human race will emerge, but an increase in the emergence of new diseases and the re-emergence of old ones such as tuberculosis (see Chapter 10) is almost inevitable. Micro-organisms previously unknown or unrecognised, or thought to only cause disease in animals can, and have, evolved to produce more **virulent** strains which can also affect humans, such as new variant CJD (Chapter 19) and avian influenza (Chapter 18). In fact, since the 1970s, more than 30 new infectious diseases have emerged worldwide[3], including Legionnaires' disease (Chapter 20) and HIV and hepatitis C (Chapter 16). An increase in the global population and global travel has led to an increasingly densely packed and mobile population, meaning that an infectious disease such as severe acute respiratory syndrome (Chapter 17), **pandemic** influenza (Chapter 18), pneumonic plague or smallpox could theoretically spread anywhere in the world within a matter of hours.

PLAGUE

Plague has been described as one of the most explosively virulent diseases[4], although it is a term that is used to describe any outbreak of a pandemic nature associated with a high *mortality rate*. The bacterial cause of plague, *Yersinia pestis,* principally affects rodents and is transmitted to humans via the bite of infected fleas. It takes one of three forms. Bubonic plague, which has a fatality rate of 50 % unless treated promptly, affects the local inguinal, cervical or axillary lymph nodes draining the area of the flea bite, causing painful swellings known as buboes[5] which can spread to other parts of the body. It is not transmissible from person to person, unlike pneumonic plague. This is spread by the respiratory droplet route, and develops as a rapidly fatal secondary pneumonia in some people with bubonic plague, although it can also be transmitted as a result of inhaling respiratory droplets containing *Y.pesti.*[4,5] Septicaemic plague commonly occurs as a complication of bubonic or pneumonic plague, although it can also be acquired as a primary infection. The septicaemic rash that develops under the skin gives this form of plague its commonly referred to name of the Black Death.[5]

The infamous Black Death which swept through Europe between 1346 and 1350 killed an estimated 50 million people.[6] Regular *epidemics* occurred and in the Great Plague of 1664–1666, which began in London and rapidly spread to other parts of the country, 70,000 people died. London in the 16th century was a hotbed of extreme poverty, squalor and social deprivation, which created the perfect environment for a large rodent population and the spread of disease. As people fled the city, plague spread to other areas of the country that had previously been unaffected. It became *endemic,* with outbreaks occurring throughout Europe, spreading across the continent via the trade routes. In an attempt to halt the spread, attempts were made to isolate infected communities and the Venetians were the first to introduce the concept of *quarantine* by making sure that incoming ships waited on an island for 40 days before entering the city. Although the number of outbreaks declined after the 17th century, plague remains one of the oldest *notifiable diseases* known to man and it is endemic in many areas of the world today, with 1,000–3,000 cases reported to the World Health Organisation (WHO) each year.[7] Areas of Africa such as the Democratic Republic of Congo, Zambia and Algeria are at risk of outbreaks of plague, together with parts of India and Asia, the former Soviet Union and the South Americas. The Democratic Republic of Congo in particular is a plague zone, and between February 2005 and October 2006 more than 1,100 suspected cases of pneumonic and bubonic plague were reported to WHO, which deployed field teams to the affected areas to provide support to the local authorities.[7]

In the wake of the September 11 2001 terrorist attacks, there are real concerns, although no actual threat as yet, that a *biological agent* could be deliberately released in the UK.[8,9] The Department of Health[10] has formulated national contingency plans detailing the public health response to the deliberate release of biological agents such as plague, smallpox, *anthrax, botulism* and *tularaemia.*

SMALLPOX

If plague is one of the oldest and most virulent infectious diseases, smallpox is one of the most devastating. Believed to have originated in India or Egypt more than

3,000 years ago, repeated epidemics swept through Europe for centuries and as late as the 18th century every 10th child born in Sweden and France, and every 7th child born in Russia died from the disease.[11] Although the last case of smallpox in the UK was in 1901, by 1967 it had threatened up to 60 % of the global population, and WHO launched a collaborative global plan that year to eradicate it. The last naturally occurring case was seen in Somalia in 1977, and WHO declared smallpox eradicated in 1979.[11] Although vaccination against smallpox was effective, it had serious adverse reactions and routine vaccination in the UK ceased in 1971 as the risks from vaccination outweighed the risk of contracting the disease.[11,12] Given that it is no longer a naturally acquired infection, outbreaks can only occur as a result of an accidental release, as in a laboratory incident in Birmingham in 1978[13] in which a medical photographer died and several other people were affected, or through a deliberate release of the virus. Following the Birmingham incident, WHO banned all research and all stocks were destroyed. The only two legitimate stocks of smallpox are held at two WHO approved high security locations – Atlanta, Georgia, USA and Koltsovo, Novosibirsk Region, Russian Federation.[14,15] The Centres for Disease Control (CDC), in Atlanta USA, declared smallpox a category A agent as it poses a potential public health threat if used as a biological weapon.[15] If there were a deliberate release of the smallpox virus, it would be catastrophic. The duration of immunity to smallpox is unknown but is thought to be no longer than 10 years so previously vaccinated individuals are unlikely to still be protected although the disease may be less severe. In response to the potential public health threat, the Department of Health published guidance in 2003[16] which details the action to be taken in the event of a deliberate release of the virus in the UK, focusing on the isolation of affected cases and the vaccination of contacts.

THE PREVENTION AND CONTROL OF INFECTION – THE CURRENT SITUATION

As medicine and healthcare have progressed immeasurably over the last 50 years, so too has the microbial world and the nature of infections and infectious diseases. With more and more patients undergoing major surgery and invasive diagnostic procedures, they are actually now more at risk from potentially life-threatening infections than ever before. An increasing elderly population, with weakened immunity and increased susceptibility to infections as a result of underlying illness and disease, represents a huge challenge to healthcare teams. Many hospitals are now no longer able to cope with the population that they were originally built to serve. Higher bed occupancy rates, patient turnaround times and increased movement of patients between wards and departments places huge demand on facilities and resources and inevitably impacts on infection rates.[17] Many NHS Trusts cover large geographical populations, with different pools of patients with different conditions and needs admitted into overcrowded environments. A lack of adequate isolation facilities has often been identified and criticised as an issue that needs to be urgently addressed[18], together with poor staff-to-patient ratios, and these factors can lead to fewer patients being isolated. The problems of competing organisms such as MRSA and *Clostridium difficile* (see Chapter 11) mean that the allocation of a side room to an infected or colonised patient has to be based on a multi-factoral risk assessment. Environmental issues around old, poorly maintained healthcare premises and concerns around poor standards of hygiene and hospital cleanliness[19] are also contributing factors. Inadequate supplies of equipment, especially equipment that is shared between patients, the lack of adequate resources for decontamination and an increase in invasive procedures and the use of invasive indwelling devices (see Chapters 6 and 7) compound the problems. Problems associated with antibiotic resistance and the emergence of multi-resistant bacteria can, to some extent, be controlled through more stringent antibiotic policies, restricted antibiotic prescribing only on the advice of a consultant microbiologist, and compliance with the basic infection control practices such as hand hygiene; but the stakes now need to be raised in terms of increasing the profile of infection prevention and control.

The political climate today, with the introduction of government targets to reduce waiting times in accident and emergency departments and on elective surgery waiting lists[20], has led to claims that there is now a 'target culture' within the NHS. The pursuit of targets at the expense of infection control, with short cuts taken in clinical practice and procedures and practices not always followed to the letter, will almost inevitably give rise to increased infection rates. The recent Healthcare Commission enquiry into an outbreak of *C.difficile* at Stoke Mandeville Hospital in 2005, in which 33 patients died[21] highlights this target culture as the main cause of the outbreak, in which the advice of the Infection Prevention and Control Team and the Health Protection Agency were ignored.

THE PROBLEM OF HEALTHCARE ASSOCIATED INFECTIONS

A healthcare associated infection (HCAI) can be defined as an infection caused by any infectious agent acquired as a consequence of a person's treatment by the NHS, or which is acquired by a healthcare worker in the course of their duties.[22] A hospital acquired infection (HAI) is one which is neither present nor incubating on admission to hospital. National *prevalence* surveys conducted in the UK in 1981 and 1996[23,24] found that 9 % of patients in hospital had an infection that was acquired in hospital, equating to 100,000 patients per year, and it has also been estimated that hospital-acquired infections kill 5,000 patients in the UK each year.[25] They are probably a contributing factor but not the primary cause in at least 15,000 other deaths[25,26] and while it is not possible to prevent all infections, there are several recognised risk factors which increase the risk to patients (see Chapter 5 Understanding the Immune System and the Nature and Pathogenesis of Infection). It is believed that at least 15–30 %, and maybe as much as 50 %, of HCAI infections can be prevented through good clinical practice[25] and applying the basic principles of infection control when undertaking patient care (see Chapter 6 The Principles of Infection Prevention and Control). As well as saving lives, potential avoidable costs could be in the region of £150 million annually.[26]

Patients with an HCAI spend on average an extra 11 days in hospital.[27] Delayed discharges equate to lost beds days for the Trust and loss of revenue, along with money spent on litigation, empirical antibiotic therapy, extra equipment, personal protective clothing and hotel services. Public confidence in the Trust is also dented as a result of adverse publicity, which may mean that patients choose to receive their treatment elsewhere if a hospital is perceived to have problems with healthcare associated infections.

HCAI impacts on a Trust's financial position. Under the new Payments by Results tariff[28] where procedures will attract a defined tariff which will not take account of additional costs incurred by the treatment of an HACI, additional costs of between £160,000 and £400,000 could be incurred in excess of tariff income for the treatment of MRSA bacteraemias, and other HCAIs could increase this figure tenfold.[29]

SAVING LIVES AND GOING FURTHER, FASTER

In 2005, the Department of Health published *Saving Lives: a delivery programme to reduce healthcare associated infection including MRSA.*[30] This programme includes an assessment tool, which is presented as nine key challenges with actions, to support acute NHS Trusts in preparing an organisation-wide action plan integral to its overall strategic direction in reducing HCAIs. In addition, *Saving Lives* also includes six high impact interventions (HIIs) which are simple evidence-based audit tools. Their use is intended to provide a systematic method of measuring and improving compliance with specific clinical procedures such as hand hygiene compliance and insertion of invasive devices, and is designed to be used electronically using ward/department based PCs.

In 2006, *Going Further Faster: Implementing the Saving Lives Delivery Programme. Sustainable Change for Cleaner Safer Health Care*[29] was published as a result of work undertaken by the DH in conjunction with a number of Trusts that have made significant sustained improvements towards the national target of a 50 % reduction in MRSA bloodstream infections (bacteraemias).[31] The main findings and key recommendations for Trusts are as follows:

- HCAI costs the NHS £1 billion per year, and between £4,000 and £10,000 per infection
- HCAI affects all aspects of a Trust's performance
- Trusts have traditionally looked to infection prevention and control teams to reduce HCAI; however, achievement of the MRSA bacteraemia target will require the engagement and active involvement of all staff working at every level of the organisation, supported by the infection prevention and control team and identified 'champions'.
- Performance management should underpin the Trust's strategy to reduce HCAI and drive improvement.

- To realise system-wide change and sustainable improvement, all managers and clinicians need to understand the impact that HCAI has on their services, and work together with the infection prevention and control team to make this everyone's responsibility.
- Reducing HCAI benefits all aspects of the quality and efficiency of patient care. Sustainable improvement in HCAI requires board-level support and endorsement, with every Trust having a prioritised action plan that is integral to its overall strategic direction.
- Trusts must work towards a culture where there are no avoidable infections.
- Trusts must utilise the mandatory enhanced surveillance data for MRSA bacteraemia to focus and prioritise the action plan.
- Each MRSA bacteraemia should be treated as an adverse clinical incident and investigated using root cause analysis.[32]
- Trusts must use individual performance review (IPR) and personal development plans (PDPs) to increase personal responsibility for HCAI.
- Trusts must ensure productive clinical engagement, which is crucial to improve performance.

THE HEALTH ACT 2006

In 2006, the Department of Health published *The Health Act 2006: Code of Practice for the Prevention and Control of Health Care Associated Infections* (also known as the Hygiene Code), the purpose of which is to help NHS organisations plan and implement actions to prevent and control HCAI under three main headings:

Management, organisation and the environment [22]

Organisations have a duty to:

- protect patients, staff and others from HCA
- have in place appropriate management systems for infection prevention and control
- assess risks of acquiring HCAI and to take action to reduce or control those risks
- provide and maintain a clean and appropriate environment for healthcare
- provide information on HCAI to patients and the public
- provide information when a patient moves from the care of one healthcare body to another
- ensure co-operation
- provide adequate isolation facilities
- ensure adequate laboratory support.

Clinical care protocols [22]

- Organisations have a duty to adhere to policies and protocols

Healthcare workers [22]

- Organisations have a duty to ensure, as far as reasonably practicable, that health-care workers are free of and are protected from exposure to, communicable infections during the course of their work, and that all staff are suitably educated in the prevention and control of HCAI.

The Code details the exact processes that NHS organisations must have in place and the specific arrangements and criteria that must be met in order to ensure that there is compliance with the Code. Each NHS body, whether it is an Acute Trust, Mental Health Trust, Ambulance Service Trust or Primary Care Trust (PCT) now has a statutory duty to put the code into practice and compliance with the Code of Practice will be assessed by the Healthcare Commission.[33] The Healthcare Commission (Commission for Healthcare Audit and Inspection) was created under the *Health and Social Care (Community Health and Standards) Act* in 2003, and replaced the Commission for Healthcare Improvement (CHI) in 2004. It has a statutory duty to assess the performance of healthcare organisations, and investigate where there have been allegations of serious failings that have a negative impact on the safety of patients, clinical effectiveness or responsiveness to patients.[21] Investigating outbreaks of serious HCAI is therefore part of its remit, and any failure to implement and comply with the Code of Practice means that the Healthcare Commission is empowered to issue an improvement notice where there has been a significant breach of the Code, or report the Trust to the Secretary of State for Health for significant failings and place it on special measures. These could include dismissal of the Trust board or individual members.[33]

THE INFECTION PREVENTION AND CONTROL TEAM

Against this background, infection prevention and control teams are facing increasing demands on their time and resources. They are the nursing and medical experts responsible for developing the Infection Control Annual Programme, the production of which has been standard practice since it became a requirement under the Controls Assurance Standards which were recently superseded by Standards for Better Health.[34] The annual programme is produced for the chief executive and the Trust board and describes the programme of work planned by the infection prevention and control team for the coming year. This may consist of the following activities, and may also identify additional work that needs to be undertaken by the Trust as a whole, as the responsibility for the prevention and control of healthcare associated infections does not rest solely with the team.

- Mandatory surveillance of MRSA bacteraemia (see Chapter 9).
- Mandatory surveillance of *Clostridium difficile* (see Chapter 11).

- Surveillance of other 'alert' organisms such as *Mycobacterium tuberculosis* (see Chapter 10) and *Streptococcus pyogenes* (see Chapter 12) resistant Acinetobacter and Vancomycin-Resistant Enterococci (VRE) (See Chapter 8).
- Reviewing and updating existing infection control polices and guidelines in line with evidence-based practice/DoH recommendations.
- Undertaking and commissioning audit projects which may be carried out solely by the team or in conjunction with the clinical audit department and/or clinical directorates, e.g. audit of *Saving Lives High Impact Interventions*; environmental ward/department audits; spot audits of IV cannula/central venous catheters and urinary catheters to ensure compliance with Trust guidelines; audit of antimicrobial prescribing.
- Education – delivering mandatory infection training for all staff who have day-to-day contact with patients; infection control training for medical staff on induction and participation in training for junior doctors; training for contracted domestic and portering staff; ad hoc training for wards/departments where required; participating in training run by other specialist teams where appropriate.
- Running an infection control link nurse programme – holding regular meeting/education sessions and an annual conference.
- Promoting the hand hygiene programme.
- Ensuring that the Trust complies with the management and monitoring of Legionella (see Chapter 20).
- Monitoring standards of cleanliness – day-to-day advice on cleaning issues; advise contractors on cleaning and domestic issues; participate in Executive PEAT visits.
- Giving infection control advice on new builds and site development, including the reconfiguration of clinical services.
- Reviewing Trust performance against the Healthcare Standards and Code of Practice.
- Continuing the day-to-day management of the infection prevention and control service – provide ad-hoc advice on the management of patients as appropriate; day-to-day management of all issues pertaining to infection prevention and control; respond to enquiries from patients and their relatives and members of the general public seeking advice; respond to media enquiries and give local television, radio and newspaper interviews as required; manage outbreaks of infection, e.g. Norovirus (see Chapter 14) and generate outbreak reports.
- Serve as members of various groups/committees e.g. infection control committee; clinical management board; risk management committee; drugs and therapeutics committee; tissue viability committee; heads of department meeting; health and safety committee; matrons forum; ward managers meetings; emergency planning group; medical devices group; consumable user review group; clinical practice forum; nutrition group; waste group.

As the only specialist nursing and medical team with responsibility for patients, staff, the public and the environment, infection prevention and control teams can find their resources stretched to the limit. In 2000, the National Audit Office[26] identified what they perceived to be as 'a growing mismatch between what is expected of infection control teams in controlling hospital infection and the resources allocated to them' (page 40). The SENIC study in the 1970s[35] recommended that there should be one infection control nurse per 250 inpatient beds and although there are no hard and fast rules in the UK, this is the figure that is widely quoted and generally accepted. The reality is that infection control as a specialty is hugely under resourced.

THE WAY FORWARD

In February 2000, the National Audit Office[26] stated that the prevention and control of HCAIs was not seen as a priority within the health service. The strategic management of hospital acquired infection needed to be strengthened nationally and at NHS Trust level as it was clear that the NHS did not have a grip on either the extent of problem or the resulting financial burden. It also clearly stated that responsibility for the prevention and control of infection did not just rest with infection prevention and control teams. While factors compounding the problem of trying to control infections were acknowledged, the message was clear; the NHS as an organisation had to get its act together, and individual NHS bodies had to accept responsibility and start to take action.

The subsequent development of initiatives and programmes such as *Saving Lives*, and *Going Further, Faster* and the publication of the Code of Practice continues to drive home the importance of the prevention and control of HCAI, and the need for all Trusts to ensure that they have in place a prioritised, targeted and sustainable action plan to specifically improve compliance with infection prevention and control and drive down rates of HCAI. Engagement at all levels has to be sought and obtained, otherwise nothing will change. As the National Audit Office identified in 2004,[36] a root and branch shift across all levels of the NHS is required if infections are to be kept under control and the burden of HCAIs reduced, and while the profile of infection control has undoubtedly increased, there is still a long way to go. Those directly involved in patient care must be responsible for their practice and ensure that they comply with infection control policies, procedures and protocols in order to reduce the risk of infection to patients and provide good quality and effective care. The prevention of HCAIs must continue to be given a high priority and practices and organisational culture must continue to change for the better.

2 Bacterial and Viral Classification, Structure and Function

INTRODUCTION

Microbiology is the study of microscopic living organisms, referred to as micro-organisms, that can only be seen with the aid of a microscope. Micro-organisms exist everywhere – in and on the body, both human and animal, in plants, soil and water. The medically important groups include bacteria, viruses, fungi, and protozoa. While the majority of bacteria are not considered to be harmful to man, there are at least 50 species that are considered to be pathogenic,[37] and therefore capable of causing a diverse spectrum of illness and disease, from colonisation to infection, and ranging from mild to life-threatening in a susceptible host. Other bacteria are opportunistic and only cause infection when the host's resistance is impaired.

Viruses are the smallest known infective agents, and are responsible for some of the pandemics of disease that we are witnessing today, such as HIV/AIDS (Chapter 16), SARS (Chapter 17) and influenza (Chapter 18).

In order to understand how the bacteria and viruses discussed in this book replicate, invade and establish themselves in the human host, resulting in colonisation or infection, a basic knowledge of their classification, structure, and function is necessary. This chapter intends to provide the reader with the necessary information to understand the basic properties and characteristics of bacteria and viruses, particularly those which act as virulence factors and increase the organism's pathogenic potential, and relate this to the disease process.

LEARNING OUTCOMES

After reading this chapter the reader will be able to:

- Describe the main structure and components of a bacterial cell
- Understand the difference between Gram-positive and Gram-negative bacteria and give examples of each
- Understand the virulence factors of bacteria
- Understand how viruses differ from bacteria and how they cause disease

BACTERIA

Bacteria are microscopically small organisms, measured in microns (1 micron = 1,000[th] of a millimetre). The surface of the human body consists of 10 times more micro-organisms on the skin than it does cells. In fact it is estimated that between 500–1,000 different species of bacteria live in and on the body[37], existing as part of the normal body flora, playing a vital role in inhibiting the growth of other bacteria with pathogenic potential.

Bacteria adopt one of three basic shapes – round, rod shaped and curved or spiral, and can occur in pairs, chains or clusters as demonstrated in Figure 2.1. Their

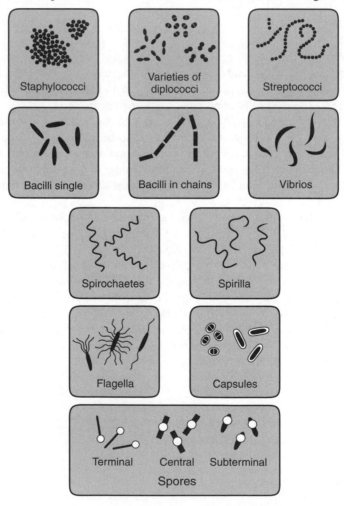

Figure 2.1 Common bacterial shapes and arrangements

Reprinted from Clinical Microbiology: An Introduction for Healthcare Professionals. Author J. Wilson, with permission from Elsevier

shape can only be revealed by Gram-staining and they need to be viewed under a compound light microscope which can magnify objects 1,000 times smaller than the smallest objects which can be seen unaided by the human eye.

Round bacteria are known as cocci, and can grow in pairs (diplococci), chains (streptococci) or grape-like clusters (staphylococci). Bacilli are rod-shaped and can also occur in pairs or chains, with very small bacilli referred to as coccobacilli, which may resemble cocci. Spiral shaped bacteria are known as spirochaetes, and curved or 'comma' shaped bacteria are called vibrios.

BACTERIAL CLASSIFICATION

The classification of bacteria is part of the process that enables rapid identification of the causative agent of illness or disease, allowing the appropriate treatment to be initiated, and the necessary preventative measures that need to be implemented to prevent the spread of infection. Bacteria are classified according to their morphology or shape, their Gram-stain reaction (which identifies the differences in their bacterial cell wall and is of life-saving importance when it comes to diagnosis and treatment), their growth requirements, and spore formation. Chapter 4 (The Microbiology Laboratory), discusses the staining of bacteria for identification and their growth requirements and reproduction in more detail. They are also classified according to their name which consists of two parts – the genus, followed by the species; for example, *Staphylococcus aureus; Streptococcus pyogenes; Clostridium difficile.*

Table 2.1 lists some common bacteria which are responsible for causing a wide range of infections, some of which are seen in healthcare settings, according to their Gram-stain reaction and shape.

BACTERIAL STRUCTURE

Cell membrane

The cell membrane, also known as the cytoplasmic or plasma membrane, is made up of proteins and lipids. It envelopes the cell, protecting its contents from the outside world, and controls the substances which enter and leave the cell.

The bacterial cell wall

The majority of bacteria have a cell wall, the exceptions being organisms called mycoplasmas, which have a cell membrane but no cell wall and so cannot be Gram-stained. The cell wall is essential for the survival of the bacteria, giving it shape, rigidity, and strength and offering protection against the host's immune response and the effects of certain groups of antibiotics.[38] This does not mean that the cell wall cannot be breached, and Chapters 5 and 8 discuss in detail how the immune system and the administration of antibiotics destroy invading bacteria.

Table 2.1 Bacteria according to their Gram-stain reaction and shape

Gram positive	Morphology	Illness/Disease
Staphylococcus *Staphylococcus aureus* *Staphylococcus epidermidis* *Staphylococcus saprophyticus*	Cocci (clusters)	Skin infections (impetigo, cellulites, abscesses, wound infection); IV line infections; pneumonia; food poisoning; osteomyelitis; acute endocarditis; septic arthritis; urinary tract infections
Streptococcus *Streptococcus pyogenes*	Cocci (chains)	Scarlet fever; 'Strep' throat; post streptococcal glomerulonephritis; skin infections; necrotising fasciitis; streptococcal toxic shock syndrome.
Group B Streptococci		Neonatal meningitis; pneumonia and sepsis.
Streptococcus pneumoniae	Diplococci	Pneumonia; meningitis; otitis media.
Bacillus *Bacillus anthracis* *Bacillus cereus*	Rods (spore forming)	Anthrax Food poisoning
Clostridium *Clostridium botulinum* *Clostridium tetani* *Clostridium perfringens* *Clostridium difficile*	Rods (spore forming)	Botulism Tetanus Gas gangrene Psuedomembranous colitis
Corynebacterium *Corynebacterium diptheriae*	Rod (non-spore forming)	Diptheria
Listeria *Listeria monocytogenes*	Rod (non-spore forming)	Food poisoning; meningitis
Gram Negative		
Neisseria *Neisseria meningitidis* *Neisseria gonorrhoea*	Diplococci	Meningitis Gonorrhoea
Enterobacteriaceae *Escherichia coli*	Rods	Diarrhoea; urinary tract infections; sepsis
Klebsiella pneumoniae		Pneumonia; urinary tract infections
Proteus mirabilis *Serratia* *Shigella* – *S.dysenteriae, S.flexneri, S.boydi* and *S.sonnei* *Salmonella* *Yersinia pestis*		Urinary tract infections Urinary tract infections Dysentry Typhoid fever; gastroenteritis Bubonic plague

Vibrionaceae	Curved rods	
Campylobacter jejuni		Food poisoning
Helicobacter pylori		Duodenal ulcer; gastritis
Pseudomonas aeruginosa	Rods	Pneumonia; osteomylitis; sepsis; urinary tract infection; endocarditis; wound infections; corneal infections
Acinetobacter baumannii	(Coccobacilli)	Pneumonia; septicaemia
Haemophilus influenzae		Meningitis; sepsis; septic arthritis
Bordetella pertussis		Whooping cough
Legionella pnemophila		Pontiac fever; Legionnaire's disease
Chlamydia		
Chlamydia trachomatis		Conjunctivitis; infant pneumonia; pelvic inflammatory disease.
Chlamydia psittaci		Atypical pneumonia
Spirochetes	Spiral	
Treponema palladium		Syphillis
Leptospira		Leptospirosis
Mycobacteria	Rods	
Mycobacterium tuberculosis		Tuberculosis
Mycobacterium leprae		Leprosy

The main component of the cell wall is peptidoglycan (or murein), which is a polymer (a long molecule consisting of structural units and repeating units) of peptidoglycan chains linked by smaller protein chains. The cross-linking of chains gives the cell wall its rigidity. The thickness of the cell wall and its composition varies according to the species of the bacteria. A Gram-positive bacterial cell consists of two layers: an inner cytoplasmic membrane, and an outer thick layer of peptidoglycan. The cell wall also contains other polymers including teichoic and lipoteichoic acids, a complex of sugar and phosphate, which act as surface *antigens*.

Gram-negative bacteria are much more complex. They also have an inner cytoplasmic membrane, but they have a much thinner layer of peptidoglycan which is covered by an outer membrane. This acts as a protective barrier, preventing or slowing the entry of antibiotics that may weaken or kill the bacteria. Coating the outer membrane is lipopolysacchaide (LPS), a complex of fatty acids, sugar and phosphate. LPS is the endotoxin component of the Gram-negative cell wall and consists of three parts – Lipid A, core polysaccharide and the O side chain. Lipid A is the most significant component of LPS, impeding the effects of many antibiotics. It is also an antigenic determinant, inducing the formation of antibodies and is toxic to the host when the cell *lyses*, and the cell membrane breaks up, releasing Lipid A into the bloodstream.

Cytoplasm

The cytoplasm consists of water, enzymes, waste products, nutrients, proteins, carbohydrates and lipids, all of which are required for the cell's metabolic functions. Embedded within the cytoplasm is the cell's chromosome, its DNA molecule, which controls and initiates cell division and other cellular activities

VIRULENCE FACTORS OF BACTERIAL CELLS

Slime and capsules

Some bacteria produce a thick layer of glycocalyx, which is secreted outside of the cell wall. This may be either in the form of slime layers, which enable bacteria to slide or glide along solid surfaces and may show as a gelatinous pus at infected wound sites, or capsules. Capsules are seen in some important pathogens such as *Neiseria meningitidis* and *Salmonella typhimurium* and their presence assists in the identification of bacteria. The capsule helps to protect the bacteria from the host's immune response as it makes it more difficult for cells of the immune system to adhere to it and inhibits phagocytosis (see Chapter 5 Understanding the Immune System and the Nature and Pathogenesis of Infection). Large numbers of encapsulated bacteria can congregate together and produce a biofilm, which consists of a matrix of thousands or millions of micro-organisms all encased in capsular material, which may be of a pure culture originating from one species of bacteria or mixed. They have been defined as 'a community of micro-organisms irreversibly attached to a surface'[39] and 'a complex, highly differentiated, multi-cultural community with a level of activity within the biofilm that resembles a city'.[40] Bacterial biofilms are medically very significant as they are notoriously difficult for the host immune system to penetrate and they have been reported to be at least 500 times more resistant to antibiotics than 'ordinary' bacterial cells[41] and highly resistant to phagocytosis.[40] While bacteria will adhere to virtually any available surface with the exception of plastic and glass, they are especially fond of indwelling devices such as intravenous cannulae and urethral catheters, as well as prosthetic implants.[39,41] They can contaminate hot water storage tanks, shower heads and air conditioning units that use water, and develop on the surfaces of endoscope tubing.[39,40,41]

Spore formation

Some pathogens, such as *Clostridium difficile* (see Chapter 11) produce spores which enhance the survival of the organism when the moisture or nutrient supply is low. A thick wall is formed which cordons off the bacteria from the outside world and protects it from the effects of heat, drying, cold and chemicals, including certain disinfectants, enabling it to survive for many years in dust and soil.[42] As seen in Figure 2.1, bacterial spores can form at the end of the cell (terminal spores) or within the cell itself.

Flagella

Flagella are essential for the bacterial cells' motility and resemble long tails which are several times the length of the bacteria.[42] They range in number from one to 20 per bacteria depending on the species.[39] They may be sited all over the cell, clustered at one end, more than one at each end of the cell, or singular, and the number and arrangement of flagella can be used to aid the identification and classification of certain bacterial species.[42,43] The movement of the flagella make the bacteria move in a tumbling motion as the flagella spin around, and they propel the cell towards or away from certain stimuli, such as movement towards a nutrient source, or away from phagocytes if the organism is attempting to evade the host immune response. This process of directed movement is known as chemotaxis, and it is not unique to bacterial cells (see Chapter 5).

Pili (fimbriae)

These are commonly seen on the surface of Gram-negative bacteria, showing up as numerous hair-like protrusions or appendages. There are two forms of pili. Common pili are important virulence factors as they enable the bacteria to adhere and attach to host cells.[44] The sex pili are involved in the transfer of genetic material through conjugation (see Chapter 8 The Problem of Antimicrobial Resistance).

The production of invasive enzymes

Some organisms produce a very potent cocktail of enzymes which facilitate penetration of the organism into the host's tissues, resulting in tissue damage. Necrotising enzymes, seen in necrotising fasciitis (see Chapter 12 Invasive Group A Streptococcal Disease) cause rapid destruction of soft tissue. Coagulase, a protein produced by *Staphylococcus aureus*, clots plasma which forms a sticky layer of fibrin around the bacteria, protecting it from phagocytes, antibodies and other host immune defences.[45] Sometimes, the host will cause a fibrin clot to form around the pathogen and wall it off in an attempt to prevent any further invasion and penetration of the tissues. Kinases have the opposite effect to coagulase, and they dissolve the fibrin clot. This means that kinase producing bacteria such as staphylococcus and streptococcus are able to escape from these clots.[45] Hyaluronidase, often referred to as 'the spreading factor' enables pathogens to spread through connective tissue by breaking down hyaluronic acid which binds connective tissue together.[45] It plays an important role in the devastating tissue damage seen in necrotising fasciitis caused by *Streptococcus pyogenes* (see Chapter 12). Streptococcus and clostridia are two pathogenic bacteria which secrete hyaluronidase. Collagenase breaks down collagen, which is found in tendons, cartilage and bone, enabling pathogens to invade tissue.[45] *Clostridium perfringens* secretes collagenase. Haemolysins damage the host's red blood cells, providing the pathogen with a source of iron and also harming the host.[45]

Toxin production

Bacteria have an impressive arsenal of weaponry at their disposal, and their ability to produce and release toxins, which are responsible for the signs, symptoms and complications of infection, are perhaps the most impressive. If the human host can survive the initial onslaught of toxins and mount an efficient immune response, they have every possibility of recovering. Endotoxins are an integral part of the Gram-negative bacterial cell wall and are secreted or released not only when the cell is lysed or destroyed, but are also shed from living bacteria.[42] Septic shock (discussed further in Chapter 5) arising from Gram-negative endotoxins carries a high mortality rate. An unfortunate consequence of the administration of antibiotics to a patient with Gram-negative sepsis is that they can initially cause the patient's condition to worsen. This is because although the antibiotics cause the destruction of the bacteria, which is obviously the desired effect, this destruction also triggers the release of large quantities of endotoxin. Exotoxins are produced within the cell and secreted by Gram-positive and Gram-negative bacteria (with the exception of *Listeria monocytogenes,* a Gram-positive rod which causes meningitis in neonates and immuno-compromised individuals, and which produces endotoxin).[42] They are often named for the target organs that they affect.[37] For example, neuro-toxins released by *Clostridium botulinum* and *Clostridium tetani* target the nervous system, blocking nerve impulses and often causing paralysis. *Clostridium difficile* and *Salmonella* and *Campylobacter* species (Chapters 11 and 15) shed enterotoxin, which bind to and colonise the gastro-intestinal tract causing diarrhoea. Entertoxin continues to be released until the pathogen is destroyed by the immune system or antibiotics, or the human host dies as a result of fluid loss, which may be severe. Entertoxin can also be released by bacteria in food which, when ingested, results in rapid onset of diarrhoea and vomiting, as seen in *Staphylococcus aureus* and *Bacillus cereus*, both of which are very unpleasant causes of food poisoning. Other types of toxic effects are also produced by bacterial species such as staphylococci and streptococci in the form of 'super-antigens', which over-stimulate the immune system, having both acute and long-term effects and causing damage to the host.[43] It is becoming increasingly apparent that it is dysregulation of the immune system that causes disease rather than a direct effect of the toxin.[44]

Plasmids

Plasmids are small, circular DNA molecules which carry genes that can render the bacteria drug resistant, give them new metabolic properties and make them pathogenic. Virulence plasmids can enable the bacteria to resist host defences or produce toxins.

BACTERIAL STRUCTURE AND FUNCTION

Figure 2.2 illustrates the main structures of a 'typical' bacterial cell.

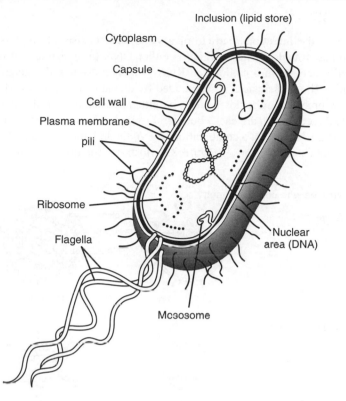

Figure 2.2 Bacterial cell structure

Reprinted from Clinical Microbiology: An Introduction for Healthcare Professionals. Author J. Wilson, with permission from Elsevier

VIRUSES

Viruses are the smallest known infective agents, approximately 100 to 1,000 times smaller than the cells they infect, and are only visible through an electron microscope. Unlike bacteria, a virus is incapable of independent replication; it needs to access a host cell so that it can substitute its own nucleic acid for the cell's DNA. They are classified according to their shape, their capsid, genetic material, and whether or not they have an envelope. They may also be classified further according to their size, the host they affect, which may be human, plant, animal or bacteria (bacteriophages), and the effect which they have on the host (cell death; transformation of the cell into a state of malignancy or latent infection which results in clinical illness at a later date). The International Committee on Taxonomy of Viruses has organised more than 4,000 plant and animal viruses into 56 families, 9 sub-families, 233 genera, and 1,550 virus species.[46,47] Of these, 24 families contain viruses that affect humans.

STRUCTURE

The virion is the infectious particle of a virus and consists of single-stranded or double-stranded nucleic acid[46], which is either DNA (a molecule that contains all of the cell's genetic information) *or* RNA, which translates the genetic material into protein. The nucleic acid is surrounded by a coat of protein, called the capsid, which is symmetrical. Capsids tend to be either icosahedral, with 12 vertices, 30 sides and 20 faces which are each equilateral triangles; helical, with the nucleic acid tightly coiled; or complex, a combination of icosahedral and helical and therefore of a more complicated structure.[46] Figure 2.3 illustrates the different viral structures.

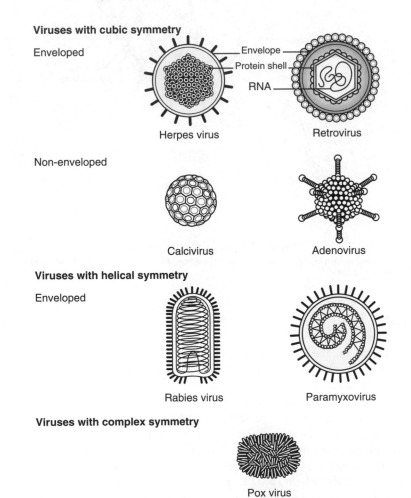

Figure 2.3 Different viral structures

Reprinted from Clinical Microbiology: An Introduction for Healthcare Professionals. Author J. Wilson, with permission from Elsevier

The capsid, made up of protein units called capsomeres, has a role to play in protecting the nucleic acid, and enabling the virus to attach to a host cell.[46] The number of capsomeres varies amongst viruses. Some viruses are surrounded by an envelope, which is acquired from the cell membrane of the host cell as the virus attaches and fuses to it. Those which do not have an envelope are referred to as non-enveloped, or naked. Viruses are host specific and have protein receptor binding sites on their outer surface, enabling them to bind or attach to other cells with the same receptor, which explains why some viruses cause illnesses which only affect the respiratory or the gastrointestinal tract. Transmission can occur as a result of inhalation or ingestion of virus particles, inoculation via blood or mucous membranes or transplacentally (from mother to fetus).

VIRAL REPLICATION

There are several stages in the viral replication and infection process. In order to initiate the beginning of the infective cycle, the virus has to 'collide' with the host cell, and virion attachment proteins on the virus and receptor molecules on the cell wall which are specific for each virus family, have to attach.[48] For example, the human immunodeficiency virus (HIV) attaches to CD4 receptors on T-lymphocytes (see Chapter 16). Because the virus–cell attachment is a highly specific reaction between the proteins and the receptors, not all collisions result in a successful infection, and collision and attachment are essentially random events.[48]

Once the virus has attached to and penetrated the cell, it is protected from the immune system, and the process of uncoating begins, where the virus dismantles and injects its genetic material. DNA viruses inject their nucleic acid into the nuclei of the host cell; RNA viruses inject into the cytoplasm. Transcription, translation and replication takes place as new virus particles are manufactured within the host cell, and the host cell then bursts, releasing new virus particles, ready to begin the process all over again in other cells.

SOME MEDICALLY IMPORTANT VIRUSES

This is not an exhaustive account of all medically important viruses, but offers a very brief description of some of the virus families and the viral infections that they result in, which may be seen within the healthcare setting. Blood-borne viruses such as hepatitis B, C and HIV, and other viral infections such as influenza and SARS are discussed in later chapters.

Adenoviridae: medium sized, non-enveloped icosahedral viruses, containing a single piece of double stranded DNA with 252 capsomeres.[49] There are thought to be more than 40 species of adenoviruses, and most individuals have been infected with several species of adenovirus by the time they reach adulthood.[50] Adenoviruses cause acute febrile respiratory illnesses such as pneumonia and bronchiolitis, particularly in young children, as well as gastroenteritis and conjunctivitis. They spread readily by droplet infection, although faecal-oral transmission can also occur.

Herpesviridae: double stranded DNA, enveloped, icosahedral viruses with 162 capsomeres.[51] Herpes viruses within this group include, amongst others, herpes simplex virus (HSV) 1 and 2, Varicella Zoster Virus (VZV), and Epstein Barr Virus (EBV). HSV produces vesicles, seen as eruptions on the surface of the skin and mucous membranes typically appearing on the lips as cold sores, and the genital mucosa. Transmission is by direct contact. VZV is the agent responsible for varicella (chicken pox) and herpes zoster (shingles) and is spread by respiratory droplets or direct contact with respiratory secretions or infected lesions or vesicles. The *incubation period* ranges from 10–20 days but is on average 14 days, with the individual infectious for two days before the onset of the rash and for at least five days afterwards while new vesicles are still appearing. The initial infection results in chicken pox, with a vesicular rash appearing on the face and then the trunk and limbs. Once the infection has resolved, the virus becomes latent within the sensory nerve ganglia. This latent state can persist for life, but the virus can be reactivated as a result of illness, including those illnesses or diseases which result in the immune system becoming compromised, and increasing age. Once reactivated, it travels along the sensory nerve pathway and erupts on the skin along that pathway, and the resulting vesicular rash is commonly known as shingles. Common sites are on the face, following the trigeminal and ophthalmic nerves, the leg following the sciatic nerve and in the thoracic area.

Patients admitted to hospital with chicken pox or shingles should be isolated until the vesicles are dry. If a patient develops the infection while they are an inpatient, either because they were incubating it on admission or because they have been exposed to an infected patient or member of staff, contact tracing of other patient and staff contacts should be initiated. Immunocompromised individuals and pregnant women are at the greatest risk of severe disease, complications and even death if they have no immunity. Vaccination with human varicella zoster immunoglobulin (VZIG) is recommended for those who have had a significant exposure[52] to chicken pox or herpes zoster *and* who have a clinical condition that increases their risk of severe disease (including immunocompromised patients, neonates and the pregnant), *and* who have no antibodies to VZV (detected by a blood test).[52] VZIG can also be administered as *prophylaxis* to healthcare workers who are unable to give a definite history of chicken pox or herpes zoster and who are VZV antibody negative.

Infection with the Epstein Barr virus (EVB) results in infectious mononucleosis or glandular fever, which has an incubation period of four to six weeks and an abrupt onset characterised by a sore throat, cervical lymphadenopathy, fever and malaise. Person-to-person spread is by the oropharyngeal route via saliva but no particular infection control precautions are required beyond normal hygiene measures, and patient isolation in a single room is not required.

Picornaviridae: small enveloped icosahedrals, with single stranded DNA and 32 capsomeres. This group consists of more than 70 enteroviruses[53], such as polioviruses, coxsackieviruses and echoviruses, and rhinoviruses. Enteroviruses are found in the intestines and excreted in the faeces, causing a variety of illnesses. Infection with poliovirus can result in asymptomatic infection or a mild flu-like illness; the added involvement of the central nervous system gives rise to symptoms of meningitis, or paralysis. Infection with coxsackieviruses and echoviruses can result in meningitis, upper respiratory tract infections, gastroenteritis, pleurisy and pericarditis. Rhinoviruses are the culprits responsible for the 'common cold'.

Hepadnaviridae: small enveloped icosahedrals with 180 capsomeres and double stranded DNA. Hepatitis B virus (HBV) is discussed in detail in Chapter 16.

Paramyxoviridae: enveloped, helical, single stranded RNA.[54] The viruses in this group include para-influenza virus, which are associated with croup and bronchiolitis in children, and minor upper respiratory tract infections, and the mumps and measles viruses. The mumps virus is generally an illness of childhood and causes pain and swelling of the parotid salivary glands. It is spread by droplet infection, with an incubation period of 14–18 days, with individuals considered to be infectious from 12–25 days after exposure. Peak *incidence* is in the winter and spring. Aseptic (viral) meningitis and orchitis are common complications, along with deafness and encephalitis.

Measles is a serious disease, responsible for one million deaths among children worldwide each year.[55] It has an incubation period of 10–12 days and begins with a flu-like *prodromal illness*, with a hacking cough and conjunctivitis. A widespread macropapular rash usually appears after four days, beginning on the forehead and spreading down the body. Although it is usually a childhood infection it can affect any age group, and complications includes pneumonia, otitis media (ear infection) and post-measles encephalitis.[54] It became a notifiable disease in England and Wales in 1940.[52]

The MMR vaccine

A single vaccine against measles became available in 1968 but it wasn't until the combined MMR (Measles, Mumps, *Rubella*) vaccine was introduced in 1988 that the number of epidemics occurring among young children of school age and under fell dramatically.[52] During the early 1990s, outbreaks of measles occurred in older children who had not been vaccinated. A vaccination campaign was launched in the UK in 1994 to vaccinate children between the ages of five and 16, and while there were limited stocks of MMR vaccine available to vaccinate against mumps, more than eight million children were successfully vaccinated against measles and rubella.[52]

MMR can be given at any age but it is recommended that the first vaccination is given at around 13 months, and the second before the child begins at school to capture those children in whom the first vaccination did not generate a full immune response.[56] Controversy in recent years over a suspected link between the MMR vaccine and autism and Crohn's disease has lead to a decrease in MMR uptake[56] and subsequent fears of a measles epidemic. Information on the safety of the vaccine and the importance of vaccination is available from the Department of Health/NHS Immunisation Information website.[57]

Caliciviridae: spherical, non-enveloped, single-stranded RNA, with 32 cup-shaped depressions on their capsid.[58] They are the main causative agents of viral diarrhoea and vomiting. Norovirus is by far the most notorious member of the caliciviruses and is discussed in detail in Chapter 14.

Coronaviridae: complex, enveloped, single-stranded RNA viruses which cause the common cold. SARS (see Chapter 17) is a new coronavirus.

Orthomyxoviridae: 80-120 nm, helical, enveloped with single stranded RNA. This group consists of the influenza viruses, which are discussed in detail in Chapter 18.

Retroviridae: 80-100 nm, complex, enveloped, single stranded RNA. Retroviruses cause HIV (see Chapter 16 Blood-borne Viruses, for more details).

Prions
Prions are not conventional viruses. They are small infectious proteins without any detectable nucleic acid, and the causative agent of a group of prion diseases called transiform spongiform encephalopathies, such as scrapie in sheep, bovine spongiform encephalopathy in cattle (BSE or mad cow disease) or new variant Creutzfeldt-Jakob disease (CJD) which occurs in humans. CJD is discussed in Chapter 19.

3 The Collection and Transportation of Specimens

INTRODUCTION

The collection of the appropriate clinical specimen is essential in order to diagnose the patient's illness/disease, and start the appropriate antibiotic treatment.[59] The quality of the result achieved from a specimen is directly related to the quality of the specimen itself, meaning that the correct specimen has to be obtained from the correct site using the correct technique in order to avoid a false-negative result.[60] Unfortunately many specimens received in the laboratory are sub-standard and therefore are not considered viable for a number of reasons that can easily be prevented. Common problems are contamination as a result of poor collection technique; leakage of the specimen in transit, representing a potential hazard to both portering and laboratory staff; inappropriate storage on the ward before reaching the laboratory rendering the organism within the specimen no longer viable; being obtained from an inappropriate body site which could give misleading results. Bearing in mind that the person collecting the specimen is responsible for its quality, it is imperative that healthcare workers posses the necessary knowledge to enable them to obtain specimens appropriately. This chapter identifies the various specimens that healthcare staff are required to collect for examination in the laboratory, and looks at the recommended methods of collection together with the health and safety issues that need to be taken into consideration in order to protect both the staff obtaining and transporting the specimen, and the laboratory staff. Chapter 4 (The Microbiology Laboratory) examines how these specimens are cultured.

LEARNING OUTCOMES

After reading this chapter the reader will:

- Understand the basic principles of specimen collection, taking into account health and safety and infection control precautions
- Be able to obtain or assist in the collection of urine, sputum, wound swabs, faecal specimens, throat swabs, nasal swabs, CSF and blood

GENERAL POINTS

A clinical specimen can be defined as any bodily substance, solid or liquid, that is obtained for the purpose of analysis. All specimens should be treated as potentially infectious and therefore careful handling and universal precautions are required when obtaining, transporting and processing specimens, particularly where there is contact with blood and body fluids. Staff should be aware of how to deal with any spillages and leakages that may represent a hazard to themselves, patients or other healthcare workers. Specimens from patients known, or strongly suspected, to have blood-borne viruses (BBV) such as HIV, hepatitis B or hepatitis C (see Chapter 16) should be labelled with a 'Danger of Infection' sticker[61] to alert the laboratory staff. Although all blood and body fluids should be treated as potentially infectious, the ward staff may know of a patient's BBV status but the laboratory staff won't unless the specimen is labelled. As they are at increased risk from an inoculation incident when the specimen is being processed in the laboratory, they may need prophylaxis in the event of an inoculation incident occurring. Sputum specimens for suspected tuberculosis should also be labelled. Portering staff who transport a specimen to the laboratory may also be at risk from a hazardous specimen, and their health and safety must be guarded.

Specimens must be collected in the appropriate sterile container. A variety of specimen containers are generally available in all wards/departments, and if staff are unsure then they should seek advice from the laboratory staff or the infection prevention and control team. The containers must be shatterproof, not overfilled, the lid secured tightly and the specimen placed in a specimen bag, which is then sealed to prevent leakage. If there is any contamination on the outside of the container this must be removed before the container is put into the bag. The request form should then be placed into a separate sleeve on the bag to prevent it from becoming contaminated.

The right specimen for the diagnosis of the illness or disease needs to be collected from the appropriate body site using an aseptic technique to avoid inadvertently contaminating the sample. This can arise from the patient's own body flora if due care isn't taken when collecting the specimen, from the flora of the person collecting the specimen, or from a non-sterile specimen container. The results of the laboratory investigation could then be misleading and the patient may not receive the correct treatment.

Where possible, specimens should be obtained before the patient commences antibiotics[60], otherwise laboratory testing could yield a misleading false negative; treatment with antibiotics before the causative organism has been identified may inhibit its growth so that it is not readily detected in the laboratory, but it may not have actually been clinically effective in treating the infection. There are some conditions however, such as meningitis (see Chapter 13 Meningococcal Disease) where antibiotic therapy needs to commence immediately, and delays in waiting for the results of any laboratory tests can mean the difference between life and death. In situations such as this, treatment with antibiotics should not be delayed or withheld.

THE SPECIMEN REQUEST FORM

Poorly completed specimen request forms, and poorly labelled specimens, may result in the specimen not being processed by the laboratory staff and the specimen being discarded. Apart from the obvious information such as the patient's name, hospital number, date of birth and the ward/department that the result needs to go back to, there is a lot of other essential information which is required but which is often incomplete.

SPECIMEN TYPE AND SITE

Sending a swab merely labelled 'wound' from a patient who may have more than one wound site is far from helpful. Different areas of the body carry different body flora (see Chapter 5 Understanding the Immune System and the Nature and Pathogenesis of Infection), and a poorly identified specimen will make it harder for the laboratory to differentiate between organisms which could normally be expected at a particular site, and those organisms which shouldn't be there. It may also make it harder for the right diagnostic investigation to be performed.

DATE AND TIME THAT THE SPECIMEN WAS COLLECTED

Some organisms are fragile and will die once they leave the body, which will obviously make their identification difficult. Additionally, if there is a mixed growth of organisms in the specimen, or the specimen was contaminated during the collection process, some organisms may overgrow, making it difficult to single out the particular organism that is causing the problem.

RELEVANT CLINICAL INFORMATION

This highly useful section is often left blank, but its completion really is essential and will help the laboratory staff and the microbiologist interpret the results. This section should include:

- any relevant clinical signs and symptoms
- recent history of foreign travel
- whether the patient is immunocompromised as a result of other illness, as immunocompromised patients are highly susceptible to infection by opportunistic and 'non-pathogenic' organisms
- whether the patient is receiving steroids and immunosuppressive drugs which can depress the inflammatory response
- current or recently completed antibiotic treatment – if antimicrobial agents are present in the specimen at the time of collection, they will inhibit the growth of any pathogens.

INVESTIGATION REQUIRED

Sometimes, requesting MC&S (Microscopy, Culture and Sensitivity) is sufficient but it will not detect all pathogens. If stool specimens are being obtained from a ward during a norovirus outbreak for example, the laboratory staff need to know what they are looking for. Giving all relevant information on the request form relating to the patient's symptoms, and a request for electron microscopy for example, will ensure that the right investigation is carried out. A different request form is normally required for specimens which have been obtained for the detection of viruses.

Finally, the specimen must be transported to the laboratory as soon as possible. Some pathogens may die rapidly when they have left the host and may not be detected if the specimen has been left sitting at room temperature on the ward for several hours waiting to be collected. Normal body flora within the specimen may proliferate and overgrow, inhibiting or killing the pathogen. Blood cultures and specimens of cerebral spinal fluid (CSF) are always treated as urgent and should be sent to the laboratory immediately. Arrangements are always in place for those specimens requiring processing and urgent analysis out of hours, as the results are often of life-threatening importance. Transportation of specimens must conform to the guidelines set out in the Health and Safety at Work Act (1974), The Management of Health and Safety at Work Regulations (1999) and the Control of Substances Hazardous to Health (COSHH) Regulations (2002).

CLINICAL SPECIMENS

- Urine
- Sputum
- Wound swabs
- Faeces
- Throat swabs
- Nasal swabs
- Blood culture
- CSF

URINE

Urine for microscopy, culture and sensitivity is one of the most requested laboratory tests[60], undertaken if a urinary tract infection is suspected, or for the investigation of a fever of unknown origin or suspected systemic infection (see Chapter 7 Types of Healthcare Associated Infection). Bladder urine is sterile but infection may arise as a result of perineal or gut flora ascending the urethra. When a urine specimen is obtained, it may become contaminated during urination by the normal flora found at the distal urethra, which is the part of the urethra furthest from the bladder. In order to reduce the risk of a contaminated sample, the urine should either be obtained as 'clean-catch' or a mid-stream specimen (MSU). There is very little evidence to suggest that meatal cleansing prior to obtaining the specimen is of any real benefit in preventing contamination of the urine sample with genital flora, although in patients with poor personal hygiene it may of some value.[62]

When an MSU is obtained, the first portion of urine is voided directly into the toilet or a bedpan, so that the organisms that normally reside within the distal urethra are flushed out. The patient must then have sufficient bladder control to be able to void the mid-stream into a sterile container, and then the remainder into the toilet or bedpan again. Collecting an uncontaminated specimen is sometimes difficult, and so the specimen request form should state the method by which the urine specimen has been obtained. If the patient is catheterised, either via a urethral or supra pubic catheter, a urine specimen should be obtained via the catheter sampling port using an aseptic technique. It should never be obtained directly from the catheter bag as the stagnant urine within the bag will be contaminated from a heavy growth of micro-organisms. Once collected, urine specimens should be sent to the laboratory within two hours of collection. If that is not possible, they should be refrigerated at 4 °C for no longer than 24 hours. If the specimen is not refrigerated, or is left at room temperature, bacteria within the sample will multiply and the detection and identification of any pathogen will be difficult.

SPUTUM

Sputum specimens are necessary for the detection of bacterial infections such as tuberculosis (Chapter 10) and pneumonia (Chapter 7).The function of sputum is to trap an inhaled foreign material, which includes bacteria, and it is produced in excess when the lower respiratory tract becomes inflamed. Sputum produced as a result of infection is generally purulent, and a good sample can yield a high bacterial load. Unfortunately however, as the mouth and pharynx are home to a large number of normal resident flora (see Chapter 5), this can make the detection of the pathogen hidden among them far from easy. Too many of the 'sputum' specimens sent to the laboratory are actually saliva, which is of no benefit at all as it will not provide any clinically relevant results. It is important that the patient is instructed to give a deep cough in order to produce a good specimen, and often the best specimen is produced first thing in the morning. If the patient has difficulty expectorating, the intervention of a physiotherapist may be required and the patient may need saline nebulisers in order to moisten the airways. Respiratory pathogens do not tend to survive for long once they have left the host and should either be sent to the laboratory immediately or refrigerated for no longer than 24 hours.

WOUNDS

Wound swabs should only be taken if there are clinical signs of infection (see Chapter 7 Types of Healthcare Associated Infection), and routine wound swabs should be avoided, particularly from chronic wounds such as leg ulcers which are often heavily colonised with skin flora. Although most wound infections do arise as a result of infection from the patient's own resident skin flora care must be taken to ensure that the specimen is obtained directly from the site of inflammation/infection and not from the surrounding skin. In order to obtain a 'good' sample, the swab should be moved over the surface of the wound in a zig-zag rolling fashion. If the wound is dry, the tip of the swab should be moistened with normal saline to make it more absorbent and increase the survival of any pathogens present prior to culture. Any loose debris on the surface of the wound should be removed as this may contain high numbers of bacteria but will not be representative of the infecting organism. If pus is present, it should be aspirated using a sterile syringe and decanted into a sterile specimen pot. As previously discussed, the site and nature of the wound should be clearly indicated on both the swab and the request form.

FAECES

The gut is home to huge numbers of **enteric** pathogens, along with resident bowel flora. Laboratory investigations are requested for bacterial infections such as *Clostridium difficile* (Chapter 11), *Salmonella, Staphylococcus aureus, Campylobacter,* and *Shigella species,* and viral infections such as norovirus. Faecal specimens may also be required if infections caused by intestinal protoza are suspected, whereby a fresh or 'hot' stool is required as the protoza are more likely to be mobile and therefore more easily identified live in a warm stool. Faecal specimens should ideally be obtained within the first 48 hours of illness as the chances of successfully identifying the pathogen diminish once the acute stage of the illness passes, and should reach the laboratory on the same day, although they can be refrigerated overnight. A 15 ml scoop of liquid faeces is sufficient, and faecal specimen pots have a handy 'scoop' attached to the inside of the lid.

THROAT

Although the majority of sore throats are due to viral infections, Group A Streptococcus (Chapter 12) is the most common bacterial cause of sore throats. *Neisseria meningitidis,* the causative agent of meningococcal meningitis (Chapter 13) is a normal inhabitant of the human nasopharynx and patients with meningitis, and their close contacts, will have throat swabs taken for the detection of meningococci. The swab should be rolled over any areas of exudate or inflammation, or over the tonsils and posterior pharynx. Care must be taken on withdrawing the swab that it does not touch the cheeks, teeth, tongue or gums as the specimen will become contaminated by the resident flora.

NASAL SWABS

The most common indication for taking a nasal swab is generally as part of MRSA screening. The tip of the swab should be moistened with the transport medium or with normal saline as the nose is normally dry. The swab should be inserted just inside the anterior nasal nares with the tip directed upwards and then gently rotated.

BLOOD CULTURE

Blood cultures are indicated if the patient displays systemic signs of infection or has pyrexia of unknown origin, and should be taken when the patient's temperature spikes, as the numbers of bacteria circulating within the bloodstream will be at their greatest then. 20–30 mL of blood is drawn which is inoculated into separate culture bottles containing liquid culture media, one for aerobic and one for anaerobic incubation, and it should be transported to the laboratory immediately.

If the skin is not decontaminated appropriately prior to drawing the blood, the culture may become contaminated with skin flora such as coagulase-negative staphylococci.[60,63] The isolation of MRSA from a blood culture is not necessarily clinically significant if the patient is systemically well, and may also indicate contamination as opposed to clinical infection. Contaminants, unfortunately, are not uncommon but can be avoided using a sound aseptic technique and optimal skin decontamination.

10 important points for taking blood cultures

- Using the correct technique will reduce the incidence of contaminated samples and false positive results.
- For safety reasons the winged blood correction set (butterfly) is recommended.
- Contamination can come from a number of sources:

  o the patient's skin
  o the equipment used to take the sample and transfer it to the culture bottle
  o the hands of the person taking the blood sample
  o the general environment.

- Only take a blood for culture when there is a clinical indication e.g.

  o core temperature out of normal range
  o focal signs of infection
  o abnormal heart rate (raised), blood pressure (low or raised) and respiratory rate (raised)
  o chills or rigors
  o raised or very low white blood cell count
  o new or worsening confusion.

- Take blood for culture before commencing antibiotics or immediately before next dose, if course in progress.
- **Always make a fresh stab** In patients with suspected bacteraemia, it is recommended that two sets of cultures are taken at separate times from separate sites. **Do not** use existing peripheral lines or sites immediately above peripheral lines. If a central line is present, blood may be taken from this and from a separate peripheral site. Identify a suitable venepuncture site before disinfecting the skin. **Avoid femoral vein puncture because of the difficulty of adequate skin cleansing and disinfection.**
- Always use 2% chlorhexidine in 70% alcohol (Chloraprop Fropp) for skin disinfection. Allow to dry.
- Wash hands with soap and water then dry. Decontaminate with alcohol hand rub.
- Always disinfect the tops of the culture bottles using 2% chlorhexidine in 70% alcohol Clinell wipe. Allow to dry.
- If blood is being collected for other tests, always collect the blood culture first.

Figure 3.1 10 important points for taking blood cultures

Reproduced by permission of East Kent Hospitals NHS Trust

CSF

Cerebral spinal fluid is obtained by lumber puncture for the diagnosis of meningitis (see Chapter 13 Meningococcal Disease), encephalitis and menigoencephalitis. A lumber puncture is performed using strict aseptic technique, and the skin is thoroughly decontaminated with chlorhexidine to prevent the introduction of organisms during the procedure, and contamination of the CSF with resident flora. It is collected into three sterile bottles and examined with regard to its appearance (which should be clear and colourless), glucose, protein, cell count and the presence of bacteria, viruses and fungi. Specimens of CSF should be dealt with by the laboratory as an emergency and maintained at room temperature and cultured within two hours of collection.

4 The Microbiology Laboratory

INTRODUCTION

In order to detect, identify and treat bacterial and viral infections, the infecting micro-organisms/viruses need to be grown under laboratory conditions which mimic the conditions in which they would grow optimally within the human host. Focusing predominantly on bacteria, this chapter looks at some of the work undertaken in the microbiology laboratory and describes how bacterial cell division and growth occurs. Techniques for culturing and identifying bacteria are described, and a brief account of how MRSA, tuberculosis and *Clostridium difficile* are isolated is given. Some other commonly used laboratory investigations are briefly described.

The reader should note that these investigations can vary according to the facilities within individual laboratories, and some specimens may have to be sent to other laboratories if certain facilities are not available on site. The techniques used to culture and stain organisms may also vary slightly.

LEARNING OUTCOMES

After reading this chapter the reader will:

- Be able to describe how bacteria grow and divide
- Understand the culture and staining techniques used to grow and identify bacteria
- Understand the basic principles of PCR, immunofluresence, serology and tissue culture in aiding bacterial and viral detection

BACTERIAL GROWTH AND CELL DIVISION

The process through which bacteria divide is known as binary fission, where one bacterial cell, called a parent cell, divides in half to produce two daughter cells. Before cell division begins, the cellular DNA is replicated so that each daughter cell will contain the same genetic material as the original parent cell. Each subsequent division of the cell should therefore result in the precise replication of the DNA. However, with millions of cell divisions occurring, it is inevitable that this process can sometimes go wrong, resulting in cell mutations.[64] Although most cell mutations will cause the cell to die, there are instances where mutations can actually make the cell more adaptable and it can thrive in circumstances that would normally destroy it. These mutations are one of the factors that contribute to antibiotic resistance, which is discussed in Chapter 8, The Problem of Antimicrobial Resistance.

The growth of bacteria is demonstrated in culture media where the number of cells increases exponentially with time, and this stage of the bacterial growth cycle is known as the exponential or log phase of growth. The amount of time taken for the cell to divide is known as the generation or doubling time, which varies among bacterial species. Bacteria such as *Pseudomonas* and *Clostridia* have a short generation time of 10 minutes, and a single cell of *Escherichia coli* can produce 10 million cells in eight hours while *Mycobacterium tuberculosis* is a slow grower and divides once within 18–24 hours. Given the short generation time of some organisms it is easy to see that if an antibiotic resistant mutant occurs during cell division, it can rapidly become the dominant organism. As the nutrient supply becomes depleted, toxic waste products build up, the culture media becomes over populated, and bacterial growth enters the stationary or lag phase as growth eventually slows down and then ceases altogether.[65] If the bacteria are inoculated onto fresh media, exponential growth will continue after a lag phase. If the stationary period is extended, the bacteria will eventually die.

Bacterial growth involves an increase in both size and the number of organisms, resulting in an increase in total mass, or biomass. This growth is dependent upon various environmental factors; if the environmental conditions are not optimal, the organism will not survive. An adequate supply of nutrients is essential for the bacteria's survival: many of these provide energy sources which the bacteria break down to derive energy from. All organisms have an optimum growth temperature, where they will be growing at their optimum rate. Temperature is important as bacteria will cease to grow below their minimum growth temperature, and will die in environments where the temperature is above the maximum. The pyrexia which often accompanies many illnesses is useful in combating infections and is actually a protective response, given that most pathogens replicate best and achieve their optimum growth at temperatures of 37 °C or below. Moisture is another essential growth requirement, as 70-95 % of the bacterial cell consists of water. The majority of bacteria will die without an adequate moisture supply, although some bacteria form spores which protect them when the moisture or nutrient supply is low (see Chapter 2 Bacterial and Viral Classification, Sturcture and Function). An example of a spore-producing organism is *Clostridium difficile* (see Chapter 11 *Clostridium difficile*). The spores enable the bacteria to survive for long periods in the environment in a dormant state, and then reactivate when the environmental conditions are right.

Oxygen is another important growth requirement, and bacteria are either aerobic, anaerobic or facultative. The human body provides a mix of aerobic and anaerobic environments, and the ability of an organism to grow and replicate in either environment is advantageous for many pathogens. Strict, or obligate, aerobic bacteria can only grow in the presence of oxygen, and can be found on the surface of wounds for example. Strict or obligate anaerobes, however, cannot grow in an oxygen-rich environment and thrive deep in wounds where the tissue is dead. They do not survive long in clinical specimens and can be difficult to isolate in the laboratory. Facultative organisms can grow with or without oxygen but achieve their optimum growth in an oxygen-rich environment.

BACTERIAL CULTURE

The principle aim of culture is to grow a population of bacterial cells which will be visible as a colony on a plate of media. This population of cells is referred to as a culture and the visible mounds of bacterial mass seen on the surface of solid (agar) culture media are called colonies, which are the product of 20–30 cell divisions of a single cell.[66] If there are different species or strains of bacteria in the culture, the colonies produced will be of different shapes and sizes as a result of different growth rates and their response to the nutrients within the media.

CULTURE MEDIA

Culture media comes in either solid or liquid form, and generally consists of water, sodium chloride and electrolytes, peptone, meat and yeast extracts and blood. Solid culture media consists of agar (which is derived from seaweed) and cultured on Petri dishes, which are 90 mm in diameter and have a vented lid. Various nutrients can be added to the agar to create the optimum environment for supporting bacterial growth. In order to select the most appropriate culture media, the laboratory staff need to be provided with the relevant information in relation to the clinical specimen which is being tested. The type of culture media used may vary widely between laboratories but broadly comes under the headings of enrichment, selective and indicator media. Enrichment media are used to encourage and amplify the growth of fastidious fragile pathogens in sufficient numbers so that they are readily detectable. These can either take the form of solid agar or nutrient broth. Blood agar, which contains nutrient agar plus 5 % horse blood, will support the growth of most Gram-positive and Gram-negative bacteria.

The upper respiratory tract and the gastro-intestinal tract have abundant resident flora (see Chapter 5 Understanding the Immune System and the Nature and Pathogenesis of Infection) and detecting a pathogen in a body site where there is a heavy population of mixed flora is not always easy. Selective media have inhibitors such as bile salts or antibiotics added, to inhibit the growth of some bacteria and therefore encourage the growth of others, and are used to culture organisms within throat swabs and faecal specimens. MacConkey agar inhibits the growth of most Gram-positive bacteria but supports the growth of most Gram-negative rods. Colonies of pathogens grown on selective media may be further identified by culture using indicator media, which differentiates between species by effecting a colour change.

INOCULATION OF CULTURE MEDIA

Petri dishes containing the nutrient agar are inoculated with the clinical specimen using a strict aseptic technique to avoid contamination.[66] A sterile inoculating loop is used to apply the specimen to the culture medium, which is dragged or streaked over the surface of the agar plate. The lid of the Petri dish is replaced to prevent airborne contamination of the plate, and the loop is then 'flamed' by passing it through the flame of a bunsen burner until the loop reaches 'red heat' to remove any residual bacteria. The lid is then removed and the plate streaked a second time, with this second streak overlapping the first but finishing independently of it. The lid is replaced, the loop flamed yet again and a third streak is made. Each streak reduces the initial inoculum. Bacteria that are well separated from others will grow as isolated colonies and can be assumed to have arisen from a single organism, or an organism cluster which is known as a colony-forming unit.

Clinical specimens that are likely to contain only small numbers of organisms, such as CSF or blood, may be cultured using nutrient broth, a liquid suspension without the addition of any setting agents. The broth is inoculated with the specimen using a sterile loop.

Once the specimen has been plated, or inoculated into a liquid medium, it is incubated either aerobically or anaerobically at 35–37 °C for 24–48 hours and then 'read' or visually observed for growth. Millions of bacterial cells will be visible on the agar plate as colonies along the inoculation lines after 24 hours, unless the organism happens to be a slow grower with a long generation time, in which case there will be no visible growth. In the case of nutrient broth, it will become increasingly cloudy or turbid due to the growth of bacteria. Obligate aerobes tend to grow on the surface of nutrient broth, while obligate anaerobes will be hidden in the depths of the media, away from the surface.

Culture plates normally grow a mix of bacteria, including normal body flora. So that a 'pure culture' of only one type of bacteria is grown, the colonies can be inoculated onto another culture plate containing a culture medium that is more selective. The colonies for sub-culture are picked out using a sterile wire or loop and plated out using the same method as before.

Bacteria grown in nutrient broth are inoculated onto solid culture medium for bacterial identification. Serial dilutions of the broth are prepared in either 0.1 mL or 1.0 mL portions and inoculated onto an agar plate and incubated overnight. The colonies are then counted and the total number of bacteria present in the original sample is calculated by multiplying the number of colonies grown by the dilution factor.

CULTURING VIRUSES

As viruses only replicate within living cells, living cell cultures that support their replication are the primary method of detecting them. Viral growth will either be shown as changes in cellular morphology or cell death.

GRAM-STAINING

When viewed under the microscope, bacteria are colourless and transparent and it is impossible to identify them. The Gram-stain[67] differentiates between Gram-positive and Gram-negative bacteria according to the make-up of their cell wall, and also reveals their shape. As prompt identification of any infecting organism is of potentially life-saving importance, Gram-staining can be used to guide the choice of antimicrobial therapy until definitive identification of the organism has been made. First of all, the specimen is 'heat fixed' onto a glass slide. Methods of heat fixing may vary but they traditionally involve passing the slide through the flame of a bunsen burner several times. The slide is flooded with a blue dye (crystal violet) and left for 30 seconds before the dye is washed off with water. The slide is then flooded with iodine, left for 30 seconds, rinsed with water and decolourised with acetone for a few seconds. The acetone is then washed off almost immediately and a counter stain is applied by flooding the slide with a red dye called safranin. After one minute, the slide is washed and blot-dried using blotting paper.

- Gram-positive bacteria retain the blue (crystal violet) dye and are stained blue/black.
- Gram-negative bacteria are stained red/pink, as they retain the red safranin dye.

PROCESSING SPECIMENS

In order to give the reader a brief insight into how meticillin-resistant *Staphylococcus aureus*, *Mycobacterium tuberculosis* and *Clostridium difficile* are detected, this next section briefly describes how wound, sputum and stool specimens are processed. It is not intended to give a definitive account, as techniques and the type of media used can vary slightly between laboratories, and the reader is advised to seek further information and guidance from their microbiology laboratory.

MRSA

Enrichment media, either solid or nutrient broth, is generally used for the culture of *Staphylococcus aureus*, either in tandem with standard culture media or on its own. Antibiotics such as oxicillin and ciprofloxacin are added to the culture media to reduce contamination and select meticillin-resistant strains of *S.aureus*. The plates are incubated aerobically at 37 °C for 18–48 hours depending on the exact method used by the laboratory. During that time they are 'read' daily. Individual colonies are 2–3 mm in diameter, circular with a smooth shiny appearance, and a golden-yellow or creamy colour. In order to distinguish MRSA from a sensitive *Staphylococcus aureus*, or *Staphylococcus epidermidis* (coagulase-negative staphylococci), further identification and sensitivity testing needs to be undertaken.

Staphylococcus aureus has the ability to clot plasma through the production of an extracellular enzyme called coagulase, and the coagulase test[68] is the definitive test for distinguishing between *S.aureus* and other staphylococci. This can be carried out using either a glass slide or a test tube, and involves the use of either human or rabbit plasma. In the slide coagulase test, a drop of distilled water is placed on the slide and the specimen is emulsified to produce a thick homogenous suspension. The plasma is added to the slide using an inoculating loop or wire. A positive result sees visible clumping of the cells within 10 minutes. The tube coagulase test gives a positive result in approximately four hours. A test tube containing 1 mL of plasma is prepared, diluted according to the manufacturer's instructions, and then a sample from the test strain is added. It is then incubated at 35–37 °C and examined hourly for four hours. If a clot forms during that time, the result is positive.

In order to determine the antibiotic susceptibility of organisms and choose the correct therapeutic agents to treat the infection, antibiotic susceptibility/sensitivity testing[69] is required. Isolated colonies are selected from the primary culture plate for testing. The most widely used technique is the disc diffusion method. An agar plate is inoculated with the test organism and paper discs containing the antibiotic are placed on the agar plate using either cooled, flamed forceps or a disc dispenser. The discs are applied no longer than 15 minutes after the agar plate has been inoculated with the specimen, otherwise the organisms may grow, which will affect the zone sizes that form around the discs. The antibiotic begins to diffuse into the agar immediately, and if it inhibits bacterial growth, a zone of inhibition will become apparent around the antibiotic disc. This means that organism is sensitive to the antibiotic, and infection can be treated with that antimicrobial agent at the therapeutic dose recommended for treatment of the organism. If it is resistant to the antibiotic, the organism will grow right up to the edge of the disc.

If the strain of *Staphylococcus aureus* grown is an MRSA, it will be resistant to the beta-lactam agents (penicillins and cephalosporins). MRSA is discussed in detail in Chapter 9 Meticillin-resistant *Staphylococcus aureus*.

SPUTUM – FOR *MYCOBACTERIUM TUBERCULOSIS*

The definitive method for detecting whether or not a patient has infectious pulmonary tuberculosis (see Chapter 10) is to examine a sputum specimen for the presence of rod-shaped bacilli. A mucolytic agent is added to the sputum to break it up, and it is then 'spun' or centrifuged to further break down any deposits and leave a 'pure' specimen. The bacterial cell walls of mycobacteria have a high lipid content and generally stain poorly as a result. However, they can be stained through the prolonged application of concentrated dyes, facilitated by heat. Once stained, the lipids in the cell wall do not dissolve when the stain is washed off with acid-alcohol, hence the name 'acid-alcohol fast bacilli', and they retain the fluorescent stain. A thin smear is placed onto a glass slide which is heat fixed, and the specimen is then stained using the ZN technique.[70] The slide is flooded with a solution of carbol-fuschin and heated gently until it starts to steam. It is then washed with water and flooded with a dilute acid, such as 3 % hydrochloric acid. The slide is washed again and a counter-stain, which is either green or blue, is applied. If red bacilli are seen against the contrasting background colour, the result is commonly reported as 'AAFB smear positive'.

A negative sputum smear does not mean that the patient does not have pulmonary tuberculosis, although it does mean that their infectivity is likely to be low. The sputum specimen will need to be sub-cultured onto special culture media to see if *M.tuberculosis* can be grown. The specimen is decontaminated in the first instance to remove any other bacteria or fungi within the sample that might overgrow any mycobacteria if they are present. It is then used to inoculate the culture media, which is incubated at 35–7 °C for 10–12 weeks and 'read' weekly. At the end of the incubation period, the ZN stain is applied to the colonies to detect the presence of AAFBs.

CLOSTRIDIUM DIFFICILE

C.difficile is cultured in the laboratory on selective and enrichment media. It is incubated anerobically at 35–37 °C for 40–48 hours. The resulting colonies are described as glossy, grey and circular, with a rough edge and a characteristic 'farmyard smell'.[71] When Gram-stained, they are identified as Gram-positive motile rods with oval spores. The colonies then undergo further testing to detect the presence of toxins.[72]

OTHER LABORATORY TECHNIQUES

There are numerous other investigations undertaken in the laboratory to aid bacterial and viral detection and identification. Some of these techniques, which can be applied to both bacterial and viral detection, are briefly described here. Others are outside the scope of this book and the reader is advised to undertake further reading to explore this area if it is one of particular interest.

Polymerase chain reaction (PCR)

PCR is a relatively new diagnostic technique which has revolutionised the detection of pathogens by amplifying fragments of DNA millions of times to such a degree that specific detection of a pathogen is possible. It is used in the detection of diseases such as HIV (see Chapter 16) and *Mycobacterium tuberculosis*, and is of particular value in detecting antimicrobial resistance genes. When DNA replicates, it 'un-zips' into two halves, with each half a template for another one. DNA fragments can be made to 'un-zip' if they are heated, which separates the strands. They are cooled down and then heated again, and this cycle is repeated approximately 10 times, amplifying the DNA logarithmically.

Latex agglutination

Antigens or antibodies (see Chapter 5 Understanding the Immune System and the Nature and Pathogenesis of Infection) can be applied to latex particles to detect antibody or antigen reactions. If antigen is added to antibody-coated latex particles, agglutination will occur and antibodies can be detected in the patient's serum.

Immunofluoresence

Antibodies specific to the antigen being detected, which may be bacterial or viral, is labelled or 'tagged' with fluorescent dye. If the antibodies and the antigen combine, in the case of bacteria a bright green fluorescent halo will be seen around the antigen; if the antigen is a virus a fluorescent clump will be seen.

Serology

During any type of infection, the host response is to form antibodies. Their production and the length of time which they take to form is dependant upon the antigenic stimulation. In the event of a severe infection, antibodies are produced early in the illness and rise sharply over the following 10–21 days. Blood serum samples collected soon after the onset of the illness, and again in the convalescent phase, can be compared for changes in antibody content. Serum dilutions can be made where pathogens are difficult to detect in culture and serological assays can be performed which focus on the interaction between antigen and specific antibodies. One of the most commonly used assays is the enzyme-linked immunosorbent assay (ELISA) which detects antibodies.[73] Plastic wells on a microtitre plate are coated with specific antigen, to which a sample from the patient's specimen is added. Any specific antibodies within the sample will bind to the antigen, effecting a colour change. Serum antibodies to HIV infection can be detected by an ELISA assay within five to seven weeks of infection.

5 Understanding the Immune System and the Nature and Pathogenesis of Infection

INTRODUCTION

In order to care for patients with an infection/infectious disease, a basic understanding of the workings of the immune system and the pathogenesis of infection are advantageous. These are complex subjects and require more than just one chapter to fully do them justice, which is beyond the scope of this book. However, this chapter aims to provide a broad and brief overview of the disease process, linking together the immune response, the chain of infection, the pathogenesis of infection, and the management of septicaemia.

LEARNING OUTCOMES

After reading this chapter the reader will:

- Understand the differences between innate and adaptive immunity, and the role played by specialised components of the immune system in fighting infection
- Understand the terms 'colonisation' and 'infection'
- Understand the chain of infection and the importance of breaking the links in the chain in order to reduce the opportunities for infection to occur
- Understand how the clinical features of infection occur by relating them to the workings of the immune response

THE IMMUNE SYSTEM

The complex and fascinating workings of the immune system are integral to our health, and indeed survival. In general 'good' health, the majority of the illnesses and infections that we are faced with are generally short lived, dispatched with ruthless efficiency by the specialised cells and organs that make up the immune system and generate an immune response, and any damage inflicted upon the body is rarely long-lasting. In diseases such as HIV (see Chapter 16) and cancer, the immune system is under sustained attack for months or years, gradually weakening until it eventually succumbs to the virus or disease and is no longer able to do its job, leaving the host at risk from overwhelming infections that it is unable to prevent.

In order to destroy invading pathogens and protect the host from infection, the immune system has to be able to differentiate between self and non-self – what is foreign to the body and what is not. There are two branches of the immune system which work both independently of each other and together; the innate or natural immune response and the adaptive/acquired immune response.

THE INNATE/NATURAL IMMUNE RESPONSE

Innate or natural immunity is quite simply the body's first line of defence; it is always 'switched on' and leaps into action as soon as a pathogen is detected. It is non-specific, meaning that its actions are directed against any pathogen the first time the pathogen is encountered, but unlike adaptive or acquired immunity the workings of the innate immune system do not confer life-long protection upon the host. It consists of physical barriers, internal and external surface secretions and cells, all of which are present in the individual from birth.

The skin

The tough horny outer layer of the skin, its generally dry condition (although some areas of the skin such as the axillae and the perineum are naturally moist), its resident bacterial population, and the natural secretion of sweat which contains a high concentration of salt, combine to provide an inhospitable living environment for many micro-organisms.[74] The shedding or desquamation of skin scales also assists in the elimination of micro-organisms[75], although this could also contribute to environmental contamination and cross-infection if an individual were to be heavily colonised with a potential pathogen such as MRSA, for example. In spite of these external defence mechanisms however, any breach in the skin resulting from a traumatic injury, surgical wound or insertion of an IV cannula for example, will create an immediate gateway into the body through which pathogens can swiftly enter and invade body tissues and the blood stream.

Resident body flora

Normal or resident (commensal) flora, the amount and type of which can vary between individuals, are present on and in various body sites, colonising the surface of the skin and the respiratory, gastrointestinal and genitourinary tracts. It is estimated that more than 1,000 distinct micro-organisms make up the total resident population, with the number of organisms in the flora outnumbering the number of cells in the body by a factor of 10.[76] Colonisation of these body sites prevents pathogens from taking up residence (known as colonisation-resistance), as they have to compete with the commensal flora, which outnumber them, for nutrients. Although they are not generally pathogenic, resident flora are often opportunists and can cause infections if they are transferred to other body sites. Bowel flora such as *E.coli* are a common cause of urinary tract and wound infections, and staphylococci can cause wound, IV site and bloodstream infections. This is known as endogenous infection because it arises from the individual's own commensal flora. Patients can sometimes cause endogenous infections themselves through the transfer of bacteria from one body site to another – on their hands if they touch their wounds or urethral catheters for example – but commensal flora can also be transferred exogenously (cross-infection) to other patients, on the hands of healthcare workers by contact with other patients or with contaminated equipment. Table 5.1 identifies some of the common commensal flora which colonise the body.

Table 5.1 Some commensals of the human body

Skin flora	Staphylococci (*S.aureus* and *S.epidermidis*)
	Micrococci
	Yeasts (especially *Candida* spp)
	Corynebacteria
	Propionibacterium
Respiratory tract (including mouth and teeth)	Staphylococci
	Actinomycetes
	Streptococcus mutans
	Streptococcus pneumoniae
	Streptococcus pyogenes
	Haemophilus influenzae
	Neisseria
	Candida
	Bacteroides spp
Gastrointestinal tract	*Escherichia coli* and other *Enterobacteriaceae*
	Enterococci
	Yeasts
	Clostridium spp
	Bacteroides spp
	Bifidobacteria
Genito-urinary tract (including the perineum and urethra)	Skin flora colonising the perineum plus *Bacteroides* spp, *Clostridium* spp and *Bifidiobacterium,* plus
	Yeasts
	Lactobacilli
	Actinomycetes
	Streptococci

Defence mechanisms of the respiratory, gastrointestinal and genitourinary tracts

Intact mucosal surfaces, which are often only one cell thick in places,[77] can be invaded by bacteria and viruses but they have their own defence mechanisms which can ward off the invaders. Tissue fluids containing enzymes called lysozymes, which are present in the lachrymal secretions of the conjunctivae, are active against the peptidoglycan layer in the bacteria cell wall, and naturally have an inhibitory effect on micro-organisms.[77] Gastric acid and peptide enzymes in the stomach account for the very few resident organisms found there because of the naturally acidic environment which is not particularly conducive to microbial life. Within the large bowel, the resident bowel flora (10^{12} organisms per gram of faeces[76]) compete for nutrients with, and inhibit the growth of, other bacteria that could become pathogenic if the balance of the microbial population is disturbed (see Chapter 11).

The ciliated epithelium and mucociliary 'blankets' which line the respiratory tract trap invading micro-organisms and waft the bacteria out. The cough reflex helps to expel them and 90 % of inhaled material is cleared from the respiratory tract within one hour.[75] While the genito-urinary tract is sterile above the distal 1 cm of the urethra, the perineum is colonised by skin and bowel flora which can gain entry into the normally sterile environment, particularly if the normal closed urethra is open because of the presence of a urethral catheter, which acts as 'the ladder to the bladder' (see Chapter 7 Types of Healthcare Associated Infection). Usually, however, the normal mechanism of emptying the bladder and the flushing effect of the urine will wash away any potential invaders.

White blood cells

White blood cells (WBCs) or leukocytes are important components of the innate immune system. There are 4,500–11,000 WBCs per cubic millimetre of blood, and that number increases in the presence of inflammation/infection. The white blood cell population consists of natural killer (NK) cells; mast cells; basophils, eosinophils and neutrophils (known as polymorphonuclear leukocytes), and the phagocytic cells (macrophages and neutrophils). Natural killer cells belong to a group of WBCs known as lymphocytes and they target abnormal cells such as those infected with viruses or cancer. They are also able to kill cells that are coated with IgG antibody (a process known as antibody-dependent cellular cytotoxicity), as they possess IgG receptors, and they primarily play a role in the adaptive immune response.[78] Mast cells line body surfaces, particularly mucosal surfaces, and they have a specific role to play in the allergic response to inhaled allergens. Basophils are present in the circulation in very low numbers, accounting for less than 0.2 % of the total leukocyte count, and along with eosinophils (1–2 % of leukocytes) they play a role in the allergic immune response, increasing in numbers and migrating to sites where an allergic reaction has taken place.[75] Neutrophils are the most abundant WBCs in the circulation, with between 2,000–7,500 neutrophils per cubic mm of blood, and they flood infected tissues within 24–48 hours of infection. They are phagocytic cells, the marauding scavengers of the immune system.

Cytokines, chemotaxis, phagocytes and phagocytosis

Although phagocytic cells are constantly on patrol, they can be attracted to pathogens by cytokines, which are small proteins or molecules released by different types of cells, including bacterial cells. Cytokines bind to cell surface receptors on pathogens and act as chemical messengers, forming part of an extra-cellular signalling network which controls every function of the innate and the adaptive immune response, including inflammation, proliferation of clones of T and B lymphocytes and regulation of their specific function.[78] Interleukins (IL), inter-ferons, and tumour necrosis factors are chemokines. The phagocytes migrate through the capillary walls and through the tissues to the affected area by the process of chemotaxis, which is a directed movement towards chemical attractants such as products of injured tissue, blood products and products produced by mast cells and neutrophils.[75,79] When the phagocytic cells encounter a pathogen, dead or dying cell debris or any foreign material, they bind to it; it is then engulfed by a pseudopod, which is an extension of the phagocytic cell membrane and killed through the combined activity of digestive enzymes and a transient increase in oxygen uptake (respiratory burst), which destroys the cell. This process is known as phagocytosis, and it plays an important role in the process of wound healing, ingesting cellular debris.

Macrophages

Macrophages are large phagocytic cells derived from monocytes, which are white blood cells formed from stem cells in the bone marrow. They reside in all body tissues at strategic locations through which blood and lymph pass, and are partic-ularly concentrated in areas such as the lungs (alveolar macrophages have a role to play in trying to ward off infection from *Mycobacterium tuberculosis*), the liver, spleen, kidneys and lymph nodes, where their role is to filter out pathogens and remove them from the circulation.[79]

THE ADAPTIVE/ACQUIRED IMMUNE RESPONSE

The adaptive/acquired immune response is uniquely remarkable for its specificity, diversity and immunologic memory[79], and can be divided into humoral (antibody) and cell-mediated (lymphocyte) responses. Its actions are targeted against specific antigens, which are molecules capable of inducing an immune response and reacting with antibodies and/or T-lymphocytes, such as bacterial toxins or bacterial cells. It takes three to five days for the adaptive immune response to be activated, so the innate immune system comes into play initially. The first encounter with the antigen generates a primary response and following this initial exposure, a more powerful and rapid response is generated on encountering the antigen/pathogen a second time.[78,79]

There a two different types of lymphocytes – T and B. They are produced in the bone marrow and found throughout the body in blood, lymph fluid and lymph tissue, where their role is to recognise and react to antigens.[79] T-lymphocytes enter the peripheral circulation and pass through the thymus gland where they mature and acquire recognition molecules, or T-cell receptors (TCRs) on their cell surface. Following maturation, they leave the thymus gland and re-enter the peripheral circulation, taking up residence in the lymph nodes and the spleen where they undertake surveillance for antigens, constantly re-circulating through the blood, lymph nodes and lymph fluid.[79] Two different types of T-cells assist in the cellular immune response. T-helper cells (TH2 cells) express CD4 molecules on their surface and assist the B-lymphocytes in generating antibody responses by secreting cytokines which signal the B-lymphocyte to differentiate into an antibody-secreting B lymphocyte.[79] Unfortunately, CD4 cells act as receptors for the HIV virus, which specifically targets the T-lymphocytes and eventually, over time, succeed in destroying the immune system and killing the host (see Chapter 16). T-suppressor cells, which express CD8 molecules on their surface (also known as cytotoxic, or killer, T-cells) target cells infected with viruses or other micro-organisms, as well as controlling the responses of the T-helper cells and suppressing their actions.[78,79]

B-lymphocytes do not pass through the thymus. It is thought that they achieve maturation and specificity in the bone marrow[79] and from there that they enter the peripheral circulation and migrate directly to the lymph nodes and the spleen. When it is exposed to an antigen, the B cell 'switches on' and differentiates into a plasma cell which secretes antibodies, forming a clone of daughter cells which secrete the same antibody as the parent cell. Plasma cells only have a short lifespan of two to three days duration, but approximately 10% of them survive to become antigen-specific B memory cells, able to respond immediately to the antigen if they encounter it a second time as they are already primed to secrete antibody.

Antibodies

Also known as immunoglobulins, antibodies are soluble globular Y-shaped proteins, some of which are carried on the surface of B-cells where they act as receptors for antigens, while others circulate freely in the peripheral blood or lymph fluid.[78,79] They also assist in triggering the complement cascade. They are antigen specific, binding to and reacting with the antigen that initiated their formation through sites called paratopes that bind with a specific part of that antigen, called the epitope. This essentially labels the antigen, effectively marking it for destruction by other components of the immune system, such as phagocytic cells which may posses particular receptors for that antibody subtype.[78,79] There are five antibody classes, or isotypes, and these are described in table 5.2.

Table 5.2 Classes of antibody

IgM	The first antibody to be produced during the primary immune response, and able to activate complement more effectively than other classes of antibody. Often associated with immune response to blood-borne organisms.
IgG	Has a long half-life of 23 days (4 to 10 times longer than other classes of antibody). Found in blood, lymph, peritoneal fluid and cerebrospinal fluid, and is the only antibody carried across the maternal placenta to the foetus. The predominant antibody produced during the secondary immune response.
IgA	Found in mucous, tears, sweat, gastric fluid and colostrums, where it prevents colonisation of areas of the body such as the GI, respiratory and genitourinary tracts.
IgD	Present in low amounts in serum. Plays a role in signalling B-cells but other host defence functions are undetermined.
IgE	Low concentrations in serum but primarily concerned with the allergic immune response, binding to allergens and triggering histamine release from mast cells. Has a role in defence against parasitic infections.

References:[74,75,78,79]

Complement

The complement system, so called because it facilitates and complements the actions of antibodies,[78,79] consists of more than 30 soluble proteins some of which, when activated by either an innate or an adaptive immune response, interact in a cascade and activate each other sequentially. There are two complement activation pathways: the classical pathway is initiated through the formation of antigen-antibody complexes, and the alternative pathway by the presence of microbial pathogens.[78] Table 5.3 describes the actions of some of the complement components.

Hypersensitivity reactions

Repeated exposure to a particular antigen or allergen can stimulate the adaptive immune response to initiate an intense reaction each time the antigen/allergen is encountered. Allergens, defined as any foreign substance that causes an immune response,[78] can be ingested, inhaled, injected or encountered through direct contact. The extent and severity of the immune response, which can cause local or systemic effects and can be so extreme that it can result in damage to the host's own tissues and even in the death of the host,[78,79] is as a result of either excessive amounts of antigen/allergen, or because the quantity of antibody to the antigen/allergen is too high. There are four types of hypersensitivity reaction – types I, II and III are antibody mediated, and type IV reactions are T-cell mediated.

Type I hypersensitivity reactions are associated with atopy and anaphylaxis. Atopic disorders such as eczema, asthma and hay fever often occur in individuals where there is a family history. Anaphylaxis (derived from the Greek

Table 5.3 Some components of the complement cascade

C1	Binds to antibody (classical pathway) and bacterial cell wall (alternative pathway).
C3	The key component, or linchpin, of the complement system involved in both the classical and alternative pathways. Splits to create C3a and Cb3.
C3a	An inflammatory mediator; increases vascular activity and activates the respiratory burst (in phagocytosis). Effects chemotaxis, attracting leukocytes to the site of tissue inflammation.
C3b	Opsonises bacteria by tagging or coating the organism; C3b is coated onto the surface of the bacteria, enhancing phagocytic activity.
C5a	An inflammatory mediator. Activates polymorphonucleocytes – enhanced phagocytic activity. Causes degranulation of mast cells and basophils, triggering the release of histamine in the allergic response.
C5b, C6, C7, C8 and C9	Create holes in the bacterial cell membrane, bringing about cell lysis (death).

References:[79,80,81,82]

words – *ana* = non, *phylaxos* = protection[78]) occurs as a response to certain foods such as peanuts, shellfish and drugs (e.g. penicillin) and is the most extreme allergic reaction of all.[83,84] IgE antibodies are generated over time in response to repeated low dose exposure to an allergen, and they bind to IgE receptors on the surface of mast cells and basophils. When the antigen is encountered the mast cells and basophils degenerate, releasing histamine, which is a potent activator of the immune response, and prostaglandins. As mast cells and basophils are situated under the skin and in the mucous membranes of the eyes, nose, lung and throat, this is where the majority of the clinical signs of an allergic response are seen.[79] In anaphylaxis, an immediate hypersensitivity reaction occurs as the allergen enters the circulation very rapidly. The release of excessive amounts of histamine stimulates an overwhelming and potentially life-threatening immune response, giving rise to the cardinal signs of anaphylaxis which are *pruritis*, *urticaria*, *angiodema*, vasodilation, hypotension, generalised 'flushing' of the skin, headache, tachycardia, and bronchoconstriction.[84] Anaphylaxis constitutes a medical allergy and individuals with known allergies to food, drugs, latex rubber and insect stings should carry a pre-loaded injectable adrenaline pen.[83]

Type II hypersensitivity reactions, involving IgM or IgG, are known as cytotoxic reactions as they damage host cells and tissues.[78] Incompatible blood transfusions fall into this class of hypersensitivity reaction, where the recipient has antibodies that react against the donor erythrocytes, hence the need for cross-matching prior to transfusion. In type III hypersensitivity reactions, an immune-complex is formed every time the antibody (IgG or IgM) meets the antigen, resulting in reactions in the bloodstream or the tissues. Immune complexes within the tissues give rise to tissue damage caused by an acute inflammatory response from the activation of complement, platelets and phagocytosis.[75]

Type IV delayed hypersensitivity reactions are slowly evolving reactions involving T-lymphocytes and macrophages that take between 24 and 72 hours to manifest after the allergen has been encountered.[75,78,79] Contact hypersensitivity reactions occur at the point of contact with the allergen, resulting in an eczema-type reaction on the skin. It takes 10–14 days[79] for the individual to become sensitised to the allergen, and when the allergen is next encountered, an immune response is directed against it. Delayed hypersensitivity reactions are also seen following the tuberculin skin test (see Chapter 10). This involves immunologic memory; a previous encounter with purified protein derivative (PPD) which acts as the antigen is remembered and an immune response involving lymphocytes and macrophages is generated at the injection site.[79]

Latex allergy

Natural rubber latex (NRL), which is found in everyday items such as rubber gloves, elastic bands, toys, balloons, condoms, adhesives, adhesive envelopes and pencil erasers as well as some items of clothing,[83,85] poses a serious problem as sensitisation to latex proteins through repeated exposure can give rise to serious allergic reactions. Healthcare workers who are repeatedly exposed to latex through the use of gloves and patients who have repeated hospital admissions/surgery (latex is found in syringes, catheters, anaesthetic mouthpieces, endotracheal tubes, oral and nasopharyngeal airways, anaesthetic masks, blood pressure cuffs, IV tubing, tourniquets and numerous other items[84,85]) are particularly at risk, as are atopic individuals. It has been estimated that up to 17 % of healthcare workers are at risk of developing allergic reactions[85] and the EPIC guidelines[86] (see Chapter 6 The Principles of Infection Prevention and Control) recommend that alternatives to NRL must be available within the clinical setting.

Latex allergy generates two types of allergic response. Non-life threatening hypersensitivity (delayed) type IV reactions occur as a result of an allergy to the chemicals that are used when processing the rubber and develop 24–48 hours after contact, presenting as contact dermatitis on the skin, with redness, itching and swelling. Type I reactions are potentially life-threatening and can lead to anaphylaxis; the culprits in these reactions are the natural proteins in the latex. Symptoms of latex allergy can become more severe on repeated exposure, so avoidance of NRL and heightened awareness among healthcare professionals is the best method of prevention.[86]

UNDERSTANDING THE CHAIN OF INFECTION

'The chain of infection' is the phrase used to describe the process by which infection can spread from one susceptible individual to another. For an infection to occur, all of the links in the chain must be intact and in the correct order. In order to break the chain, it is important that healthcare workers understand how the different components of the chain interact and facilitate the spread of infection. Then, the basic principles of infection prevention and control can be applied to clinical practice to break the chain (see Chapter 6 The Principles of Infection Prevention and Control).

Link 1. Causative organism

This can be any organism that demonstrates pathogenicity and/or virulence, which are not necessarily one and the same thing. Pathogenicity is the ability of the organism to cause infection. Not all organisms are pathogenic, and those that are may cause infections that range from asymptomatic or mild, to severe. Virulence refers to the organism's ability to cause severe disease, and while all pathogens are able to cause disease, some are more virulent than others. The degree of virulence is dependent on the host's susceptibility and the virulence factors that the organism possess (see Chapter 2 Bacterial and Viral Classification, Structure and Function). An example of virulence can be demonstrated by looking at shigella and salmonella, two medically important bacteria which cause severe diarrhoea. While 10–1,000 salmonella cells are required to cause salmonellosis (see Chapter 15 Campylobacter and Salmonella), only 10 shigella cells will cause diarrhoea, making shigella a more virulent organism than salmonella.[45] The organism's infectiveness, or ease with which it can spread to other people, its invasiveness, which is related to its ability to spread through the body, and its toxigenicity, or toxin producing properties, are other important contributing factors.[77,87]

Link 2. Reservoir/source

The reservoir is the site where the organism usually lives, and where it will find the nutrient and moisture supply necessary for its growth and survival. It may be environmental, human or animal, and in the healthcare setting, environmental and human reservoirs are commonly the most problematic and difficult to control. As discussed earlier in this chapter, the human body is the reservoir for the bacteria that colonise the skin, bowel and respiratory tract. They generally do not harm the host unless the immune system is impaired, when they can cause opportunistic infections in immunocompromised patients. The hospital environment can serve as a reservoir for organisms if standards of cleanliness are not adhered to.

Patients can become a source of infection if they have infected skin lesions, skin scales, secretions and excretions which can easily be transferred to other people. Organic material such as dirt, blood and body fluids can harbour bacteria, and any equipment that has been in contact with the patient can serve as both a reservoir and a source of infection. Bed frames, mattresses and manual handling equipment have all been implicated in the spread of infection.[88]

Link 3. Portal of exit

There are many different portals of exit, which are the routes by which the organism leaves the reservoir. These include the respiratory and alimentary tracts and the skin and mucosa, with organisms carried in blood and body fluids, respiratory droplets and on the surface of the skin. In some organisms, the portal of exit can be the same as the portal of entry, such as the respiratory tract in tuberculosis, or it may be different; in salmonella infections, the route of entry is usually the mouth as salmonella has to be ingested, and the exit route is in the faeces.

Link 4. Mode of transmission

This refers to the way in which the organism is spread and acquired. Direct contact with infected body fluids, secretions and lesions can transmit infections such as HIV, the common cold and impetigo. The hands of healthcare workers are the most important source of cross-infection, transferring resident and transient skin flora. Fomites are objects which can become contaminated with organisms from patients or staff, and subsequently become a source of cross-infection. They include IV stands, pumps and monitors, bed linen, computer keyboards and telephones. The risk that these pose depends largely on the degree or extent to which the object/piece of equipment is contaminated, the microbial load and the amount of direct contact that it has with the patient. However, even if it does not come into contact with the patient, the hands of any healthcare workers who may have had contact with it could serve as vehicles for cross-infection.

Airborne transmission of particles such as dust, water and respiratory droplets, which can all contain micro-organisms, can result in infection if they are inhaled or settle on equipment or on wounds. Legionella (see Chapter 20) is present in aerosols which can, depending on wind speed, travel up to 500 metres and infect large numbers of people. Pathogens may be expelled from the respiratory tract during coughing, sneezing and talking. These droplets partially evaporate to form droplet nuclei, where they remain suspended in the air for long periods of time and can subsequently be inhaled. Other droplets, or large dust particles, may fall rather rapidly, and settle on furniture, bedding or equipment and although they are unlikely to become airborne again, they can still cause infection.

Bacteria may be ingested through consuming contaminated food or water (for example cholera, campylobacter and salmonella). Patients may also acquire some infections as a result of faecal-oral transmission, whereby their hands have become contaminated and they subsequently move their hands to their mouth. Norovirus can be spread by both the airborne and the faecal-oral routes.

Transmission of blood-borne viruses such as HIV and hepatitis B and C via inoculation injury, either from a contaminated sharp (see Chapter 6) or a splash of blood or body fluids into the mucosa, can pose a big risk to healthcare workers.

Some infections may also be spread endogenously – they are acquired as the result of the patient's own body flora being transferred from one body site to another.

Link 5. The susceptible patient

Any patient in a hospital bed is potentially at risk from contracting an infection during their inpatient stay, but there are many factors which significantly increase that risk. These risk factors are summarised in Table 5.4.

Table 5.4 Factors influencing susceptibility to infection

Age
Any pre-existing underlying illness/disease
Patients who are immunocompromised – through illness or medication
Surgery – including anaesthesia, mechanical ventilation, the insertion of foreign material
    such as prosthetic implants
The presence of any indwelling invasive devices
Medication – steroids alter the immune response; antibiotics disrupt the normal body flora

---

COLONISATION, INFECTION AND THE INFLAMMATORY RESPONSE

Not all patients with an 'infection' are genuinely infected, so the isolation of an organism from a body site is not necessarily clinically significant. Once an organism has made contact with the host and adhered to the skin or mucosal surfaces, it often establishes itself at that site and colonises it, without causing any adverse effects or harm. Meticillin-resistant *Staphylococcus aureus* for example colonises the nose, throat and perineum with the majority of patients having asymptomatic carriage. The length of time that a site may be colonised is variable and depends on both host factors and the properties of the organism involved. The host may go on to develop immunity to the organism by developing specific T-cell or antibody responses. Immunity to *Neisseria meningitidis*, the potentially pathogenic organism that inhabits the nasopharynx of 10 % of the normal healthy population as part of their nasopharyngeal flora, is acquired this way (see Chapter 13). Streptococci, which have the ability to cause devastatingly invasive infections such as necrotising fasciitis and toxic shock syndrome (see Chapter 12 Invasive Group A Streptococcal Disease) are part of the resident flora of the upper respiratory tract. The status quo may change however if the relationship between the host and the organism alters to the extent that the organism can extend beyond colonisation to local invasion of the tissues, or even the whole body.[77]

Infection is the process of microbial invasion which results in tissue damage at the site of the infection or, in the worst case scenario, the death of the host. Unlike colonisation, infection manifests itself both physically and physiologically. These signs may be either localised, or ***systemic.***

There are several stages in the pathogenesis of infection:

- Entry of the organism: as seen in the chain of infection, there are a number of ways in which the organism can enter the host.
- Attachment: the organism needs to attach itself to the tissues so that it can penetrate them.
- Multiplication, invasion and spread: once attached, and providing that the environmental conditions required for the organism's growth and survival are right, it will begin to multiply. It can do this locally at the site of attachment, or it

may invade the bloodstream and be carried to other body sites. Clinical signs of infection then become apparent.

- Evasion of host defences: the organism will try to avoid the effects of the host's immune system.
- Damage to tissues/the host: in some cases, the damage resulting from the infection may be so severe that it leads to the death of the host.

When the body suffers a traumatic injury, or is invaded by micro-organisms, it generates an inflammatory response, which is designed to localise the infection and limit its spread. The success of the inflammatory response, however, depends on the strength of the host's immune system and the pathogenicity, virulence and toxigenicity of the organism involved. The physiological events that subsequently take place give rise to the cardinal signs of infection, or inflammation:

- redness or erythema (rubor)
- heat (calor)
- swelling (tumor)
- pain (dolor)
- loss of function.

Vasodilation occurs at the site of 'injury', caused by the release of histamines and prostaglandins from damaged cells. This results in an increased blood flow, which contains plasma proteins, neutrophils and phagocytes, to the affected site. The temperature of the skin rises as a result of the increased blood supply and an increase in the metabolic activities in the cells of the tissues at the damaged site. An increase in body temperature, which is regulated by the hypothalamus and 'set' at 37 °C, often occurs and is generated by activated macrophages, which release cytokines and basically 'reset' the hypothalamus. As most bacteria replicate at, or below, 37 °C, an increase in body temperature may adversely affect the pathogen, as it will lead to an increase in the production of phagocytes and antibodies.

The capillaries that line the epithelial cells dilate, releasing plasma which causes swelling; depending on the site involved and the severity of the swelling this may lead to loss of function. The process of phagocytosis begins with the release of chemokines, which attract the phagocytes to the area where they are needed. The phagocyte then attaches itself to the bacteria, surrounds it and ingests it. Some pathogens are able to evade phagocytosis, either by producing a toxin (leukocidin) which destroys the phagocyte, or because the pathogen has the ability to survive within it and multiply, and yet remain in a dormant state, resulting in disease months or even years later.

An inflammatory exudate forms at the site of inflammation, consisting of fluid, cells and cellular debris. Purulent discharge or pus, often seen in wound infections or at infected intravascular cannula sites, contains living and dead organisms, phagocytes and cell debris. With some organisms such as staphylococci and streptococci, the inflammatory exudate may be excessive. *Pseudomonas aeruginosa* produces a distinctive blue-green exudate on wound dressings caused by green fluorescent pigment (fluorescein) and a blue pigment (pyocyanin), and has a slightly sweet, sickly smell. Once the invading bacteria have been dealt with, the damaged tissues and cells begin the process of repair. However, if the immune response has been weak or the infection overwhelming, the host may die.

BACTERAEMIA, SEPTICAEMIA AND THE SYSTEMIC INFLAMMATORY RESPONSE SYNDROME

Although blood is sterile, bacteria can enter the blood in large numbers in three main ways.[89] They can escape from a site of natural occurrence if the integrity of the tissue is damaged, which may occur as a result of trauma, inflammation or malignancy. They may then colonise a surface, invade the epithelium and then enter the bloodstream. If there is a deep cavity or site of sepsis, such as an abscess, or an area of necrotic tissue, the network of tiny blood vessels within that cavity may be invaded. Bacteria can also be inoculated into the blood stream via a bite, scratch, trauma or *iatrogenic* injury.

The presence of viable blood circulating in the bloodstream is called bacteraemia, and it is not always associated with fever and signs of illness. The bactericidal properties of the blood, including phagocytes, the complement pathway and antibodies help to resolve many episodes of *transient* bacteraemia, which can arise following dental work, childbirth and procedures such as bronchoscopy and sigmoidoscopy. The organisms responsible for these transient bacteraemias are normally the flora that reside at that particular site, and are of low virulence.[89] However, there are four general categories of clinically important organisms[89] causing bacteraemia, which can be classified as:

- staphylococci and streptococci, both community- and hospital-acquired
- members of the genus *Enterobacteriaceae*, which are commonly hospital-acquired
- anaerobic and aerobic opportunists, mainly hospital-acquired
- community acquired organisms such as *N.meningitidis* and *Haemophilus spp*s.

The inflammatory response generated by the immune system against the invading bacteria may be so strong that it triggers an extremely potent immunological cascade that may be overwhelming for the patient. Sepsis is the 'umbrella' word frequently used to describe systemic infection, and 18 million people die from sepsis worldwide each year.[90] Septicaemia is the systemic illness which arises as a result of the uncontrolled spread of bacteria or their toxins through the bloodstream, and is the leading cause of death of death in intensive care units.[91,92] There has been confusion over the definition of the word sepsis,[93] which is often used interchangeably with septicaemia and septic shock, and historically there has been a general lack of consensus in actually agreeing these definitions. However, in 1991 clear and concise definitions were agreed[93,94] for the terms sepsis, severe sepsis and septic shock, together with the introduction of a new term known as systemic inflammatory response syndrome (SIRS).

SIRS is defined as a clinical response arising from a non-specific insult and which includes more than two of the following[93]:

- temperature greater than 38 °C or less than 36 °C
- tachycardic, with heart rate >90 beats/minute
- tachyapnoeic – respiratory rate >20 breaths/minute
- white cell count >12,000 per mm^3 or < 4,000 per mm^3.

Sepsis is defined as SIRS with a presumed or confirmed infection and accompanied by two or more of the SIRS criteria.[93] Severe sepsis is said to occur if there is a known or suspected infection, along with two or more SIRS criteria plus more than one sign of acute organ dysfunction, which can involve any of the major body organs.[93] Signs of organ dysfunction may manifest themselves as altered mental state; hyperglycaemia (in the absence of diabetes); hypoxia (oxygen saturation <93 % or arterial blood gas <9kPa); urine output <0.5ml/kg/hr, and/or raised urea and creatinine; coagulopathy (INR >1.5 activated partial thromboplastin time >60 seconds, or platelets <100). Table 5.5 summarises the patient risk factors for developing sepsis.

Septic shock is defined as severe sepsis together with cardiovascular dysfunction, and is characterised by hypotension which does not respond to fluid resuscitation.[94,95]

It is commonly seen as a complication of septicaemia caused by Gram-negative endotoxins, (or Gram-positive toxins such as staphylococcal enterotoxins) which initiate a cascade of events, leading to hypotension and *disseminated intra-vascular coagulation* (DIC) which may be irreversible. The release of toxins trigger the release of inflammatory mediators into the bloodstream, such as histamine, serotonin, noradrenalin and plasmakinins, along with tumor necrosis factor (TNF) and

Table 5.5 Risk factors for developing sepsis

Age
Obesity
ITU patients
Patients with invasive indwelling devices
Underlying chronic diseases – chronic obstructive pulmonary disease (COPD), heart failure, chronic renal failure
Immunocompromised – drugs or disease
Cellulitis
Urinary tract infections
Meningitis
Abdominal surgery
Infection with antibiotic resistant organism

---

inter-leukin 1 (IL-1), which are released from macrophages. These inflammatory mediators cause the blood vessels to dilate. TNF and IL-1 also cause disturbances in the temperature regulation giving rise to signs of fever.

The macrophages activate the complement system and release other inflammatory cytokines, which have an effect on vascular endothelial cell function and integrity. As the blood capillaries become more permeable and fluid leaks out of the general circulation, the blood pressure falls due to the drop in circulating volume, and the patient becomes hypovolaemic. The coagulation pathway becomes activated, triggering clotting abnormalities, and disseminated intravascular coagulation (DIC) may develop. As a result of bloodclotting abnormalities, purpuric lesions may develop and manifest as areas of petechiae on the skin, as seen in meningococcal septicaemia. Small blood clots develop in the blood vessels which result in poor tissue and organ perfusion, and can affect digits or an entire limb. The affected limb will initially appear ice cold, white and bloodless and will eventually become blackened and necrosed as arterial and venous occlusion progresses.

Multi-organ dysfunction swiftly develops. An increasing respiratory rate heralds the onset of impending respiratory failure; impaired cerebral confusion and metabolism attributed to hypotension, *hypoxia* and *acidosis* leads to decreased neurological function and may result in coma; reduced renal perfusion will contribute to renal failure.

Management of sepsis and septic shock

Aggressive treatment influences survival and the severity of the illness[95,96] and should begin immediately sepsis is recognised. The Surviving Sepsis Campaign[95] guidelines for the management of severe sepsis and septic shock are a series of evidence-based recommendations intended to improve survival outcomes for critically ill patients, beginning with the establishment of vascular access and aggressive fluid resuscitation as the first priority. Patients will require ventilatory support to reduce the respiratory workload, and are at risk of developing acute respiratory

Table 5.6 Investigations to determine the cause of sepsis

Blood culture
Arterial blood gas
Full blood count (FBC)
Urea and electrolytes
Clotting screen
Glucose
Chest x-ray
ECG
Culture – urine, sputum, CSF
Swabs – wounds, peripheral IV/CVC lines, wound drainage sites, pressure sores
Remove invasive indwelling devices
Surgical debridement/drainage of abscesses if appropriate

distress syndrome (ARDS) which can arise from pulmonary capillary leak, or pulmonary oedema secondary to left ventricular failure. The administration of inotropes in the form of dopamine and dobutamine are required to help restore renal perfusion and cardiac function, along with adrenaline and noradrenaline to restore blood pressure.[95]

From an infection control perspective, blood cultures should be taken together with cultures of urine, wounds, sputum and invasive devices, and antibiotics should be commenced as soon as the cultures have been obtained. The choice of antibiotic, which may necessitate combination therapy, should be guided by the susceptible patterns of micro-organisms both in the community and the hospital, should have activity against likely bacterial and fungal pathogens, and penetrate to the presumed source of sepsis.[92,96] Attempts should also be made to control the source of sepsis, such as removing potentially infected invasive devices, debriding any necrotic tissue and draining of any abscesses if present. Table 5.6 summarises the investigations that should be carried out in order to determine the source of sepsis.

6 The Principles of Infection Prevention and Control

INTRODUCTION

To prevent the risk of cross-infection to patients and staff, certain basic infection control actions need to be implemented by healthcare workers in all healthcare settings all of the time, bearing in mind that infected or colonised patients are not always known. Failure to stringently apply these actions provides numerous opportunities for cross-infection to occur.

This chapter explains the principles of infection control and the standard precautions that need to be taken in line with the recommendations contained within the EPIC guidelines.[86] It looks at the importance of hand hygiene; the use of personal protective equipment and clothing; the safe handling and disposal of sharps; the management of waste and linen, and decontamination of both equipment and the environment; the decontamination and re-use of medical devices; and patient isolation.

LEARNING OUTCOMES

After reading this chapter the reader will:

- Understand the importance of hand hygiene, the wearing of personal protective equipment and clothing, and the safe handling and disposal of sharps
- Understand the principles of cleaning, disinfection and sterilisation

BACKGROUND

Most healthcare workers are familiar with the phrase 'universal precautions', or 'standard precautions' to describe the infection control actions (hand hygiene, the safe handling and disposal of sharps, the use of personal protective equipment and clothing, and decontamination) that healthcare workers take to prevent the spread of healthcare associated infections. These terms have their origins back in the 1970s in the USA, when seven categories of different isolation precautions were devised[97] – strict isolation; respiratory isolation; protective isolation (later removed as it was not considered to be of any proven value); enteric precautions; wound and skin precautions; discharge precautions (later to become drainage and secretions precautions), and blood precautions. Tuberculosis precautions were added to the list, and in the 1980s, blood precautions were expanded to include patients with AIDS as well as other body fluids, and became known as blood and body fluid precautions. In 1985, in response to the mounting problems with HIV and growing concerns over the risks that occupational exposure to HIV posed to healthcare workers, the Centres for Disease Control (CDC), Atlanta, USA, introduced the term 'universal precautions'. This was in recognition of the fact that not all patients with a blood-borne virus have their infection diagnosed, and included within universal precautions were blood and body fluid precautions which incorporated the use of masks and face protection in order to protect healthcare workers against mucous membrane exposures. In 1987[97], another category of precautions called body substance isolation was developed; this latest set of precautions highlighted the need to protect healthcare workers, and other patients, from the cross-infection risks potentially posed from other pathogens apart from blood-borne viruses, isolated from moist body sites such as faeces, urine, sputum and other body fluids and secretions. Then, in 1996, the CDC replaced universal precautions with standard principles[97], incorporating infection control measures to protect against blood-borne viruses as well as other pathogens, and transmission based precautions focusing on preventing the spread of infection from airborne, droplet and direct contact.

The Department of Health commissioned the development of national evidence-based guidelines for the prevention of healthcare associated infections (known as the EPIC guidelines) which were published in 2001 and revised in 2006.[98,86] These guidelines on the standard principles for preventing healthcare associated infection aim to inform best practice in relation to preventing the spread of HCAI based on the best evidence currently available. The recommendations from the 2006 revised guidance, known as EPIC 2, are referred to throughout this book.

HAND HYGIENE

Within the healthcare setting it is crucial to patient care that micro-organisms are removed from the hands of healthcare workers in order to prevent their potential transfer to patients, since hands are the principle route by which cross-infection occurs.[99,100,101] The transmission of micro-organisms from one patient to another via the hands, or from hands that have been contaminated from the environment can occur:

a) **Directly**

When micro-organisms are introduced into susceptible sites such as surgical wounds and intravenous cannula sites.

b) **Indirectly**

Where micro-organisms transferred by the hands become established on a patient and subsequently cause infection at susceptible sites.

The microbial flora of the skin consists of both resident and transient micro-organisms. Resident skin flora, with a population density of between 10^2 and 10^3 colony forming units (CFU) per cm^2 of skin, are deep-seated within skin crevices, sweat glands, hair follicles and beneath the finger nails, and are more resistant to mechanical removal with soap and water than transient organisms.[102] Although they are generally of lower pathogenicity and they have a role to play in protecting the skin from colonisation by other more potentially pathogenic bacteria (colonisation-resistance), they can themselves be pathogenic if they are transferred into susceptible sites in vulnerable patients, such as wounds or cannulae sites. Transient micro-organisms are more of a problem within the healthcare setting and they are frequently associated with infections in hospital. They are readily acquired through contact with other people, equipment or body sites, and although they do not survive on the skin for more than a few hours due to the skin's inherent antibacterial properties, there is sufficient time for them to be transferred to other patients and equipment.[103,104,105,106] While most transient micro-organisms are likely to be acquired from heavily contaminated material such as body fluids, they can also be acquired from contact with apparently clean objects or surfaces such as patients' skin, bed linen and work surfaces. MRSA and *C.difficile* are examples of micro-organisms that can be carried on the hands transiently.

Hand hygiene has a dual role in protecting both patients and healthcare workers from acquiring micro-organisms which may cause them harm, and it results in a significant reduction in the carriage of potential pathogens on the hands. This can be readily achieved by using liquid soap and water with an effective technique, or using an alcohol hand rub on visibly clean hands. Hands should be cleaned or decontaminated before every episode of patient care that involves direct contact with:

- a patient's skin
- a patient's food
- any invasive device
- when dressing a wound.

Hands should also be decontaminated after completing an episode of patient care to minimise cross-contamination of the environment.

HAND WASHING

Hand washing has been defined as '. . . a vigorous, brief rubbing together of all surfaces of lathered hands followed by rinsing under a stream of water'[107] and the mechanical action of lathering and rubbing the hands together along with rinsing under running water will remove transient micro-organisms from the skin. Table 6.1 describes the technique for routine/social hand washing.

While washing hands with liquid soap and water suspends micro-organisms in solution, enabling them to be washed off, ordinary soap has minimal or no antimicrobial activity, and does not reduce the microbial load on the skin. Hands can become contaminated by the soap (communal bars of soap should be avoided), taps and sinks,[108] the removal of contaminated personal protective equipment such as gloves, aprons and masks, and the presence of rings, which can cause the skin underneath the ring to become colonised by Gram-negative bacteria, which would normally be found as transient skin flora.[109] Deep-seated resident skin flora is not removed by social hand washing, and requires the use of preparations that contain antiseptics, which have a residual action on the skin flora.

In 1847, Ignaz Semmelweiss demonstrated a convincing reduction in mortality from puerperal sepsis (group A streptococcal infection) following childbirth after the introduction of chlorinated lime as a method for decontaminating the hands prior to examining women in labour.[110] Since then, hand hygiene has been widely acknowledged to be the single most important factor in the control of infection,[86,98,106] and the National Audit Office Report published in 2004[36] suggested that good hand hygiene practice could contribute to the reduction of healthcare associated

Table 6.1 Hand washing technique[107]

---

1. Remove all wrist and hand jewellery at the beginning of each clinical shift so that it does not inhibit hand washing.
2. Wet hands under warm running water before applying liquid soap.
3. Apply liquid soap to wet hands, ensuring that it comes into contact with all surfaces of the hand.

NB: The hands must be rubbed together vigorously for a minimum of 10–15 seconds, with the liquid soap in contact with all surfaces of the hands.

4. Rub hands palm to palm.
5. Rub right palm over left dorsum and left palm over right dorsum.
6. Rub palm to palm with fingers interlaced.
7. Rub backs of fingers to opposing palm with the fingers interlocked.
8. Rotational rubbing of the right thumb clasped in the left palm.
9. Rotational rubbing of the left thumb in the right palm.
10. Rotational rubbing with clasped fingers of the right hand in the left palm.
11. Rotational rubbing with clasped fingers of the left hand in the right palm.
12. Rinse thoroughly under clear running water.
13. Dry well using disposable paper towels.
14. Apply hand cream regularly to protect the skin from the drying effects of regular hand washing.

Table 6.2 Factors contributing to poor hand washing compliance

---

Lack of time – too busy, staff shortages, patient needs take priority over hand washing.
Inadequate facilities – shortage of clinical hand wash basins, liquid soap and paper towels.
Inconvenience.
Lack of knowledge about how infections are spread, scepticism about the value of hand
washing and poor motivation.
Hands don't need washing if they don't look dirty.
Lack of knowledge of infection control guidelines.
Not thinking about it.
Belief that wearing gloves is a substitute for hand washing.
Lack of institutional priority.
Complications associated with frequent handwashing – skin irritation.

Refs: [102,111,114,115]

infections by 15 %. Although it is accepted throughout the healthcare community as a basic clinical procedure essential for the prevention of infections in patients and healthcare workers alike, the vast amount of literature published on the importance of hand washing over the last 30 years shows that hands are either inadequately, infrequently or inappropriately washed and that compliance is poor.[102,104,111,112,113] Factors contributing to poor hand washing compliance are highlighted in Table 6.2.

A study by Larson and Kretzer[114] which reviewed 37 other studies published between 1989 and 1994 on hand washing compliance by healthcare workers revealed, among other things, that hand washing occurred after only 50 % of patient contacts. This is of concern as recent studies have demonstrated that this level of compliance will not reduce the risk of transmission of multi-drug resistant bacteria in hospitals.[115]

ALCOHOL HAND RUBS

Hand hygiene is, however, currently undergoing something of a global renaissance which may in part be due to the widespread introduction of alcohol hand rubs which are providing a novel and pragmatic approach to this important but still low profile aspect of healthcare. In 2002, the Centres for Disease Control and Prevention (CDC) released guidelines for hand hygiene in healthcare institutions that supported the use of alcohol based sanitisers.[116] The recommendation to use alcohol hand rubs for routine hand decontamination had previously been made within the 2001 EPIC guidelines[98], and the recommendation made by the CDC provided added weight to the argument of promoting alcohol based hand rub as the primary method for hand decontamination. The rapid efficacy of alcohol based solutions, as opposed to the more traditional methods of hand washing using liquid soap and water, or disinfectants such as hydrex or betadine, and their availability at the patient's bedside and point of use, make these products an ideal substitute for conventional hand washing, addressing the real and perceived constraints associated with handwashing, and substantially increasing hand hygiene compliance rates.[117,118] Alcohol based hand rubs are active immediately against a wide range of organisms and are approximately 100 times more effective against viruses than any other form of hand washing product.[119] They should be applied to visibly clean hands in sufficient amounts (as recommended by the manufacturer – amounts can vary between products) to cover all areas of the hands and rubbed in for approximately 30 seconds until the hands are dry. This can be done on the move, a distinct advantage in environments where hand washing facilities are lacking. Alcohol based hand rubs do not require access to a sink, running water or paper towels, are kinder to the skin due to added emollients, useful for rapid bedside hand decontamination in between patients and/or procedures, and are useful for clinical areas where access to hand washing facilities may be lacking.[106] However, they are not cleansing agents and they do not work in the presence of organic material such as dirt or blood, and they are ineffective against *Clostridium difficile* spores (see Chapter 11), so hand washing with liquid soap and water is absolutely essential in these situations.

CHOICE OF AGENT FOR HAND CLEANSING/DECONTAMINATION

There are a range of products available for hand cleansing/decontamination and the wide choice can be confusing for the healthcare worker. The selection of the correct agent will depend on whether the removal of resident or transient micro-organisms is required.

Soap and water

Soap and water is not suitable for hand decontamination where a higher level of skin disinfection is required, i.e. prior to surgery or other highly invasive procedures. Liquid soap dispensers with individual replacement cartridges are the preferred option in clinical settings. Bar soap is not recommended as it becomes contaminated during communal use and frequently grows micro-organisms.

Advantages of soap and water

- Cheap and readily available.
- Effectively removes transient micro-organisms.

Disadvantages of soap and water

- Time consuming.
- Requires facilities for washing and drying.
- Can damage the skin.

Alcohol hand rubs

The use of alcohol hand rubs has now become the gold standard for routine hand decontamination[86,98] and should be used routinely when hands are not visibly soiled (i.e. most of the time).

Advantages of alcohol hand rubs

- More effective in destroying transient micro-organisms than antiseptic hand washing agents or soap and water.
- Active immediately against a wide range of micro-organisms.
- Requires no facilities such as a sink, running water or paper towels.
- Kinder to the skin due to added emollients.
- Can be packed into bag/pocket sized containers.
- Useful for rapid bedside hand decontamination between patients or procedures.
- Useful for community based healthcare workers where access to handwashing facilities may be lacking.

Disadvantages of alcohol hand rub

- Not a cleansing agent.
- Astringent – makes the skin sting if minor abrasions are present.
- Limited activity against bacterial spores (i.e. *Clostridium difficile*).

Aqueous antiseptic solutions

Antiseptic hand washing solutions used with water will both remove and destroy micro-organisms on the hands, a process referred to as chemical removal of micro-organisms. Some antiseptic agents have a residual activity and provide continued anti-microbial activity which is of benefit during surgical procedures. A range of aqueous antiseptic solutions are available in the UK but only a few are routinely used. These include Chlorhexidine, Iodophors (Betadine) and Triclosan (Aquasept).

THE 'CLEANYOURHANDS' CAMPAIGN

In September 2004, the National Patient Safety Agency (NPSA) issued a Patient Safety Alert[120,121], announcing the phased rollout of the 'cleanyourhands' campaign during 2004/05. The aim of the campaign, which is ongoing, is to minimise the risk to patient safety posed by poor hand hygiene compliance amongst healthcare professionals through a national strategy of improvement. This involves the placement of alcohol hand rub at the patient's bedside, the use of posters and other promotional material to inform and influence healthcare staff and patients,

Table 6.3 Practical benefits of placing alcohol hand rub at the point of care[122]

Quick to use and can be used without interrupting work.
Patients can see that staff are decontaminating their hands – increases patient confidence.
Reduces bacteria at a greater rate than soap and water, and does not need to be placed by a
   sink.
It causes less irritation to the skin than soap.

and the involvement of patients themselves by encouraging them to ask healthcare workers if they have cleaned their hands. Full details of the campaign
can be found on the NPSA website.[122] Following the implementation of the
pilot campaign in six acute trusts in which an alcohol based rub was made
available at the point of care, an economic evaluation of the 'cleanyourhands'
pilot suggested that successful implementation of the campaign might release
cash savings to the NHS of around £140 million per year and save 450 lives
in a 500 bedded hospital once target compliance rates have been reached.[123]
The practical benefits of placing alcohol hand rub at the point of care are
described in Table 6.3.

In July 2004, the NHS Purchasing and Supply Agency (PASA) announced
a new national contract for alcohol hand rub products.[124] All of the products
available on the current NHS supplies contract were rigorously and independently tested against the European standard (EN: 1500) to ensure that they
were fully effective, and subjected to a range of skin acceptability tests by
leading dermatologists. As a result, PASA recommended that three products were
available for order on the national contract (Ecolab Ltd, B-Braun Medical and
Gojo Europe Ltd), although there was no obligation for Trusts and their infection prevention and control teams to change to one of these products from
their existing product.

While much of the focus is, quite rightly, on the compliance with hand
washing/hand decontamination among healthcare workers in preventing the spread
of infection, the role of patients' hands in the spread of infection should not
be ignored.[125] They can acquire micro-organisms on their hands from the environment, and they can auto-infect themselves, moving commensal flora from
one body site to another. Patients should be encouraged to wash their hands
or use alcohol hand rub. If this is not possible, they should be provided with
disposable hand wipes.

HAND HYGIENE – RECOMMENDATIONS FOR PRACTICE

Table 6.4 summarises the recommendations in relation to hand hygiene contained
within the EPIC 2 guidelines.[86]

Table 6.4 Hand hygiene recommendations for clinical practice[86,98]

Decontaminate hands immediately before each episode of direct patient contact and after any activity or contact that potentially results in hands becoming contaminated. Alcohol hand rub is preferable unless hands are visibly soiled.

If hands are visibly soiled or potentially grossly contaminated, they must be washed with liquid soap and water

Jewellery on the wrists and hands should be removed at the beginning of a clinical shift.

Cuts and abrasions on the hands must be covered with waterproof dressings.

Fingernails should be kept short and clean; nail polish and nail extensions must not be worn.

When hands are washed, an effective technique consisting of three stages (preparation, washing and rinsing, and drying) must be used.

When alcohol hand rub is used, it must only be used on visibly clean hands and must come into contact with all surfaces of the hands. It should be rubbed into the skin until the solution has evaporated and the hands are dry.

Staff should use hand creams to help counter-balance the effects of liquid soap/alcohol hand rub and maintain the integrity of the skin.

In the event of skin irritation developing, the occupational health department should be contacted for advice.

Alcohol hand rub should be available at the point of use.

All healthcare workers should receive an annual update in effective hand hygiene technique.

Compliance/practice should be audited and fed back to healthcare workers.

PERSONAL PROTECTIVE EQUIPMENT AND CLOTHING

The main purpose of wearing personal equipment and clothing, such as gloves, aprons, masks and eye protection, is to protect healthcare workers from blood-borne pathogens and prevent the transmission of micro-organisms to both patients and staff. The EPIC 2 guidelines[86,98] clearly state that the selection of protective equipment must be based on a risk assessment of the risk of transmission of micro-organisms to the patient or carer, and the risk of contamination with blood, body fluids, secretions and excretions, but healthcare workers are often unsure when to wear PPE, and haphazard and inconsistent practices can place both staff and patients at risk.

GLOVES

The wearing of gloves has two main purposes; they act as a protective barrier, preventing contamination of the healthcare worker's hands with organic material such as blood and faeces as well as from micro-organisms, and they prevent the transmission of micro-organisms to patients during invasive procedures.[126] Glove use can be a ritualistic rather than evidence-based practice and sensitivity reactions associated with frequent glove use such as irritant contact dermatitis, which tends to resolve once the healthcare worker stops wearing them, may influence whether or not the healthcare worker wears gloves for certain procedures, potentially increasing the risk of cross-infection.

The EPIC 2 guidelines[86] recommend that healthcare workers wear gloves for the following activities:

- all invasive procedures
- contact with sterile sites and non-intact skin or mucous membranes
- where there is a risk of exposure to blood, body fluids, secretions or excretions
- when handling sharp or contaminated instruments.

Gloves are not necessary for other activities involving contact with the patient such as bed making, assistance with mobility, recording the patient's temperature, pulse or blood pressure, or taking items into the patient's room. This is because hands are less likely to become heavily contaminated with micro-organisms during these activities and the bacteria that do get picked up are easily removed through hand washing, or decontaminated with the use of alcohol hand rub as long as there is no visible contamination. Gloves must be changed in between patients and in between different procedures on the same patient, otherwise bacteria will be spread from patient to patient or transferred from a colonised site on a patient to a susceptible site such as a wound or a urinary catheter. They should be disposed of promptly after use to avoid contaminating clean surfaces, equipment or other patients.

Gloves are not a substitute for handwashing, and yet all too often staff wear the same pair of gloves from patient to patient, assuming that the wearing of gloves means that their hands are clean. They should be worn as single-use items (not rinsed under the tap or decontaminated with alcohol hand rub in between healthcare interventions) and disposed of as clinical waste after use. They will become heavily contaminated during use, and the healthcare worker's hands will become contaminated on removing the gloves. Staff must ensure that they decontaminate their hands once gloves have been disposed of, either with soap and water if they are visibly contaminated or with alcohol hand rub, depending on the product available.

Disposable gloves are manufactured from both natural and synthetic materials, such as natural rubber latex (NRL), vinyl (polyvinyl chloride) and nitrile (acrylonitrile). Natural rubber latex is increasingly associated with latex sensitisation and latex allergy, which can vary between mild skin irritation to urticaria and potentially life threatening anaphylaxis (see Chapter 5) and other alternatives to latex such as nitrile must be available to staff with latex allergy.[86,98,126,127] Gloves containing powder are no longer recommended for use within healthcare settings as they present potential hazards.[98] Powder was originally introduced as a lubricant to facilitate the donning and removal of gloves[128], but it can contaminate the environment and if powdered latex gloves are worn, the corn starch powder can act as a vector for the latex proteins and increase the level of latex exposure to latex-sensitive individuals.[129] While all gloves have the potential to fail during use if they are torn or punctured, polythene gloves can leak and are not recommended for use when dealing with blood or body fluids[98]; latex/nitrile non-sterile gloves offer better protection against blood-borne viruses.

DISPOSABLE APRONS

Uniforms can become heavily contaminated during direct patient contact, or contact with contaminated equipment, and disposable plastic aprons protect the part of the uniform that is in the closest contact with the patient. Aprons should be worn:

- for potential direct contact with an infectious patient and their environment when it is anticipated that clothing may become contaminated with micro-organisms, or blood, body fluids, secretions and excretions during healthcare interventions
- for direct contact with an infectious patient and their environment
- when clothing is likely to become wet or soiled
- bed making.

They must be discarded as clinical waste after each task or episode of patient care and not worn from patient to patient.

Full-body fluid-repellent gowns should be worn for any activity where there is the risk of extensive splashing of blood or body fluids, secretions or excretions, and are not required for the majority of patient contacts.

FACE AND RESPIRATORY PROTECTION

Masks, visors and goggles protect the mucous membranes of the eyes and mouth from exposure to blood and body fluids in situations where splashes can occur. Some healthcare workers may wear standard face masks as protection against respiratory droplets, or in outbreak situations, but the main purpose of wearing a mask is to prevent the expulsion of respiratory droplets into the environment by the wearer, or to protect the wearer from exposure to blood or body fluids. Where protection against respiratory droplets is required (for example, multi-drug resistant tuberculosis, severe acute respiratory syndrome, or pandemic influenza), disposable respirator masks that conform to the European Standard EN149:2001 are required. EN149 is the European Respiratory Protection Standard for dispos-able filtering respirators, which are worn as face masks covering the nose, mouth and chin, and filter particles including bacteria and viruses. The FFP3 respi-rator provides 99 % particle filtration efficiency, and affords the highest level of protection. The use of masks is discussed further in Chapter 10 (Tuberculosis). Table 6.5 summarises some important considerations with regard to the use of these respirators.

Table 6.5 Respiratory masks

Disposable respirators help reduce exposure to airborne particles and must seal tightly to the face/against the skin to prevent air from entering from the sides.

Respirators will not seal against the skin if the wearer has stubble, a beard or long moustache.

The respirator must be fitted exactly as per the instructions that are provided with each box of respirators:

- the metal strip must be moulded to the bridge of the nose
- one of the elastic bands attached to the respirator must be fitted to the top of the head, and the other to the back of the head to ensure that the fit is snug.

The healthcare worker must be fit-tested to ensure that there are no leaks, and a fit-test performed each time a new respirator is worn.

Although they can be worn for a maximum of eight hours, they should be disposed of after use as clinical waste.

THE SAFE HANDLING AND DISPOSAL OF SHARPS

Sharps include needles, scalpels, stitch cutters, ampoules, sharp instruments, broken glass and crockery. Not only are healthcare workers at risk from injury from sharps, particularly needles and scalpel blades, but so too are patients if sharps are inappropriately used and carelessly discarded (for example, used needles left amongst the bedclothes, on bedside lockers, or if sharps bins are easily accessible).[130] Exposure to blood-borne viruses through sharps-related injuries is largely preventable and healthcare workers have to accept responsibility for the sharps that they use and the method of handling and exposure (see Chapter 16 Blood-borne Viruses). Figure 6.1 summarises some important points in relation to the safe handling and disposal of sharps.

THE DISPOSAL OF WASTE

Hospitals generate two types of waste; household waste, which includes items that are not contaminated with potentially infectious material, such as paper and packaging, paper towels, dead flowers, disposed of in black sacks and sent for landfill, and clinical waste. The Controlled Waste Regulations (1992)[131] define clinical waste as any waste that wholly or partly consists of blood or other body fluids, excretions, human or animal tissue, swabs or dressings, sharps (needles or instruments) and drugs or other pharmaceutical products. Waste must be segregated properly to comply with regulations and prevent any cross-contamination risk to waste handlers. Failure to comply with waste regulations with regard to the collection,

1. The PERSON USING the sharp is responsible for the DISPOSING of it.

2. SHARPS must be DISCARDED into a sharps box at the POINT OF USE.

3. SHARPS MUST NOT be passed directly from HAND TO HAND.

4. USED NEEDLES must NEVER be resheathed.

5. NEEDLES and SYRINGES must NOT BE DISASSEMBLED by HAND prior to disposal.

6. Ensure SHARPS BOXES are ASSEMBLED CORRECTLY.

7. SHARPS BOXES must not be FILLED above the FILL LINE.

8. NEVER place your hands INSIDE or FORCE sharps into a sharps box.

9. Sharps boxes must be kept OUT OF THE REACH of CHILDREN/ CONFUSED PATIENTS. Where this is not possible temporarily close the lid between uses.

10. BLOOD COLLECTION SYSTEMS (vacutainers) should be used for taking blood. Needles and syringes should be AVOIDED wherever possible.

The average risk of transmission of blood-borne viruses following a single needlestick injury has been estimated to be:

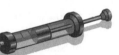

Hepatitis B Virus (HBV) 1 in 3
Hepatitis C Virus (HCV) 1 in 30
Human Immunodeficiency Virus (HIV) 1 in 300

Figure 6.1 Important points for the safe use/disposal of sharps
Reproduced with permission from East Kent Hospitals NHS Trust

segregation, storage and transportation of waste can result in severe financial penalties.

In 2006, the Department of Health published Health Technical Memorandum (HTM) 07-01: Safe Management of Healthcare Waste[132], as a best practice guide to the management of healthcare waste. This document identifies new methodology for identifying and classifying infectious and clinical waste; a new colour coding system involving the use of different coloured containers/waste sacks to assist in the identification and segregation of waste; the use of European Waste Catalogue Codes (EWC) which replace the A–E classification system currently in use, and an offensive/hygiene waste stream that includes non-infectious human hygiene waste such as nappies, incontinence pads and sanitary napkins. Healthcare organisations are advised to comply with relevant legislation and while the recommendations within HTM 07-01 are not in themselves mandatory, healthcare organisations have been requested to ensure that they have alternative arrangements in place that will ensure their compliance with relevant legislation.

LAUNDRY

Linen can be heavily contaminated with micro-organisms, presenting an infection risk to staff who have to handle or launder it, and guidance on the laundry arrangements for used and infected linen were published in 1995.[133] Infected linen should be placed directly into a water-soluble bag, which is then placed into a red laundry bag, and at the laundry both bags are placed straight into the thermal washer where the water-soluble bag dissolves. Used linen, which consists of items soiled with excretions and secretions and accounts for 90% of all hospital linen[134], should be disposed of into a white linen bag. Clean linen should not be carried by staff as it can become contaminated with micro-organisms if it comes into direct contact with the healthcare worker's uniform or disposable plastic apron if one is worn; it should be taken to the patient's bedside on a clean trolley. Used linen should be disposed of directly into the appropriate coloured linen bag and not carried – it will contaminate the healthcare worker's uniform and micro-organisms may be shed from the linen into the environment.

UNIFORMS

The infection control risk associated with healthcare workers' uniforms, including white coats worn by medical staff, has been a contentious issue for many years.[135,136,137] Given the high media profile surrounding the topic of healthcare associated infections and the lack of public confidence in the ability of the NHS to tackle the problem, reports of staff wearing their uniform to and from work and while shopping in the supermarket have come to be viewed by the public and the media as significantly contributing to the problems with MRSA and *C.difficile*. Historically, the supply and provision of uniforms to healthcare workers has been a bone of contention, as inadequate numbers of uniforms are often supplied (the recommended number of uniforms that staff should be provided with is nine[137]) and changing facilities and on-site laundry facilities are generally inadequate, with slow laundry turnaround times. Consequently, many staff launder their uniforms at home and wear them to and from work. However, in spite of the public concern, *robust* evidence to suggest that uniforms are a cross-infection risk has always been lacking. This has been supported by a recent review of the evidence base, commissioned and funded by the Department of Health[1], which looked at the epidemiological link between contaminants on uniforms and cases of HCAI, along with all aspects of the laundry cycle (including hospital v home laundry). The review found that even though uniforms do become contaminated with pathogenic organisms acquired both

[1] Wilson J.A, Loveday H.P, Hoffman P.N, Pratt R.J (2007). Uniform: an evidence review of the microbiological significance of uniforms and uniform policy in the prevention and control of healthcare associated infections. Report to the Department of Health (England). *J Hosp Infect* (2007), doi:10.1016/j/jhin.2007.03.026

from the wearer, patients and the environment, there is no evidence to support the belief that they act as vehicles of cross-infection. The review emphasises the importance of staff adhering to the EPIC 2 guidelines[86] with regard to the wearing of protective clothing during any patient-related activity whereby their uniform may be contaminated, and it should go without saying that if the uniform becomes heavily contaminated with dirt, blood or body fluids, it must be substituted for a clean uniform. Where uniforms are washed in a domestic washing machine, they should be washed according to the manufacturer's instructions and the machine should not be overloaded. Staff should adhere to the recommendations made within their own local uniform policy, and guidance on the wearing and laundering of uniforms is also available from the Royal College of Nursing (RCN).[138,139]

SPILLAGES OF BLOOD/BODY FLUIDS

Blood and body fluids can contain bacterial or viral pathogens, and spillages should be dealt with immediately.

Table 6.6 Procedure for dealing with spillages of blood and body fluid

---

Cordon off the area where the spill has occurred.

Gather together disposable non-sterile gloves and a disposable plastic apron, plus eye/facewear if required, paper towels a yellow clinical waste sack, sodium dichlorisocyanurate solution 10,000 ppm, and sodium dichlorisocyanurate granules.

Wearing protective clothing, cover the surface of the spill either with dichlorisocyanurate granules, or cover the spill with paper towels and gently pour a solution of 10,000 ppm sodium dichlorisocyanurate over the towels.

Wait until the granules solidify, or leave the solution for two minutes to take effect, and then gather up the towels and put them into the clinical waste sack.

Wipe over the area with detergent and warm water.

Dispose of gloves and apron as clinical waste and decontaminate/wash hands.

DECONTAMINATION OF EQUIPMENT, THE ENVIRONMENT AND MEDICAL DEVICES

Decontamination is a general term used to describe cleaning, disinfection and sterilisation – the combination of processes used to make a re-usable item safe for further use on patients and for handling by staff[140], and within the health-care setting it relates to both the environment and medical equipment/devices. The exact process, or combination of processes, used depends very much upon the item in question and the level of risk associated with its use. Medical equipment and invasive devices, for example, are often designed for re-use, and require a combination of cleaning, disinfection and sterilisation to render them safe. Inadequate decontamination will potentially expose the patient to infection from pathogenic bacteria, blood-borne viruses (HIV, hepatitis B and C) and prion disease, and if

Table 6.7 Classification of infection risk associated with the decontamination of medical devices

Risk	Application of item	Recommendation
High	• In close contact with a break in the skin or mucous membranes • Introduced into sterile body area	Sterilisation
Intermediate	• In contact with mucous membranes • Contaminated with particularly virulent or readily transmissible organisms • Prior to use on an immunocompromised patient	Sterilisation or disinfection required Cleaning may be acceptable in some situations
Low	• In contact with healthy skin • Not in contact with patient	Cleaning

MAC Manual. *Sterilisation, Disinfection and Cleaning of Medical Equipment: Guidance from the Microbiology Advisory Committee of the Department of Health. Crown Copyright*

medical equipment/devices that are not designed for re-use *are* decontaminated for use on another patient, whatever method of decontamination is used will not be appropriate. Poor standards of hospital hygiene in relation to the environment create a reservoir for infection, harbouring organisms such as MRSA and *C.difficile* and increasing the risk of cross-infection. Environmental cleanliness is very much in the public, media and political arena, leading to the publication of documents such as *A matron's charter: an action plan for cleaner hospitals*[141], and *Towards cleaner hospitals and lower rates of infection.*[19] *Winning ways: working together to reduce healthcare associated infection in England*[142] highlighted environmental cleanliness and the decontamination of instruments and other devices as action areas for the NHS.

Table 6.7 details the decontamination methods that should be used for the decontamination of medical equipment and devices dependent upon the infection control risks.

CLEANING

Cleaning is the process that physically removes contamination with organic material such as blood and body fluids, along with dirt and dust, reducing the bacterial bio-burden by removing, but not destroying, micro-organisms from the surface of the item that is being cleaned. It is the essential prerequisite to disinfection and sterilisation, as failure to remove surface contamination means that micro-organisms will be trapped within organic material, and may survive disinfection and sterilisation. The presence of organic material can also reduce the effectiveness of disinfectants, so if it is removed there will be better physical and chemical contact with the disinfecting/sterilising agent. Cleaning on its own without disinfection is sufficient for the decontamination of low risk items such as bedside tables and lockers, high and low surfaces within the ward environment, including floors and walls, wash bowls, and mattresses. Cleaning can be either a manual process, or automated via a thermal washer-disinfector or ultrasonic cleaner. Manual cleaning requires the use of hot water and detergent at the correct temperature and dilution, and can remove 80 % of the microbial bio-burden from the item being cleaned if it is carried out properly, but poor cleaning technique will merely redistribute, rather than remove, dirt and micro-organisms.

CLEANLINESS IN HOSPITALS

There is a general lack of public confidence that hospitals in the UK are clean, and concerns have been expressed about the deteriorating standards of cleanliness ever since the provision of in-house domestic services ceased and was contracted out to external companies. HCAI in general has a huge media profile and the continuing problems with organisms such as MRSA and *Clostridium difficile* have been largely, although not solely, attributed to dirty hospital wards. The constant turnover of patients and high bed occupancy rates, poor hospital/ward design and layout, poor maintenance of ward areas with decaying fabric and peeling and cracked paint and plaster work, lack of adequate isolation facilities, lack of storage space for supplies and equipment, and staffing shortages (both nursing and hotel services/domestic) all contribute to the problem of cleanliness, making it a challenge to keep the environment clean. However, these factors aside, it goes without saying that the patients and the public have a basic right to expect to be cared for in a clean environment, and dirt and dust will harbour micro-organisms. In July 2000, as part of the NHS Plan[20], £30 million was allocated to NHS trusts to improve hospital cleaning, and more than £68 million has been invested to make improvements to the hospital environment. Patient environment action teams (PEATs), consisting of nursing, catering and medical staff, executive and non-executive directors, estates, domestic/hotel services staff and patient representatives, were established in 2000 to assess NHS hospitals, examining environmental cleanliness from a patient perspective. Under the PEAT programme[143], which as of 2006 has been managed by the National Patient Safety Agency, every healthcare facility which has more than 10 inpatient beds is assessed annually and rated excellent, good, acceptable or poor in terms of hospital cleanliness. The programme has expanded since its inception, with the inclusion of the monitoring of patient food, as well as patient privacy and dignity. PEAT is now undertaken through self-assessment but the scores are subjected to a validation process in the form of an external validation visit by unannounced independent teams.

In 2001, National Cleaning Standards for the NHS[144] were introduced and these are used by domestic services teams in conjunction with the Healthcare Facilities

Cleaning Manual[140] to ensure that best practice is adhered to in relation to the effective cleaning of healthcare premises. The manual recommends the use of a colour coding system (red, blue, green, white and yellow) for cleaning materials, based upon that recommended by the British Institute of Cleaning Standards[145] in order to prevent cross-contamination of cleaning equipment. But while most hospitals have instituted a colour coding scheme, the NPSA has highlighted that there is no consistency with regard to the type of colour coding used.[146] It estimates that there are approximately 50 different colour coding schemes in use and although they revolve around the core colours, their meaning varies amongst Trusts, posing a potential risk as there is no consistency among hospitals.

Many hospitals are now using microfibre cloths and mopheads for cleaning, as opposed to the more traditional methods of mops, buckets and detergent. Microfibre traps and lifts dirt and dust, and can be used dry or with water for cleaning large surface areas such as floors. There are several microfibre systems available, and these were trialled in the UK in 2004. More information on microfibre is available from the Association of Healthcare Cleaning Professionals.[147]

Cleaning should not just be seen as the responsibility of domestic services staff – all healthcare staff have an equally important role to play in making sure that the patient environment is kept clean. Contaminated patient equipment will potentially contaminate the environment, and increase the risk of cross-infection to patients and staff, serving as a vector for the transmission of bacteria such as MRSA. The use of detergent wipes to clean the surfaces of equipment in between patient use, particularly equipment that is shared such as IV stands, dynamaps and monitors, makes the cleaning process quick and easy to do. Bed frames, mattresses and pillows should be cleaned in between patients – sometimes a challenge when there is a high turnover of patients – but these items can be heavily contaminated.[148] Ward sluices and store rooms should be kept tidy and equipment stored appropriately (i.e. off of the floor) in designated areas. In outbreak situations, increased levels of cleaning are required in order to reduce environmental reservoirs of infection, and the EPIC 2 guidelines[86] recommend the use of hypochlorite and detergent for cleaning on these occasions.

DISINFECTION

Disinfection is the process used to reduce the number of viable micro-organisms (but not bacterial spores) to a level that it is not harmful to health, and heat, using thermal washer disinfectors, is the most effective method of disinfection, although chemical disinfectants are often used. Items that come into direct contact with mucous membranes require disinfection as opposed to cleaning because of the risk of contamination. Chemical disinfectants are used in areas where there is no access to a thermal washer disinfector or the equipment for disinfection is heat labile, but their use is fraught with potential pitfalls and it is important that staff who use chemical disinfectants for the decontamination of equipment receive training in how to use them safely and effectively. Blood and body fluids have to be manually removed before the equipment is immersed in the disinfectant; the chemical disinfectant used has to be a suitable disinfectant for that particular item of equipment and the dilution of chemical to water ratio has to be exact – too dilute and the disinfection process will not be effective, too great and it may be corrosive and toxic, damaging the item and also the user; it may also affect the patient, as the chemical may leach out of the item during use, causing chemical burns; the disinfectant must come into contact with all parts of the item and it must be immersed in the disinfectant for the recommended amount of time, not just 'dunked' in and out. Thorough rinsing is essential in order to remove all traces of the disinfectant which can cause irritation to the mucous membranes when the equipment is next used on a patient. Endoscopes are examples of equipment that require a high level of disinfection.

THE DECONTAMINATION OF ENDOSCOPES

Endoscopic procedures are routinely performed in hospitals for diagnostic purposes and are used to internally visualise organs, tissues and sterile body cavities but, as with any procedure, there are associated risks. Infectious agents such as microorganisms, blood-borne viruses or other agents such as abnormal prior protein (CJD) can be transmitted to other patients, and any patient undergoing an endoscopic procedure must be viewed as a potential infection risk, although the risk of transmission of infection from patient to patient has been estimated to be as low as 1: 1.8 million procedures.[149] Failure in the decontamination process may not only transmit infection, it may also lead to the patient being incorrectly diagnosed if any specimens taken from the patient during the procedure become contaminated. Table 6.8 highlights the infection risks associated with the use of endoscopes.

Guidance on the decontamination of endoscopes has been issued by the Medical Devices Agency and the British Society of Gastroenterology.[150,151] Rigid scopes are used for invasive procedures such as laparoscopy and arthroscopy, and ideally require sterilisation by steam or gas following use. Flexible scopes, such as gastroscopes and nasendoscopes come into contact with intact mucous membranes and are exposed to pathogens within mucous, blood (blood-borne viruses), pus, secretions and faeces (enteric pathogens). Regardless of whether the endoscope is rigid or flexible, they are complex pieces of equipment, consisting of numerous working channels and ports, and detachable attachments and accessories such as snares and biopsy forceps. The risk of infection is associated with the type of endoscopic procedure, the presence of any infective agent (bacterial or viral pathogen), the effectiveness of the endoscopic decontamination process, the recontamination of the endoscope during and after re-processing and storage, and the susceptibility of the patient to infection.[150] Flexible endoscopes are heat labile and require high level disinfection as they are unable to withstand the sterilisation process. The decontamination process consists of two parts – manual cleaning and high level disinfection.

Table 6.8 Infection risks associated with endoscopes[150]

The type of procedure undertaken: procedures that penetrate mucosal membranes such as endoscopic retrograde cholangiopancreatography (ERCP).

The susceptibility of the individual patient to infection: patients who are immunocompromised through underlying illness such as HIV or chronic pulmonary disease are susceptible to infections from opportunistic organisms that are of low pathogenicity. These include the environmental mycobacteria such as *M.chelonae*, which can contaminate bronchoscopes if the quality of the rinse water during the decontamination process is not of good quality.

Bacteria/viruses or other infectious agents present in the secretions of the previous patient: these include the blood borne viruses *Mycobacterium tuberculosis* and environmental opportunists; Gram-negative pathogens such as *Pseudomonas aeruginosa*, *Klebsiella species, Enterobacter* species and *Serratia marcescens.*

The effectiveness of the decontamination process, including storage and aftercare: inadequate manual cleaning prior to high level disinfection, the use of chemical disinfectant at the wrong dilution and insufficient contact time with the scope, poor quality rinse water, and poor storage and handling of the scope after decontamination will all negate the efficiency of the decontamination process and expose subsequent patients at risk of infection.

Staff need to be competent in the decontamination of these pieces of equipment and undergo training in both the manual and the automated processes of cleaning and high level disinfection. The BSG guidelines[151] describe the various stages in the decontamination process of flexible scopes, which begins as soon as it is removed from the patient. Water is manually sucked through the working channels to ensure that all debris is removed and the channels are not blocked, and the air and water channels are irrigated to ensure that they are not blocked with blood and mucous. The external surfaces are then wiped down and visually inspected for damage, and the scope is detached from the light source. It is then subjected to leak testing as it is important to check the integrity of the channels and ensure that the scope has not been damaged in any way. If the leak test is satisfactory and no damage to the scope is detected, all detachable parts are then removed and it is manually cleaned using a foaming enzymatic agent, which breaks down organic material and assists in the removal of blood, tissue debris and bacterial biofilm (see Chapter 2). Single use disposable wire brushes are used to clean the accessible ports and channels. The scope is then subjected to high-level disinfection in an automated washer-disinfector, rinsed, purged with 70 % alcohol and dried. It is important that the scope is stored appropriately to prevent it sustaining damage and also to prevent contamination arising from accidental contact with a used scope that has not been through the decontamination process. As with all instruments that are re-used, it is absolutely essential to ensure that the scope can be traced back to the patients that it has been used on. All endoscopes have a unique serial number which has to be documented in the patient's medical notes when the procedure is formed. Traceability and tracking systems can be either be automated or manually undertaken, and provide a record of the serial number of the scope, the type of scope used, the patient's details, as well as the decontamination process.

STERILISATION

Sterilisation is the complete destruction of all micro-organisms, inactivating viruses, vegetative bacteria and bacterial spores, and is used for high risk items that penetrate the skin or mucous membranes or enter a sterile body area that is usually free from bacteria. Although it can be carried out using chemicals and radiation, the best method of sterilisation is by steam under pressure (autoclaving), which is the method used in healthcare premises for the sterilisation of re-usable surgical instruments or other items. If the sterilisation process has been effective, there is a less than 1 in 10^2 that there are any viable micro-organisms remaining on that item.[152]

SINGLE USE DEVICES

Historically within the NHS many items and devices have been reprocessed and re-used on other patients as a cost-saving exercise, a practice which increases the risk of infection. The Medicines and Healthcare Products Regulatory Agency (MHRA) issued a bulletin in 2000 alerting healthcare staff to the implications and consequences of reusing single-use devices, and this guidance was re-issued in 2006.[153,154] The main points are summarised in Table 6.9.

Table 6.9 Implications and consequences of the re-use of single-use medical devices[153,154]

Reprocessing of a single-use device may render it not fit for purpose, as its intended function may be compromised.

Single-use items may not be designed to withstand the decontamination process – either by cleaning, disinfection or sterilisation.

The characteristics of the device may be altered by reprocessing, compromising its function and rendering the device non-compliant with the manufacturer's original specification.

Single-use devices will not have undergone extensive testing and validation to ensure that they are safe to re-use.

Reprocessing of a single-use device may alter or damage it.

There is a risk of cross-infection to other patients as the design of the device may mean that the reprocessing system will not sufficiently remove all viable micro-organisms; the presence of coils, acute angles and narrow and long lumens mean that thorough cleaning is difficult.

Table 6.9 (Continued)

Residue from chemical agents used in the decontamination process may be absorbed by materials such as plastic and cause chemical burns or sensitisation to the patient or user.

Exposure to chemical agents or elevated temperatures as part of the decontamination process may cause the device to soften, crack or become brittle.

Reprocessing may result in fatigue-induced failure of the device.

If the device is heavily contaminated with a high bacterial load which cannot be adequately removed by cleaning, the sterilisation process will not inactivate bacterial toxins.

Abnormal prion protein (CJD/v CJD) is resistant to all conventional methods of decontamination.

Anyone who reuses a device that is designated single-use is responsible for its effectiveness and safety.

Single-use devices differ from those which are single-patient use. If an item is designated single-patient use, it can be used again on that patient and can undergo the decontamination process. Singe-use items, however, must never be reprocessed and must be used just once and then discarded. The symbol for single use, which is clearly marked on the packaging, isillustrated here.

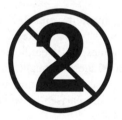

Figure 6.2 Single use mark
Reproduced from BS EN:980:2003 with permission of the British Standards Institute

ISOLATION OF PATIENTS WITH INFECTIONS/INFECTIOUS DISEASES

In addition to the use of standard principles in preventing the spread of infection, patients may also be isolated in a single room on a ward or in a designated isolation unit. This is known as source isolation (also often referred to as standard isolation) and aims to prevent the transfer of micro-organisms from infected or colonised patients who may act as a source of infection for other patients or staff. Other categories include:

- Strict isolation: used for very rare infectious diseases such as viral haemorrhagic fever, plague, diptheria and pulmonary anthrax. Patients requiring strict isolation precautions are cared for in a designated high security infectious disease unit.
- Protective isolation: patients who are neutopenic and consequently are highly susceptible to, and need protection from, infection.

As the availability of isolation facilities varies between hospitals (either 'ordinary' single rooms on wards, designated isolation wards, or purpose-built units), isolating patients can prove to be a challenge. Other factors may compound the problem; the patient's overall condition may mean that they will be unsafe in a single room where direct observation is difficult; staffing shortages may mean that the patient cannot be adequately supervised; there may be more than one patient on a ward who requires isolating, with pressure from competing organisms. In these situations, a careful risk assessment must be undertaken, taking into account the organism causing the infection, its route of transmission, the risk to other patients and staff and the patient's overall condition, and the advice of the infection prevention and control team should be sought. In some circumstances patients requiring standard source isolation may have to be nursed on the main ward according to local policy.

7 Types of Healthcare Associated Infection

INTRODUCTION

The first and second national prevalence surveys of hospital acquired infections in 1981 [23] and 1996 [24] found that 9.2 % and 9 % of patients respectively had an infection that was not present on admission. In 2006, the Hospital Infection Society (HIS) and the Infection Control Nurses Association (ICNA), funded by the Department of Health, conducted the third national prevalence survey[155], assisted by infection prevention and control teams across England. This involved more than 58,000 patients in 190 hospitals, with parallel surveys carried out in Wales, Northern Ireland and the Republic of Ireland. The survey found that 8.2 % of patients in hospitals in England have a healthcare associated, or hospital acquired, infection, and that surgical site infections, urinary tract infections, pneumonia and gastro-intestinal infections were the most predominant.

Surgical site infections, urinary tract infections, bloodstream infections and pneumonia have historically accounted for the major types of healthcare associated infections in hospitals in England, and this chapter focuses on the risk factors for, and the prevention and management of, each of these.

LEARNING OUTCOMES

After reading this chapter the reader will:

- Understand the pathogenesis of urinary tract infections and how to manage urethral catheters appropriately to reduce the risk of infection
- Understand the risk factors contributing to surgical site infection
- Understand the principles of line management associated with peripheral venous and central venous catheters
- Understand the risk factors associated with hospital acquired pneumonia

The *Saving Lives* [30] programme contains six high impact interventions, of which four are designed to audit compliance with key processes and clinical procedures associated with the management of invasive devices and the prevention of surgical site and urinary tract infections and pneumonia. The reader is advised to familiarise themself with these tools.

URINARY TRACT INFECTIONS

Urinary tract infections accounted for 19.7 % of healthcare associated infections in the 2006 prevalence survey[155], as opposed to 23.2 % in the second prevalence survey back in 1996[24] – still a significant number and an ever-present contributing factor to the economic burden of healthcare associated infections. Infection of the upper urinary tract involves the kidney and the renal pelvis (pyelonephritis), while lower urinary tract infections can involve the bladder (cystitis, which commonly affects women), the urethra (urethritis) and, in men, the prostate gland (prostatitis) because of its close proximity to the male urethra.[156] In 2001, Plowman et al[27] estimated that UTIs cost the NHS an estimated £124 million per annum which equates to 800,000 lost bed days and incurs an additional cost of £1,327 per patient, blocking a hospital bed for an extra six days, a huge drain on NHS resources as well as patient care. Although there are various risk factors that predispose individuals to develop a UTI (see Table 7.1) urinary tract infections among patients in hospital are strongly associated with indwelling urinary catheters, with the risk of infection associated with the method and duration of catheterisation and the susceptibility of the patient.[86,98]

Catheterisation is an accepted and commonplace healthcare intervention and the prevalence of catheterised patients in UK hospitals has been estimated at 12.6 %.[157] While there are many clinical indications for catheterisation (see Table 7.2), in some instances it can be a practice which is difficult to justify; also, once it has been inserted, the catheter may be forgotten and catheter care subsequently neglected.[158]

Of those catheterised patients who have had a catheter in situ for longer than seven to ten days, 50 % will develop bacteria in their urine (bacteriuria, or bacterial colonisation of the urine). Although bacteriuria is often symptomatic, it can lead to microbial invasion of the tissues, with 20–30 % of patients going on to develop a symptomatic urinary tract infection. Of those, 1–4 % will develop a bacteraemia (bacteria in the blood stream but without systemic signs of infection) and 13–30 %

Table 7.1 Predisposing risk factors for urinary tract infections

Catheterisation
Patient age
Renal tract abnormalities
Immunosupression
Diabetes mellitus
Sexual intercourse
Pregnancy

Table 7.2 Indications for catheterisation

Convenience
Management of incontinence
Fluid balance
Acutely ill patient (e.g. ITU care)
Inserted post-operatively
Poor patient mobility
Urinary retention
Bladder irrigation
Prior to investigations/procedures
During labour
The administration of chemotherapy

will subsequently die.[98,159,160] As two-thirds of bacteraemias of known source are associated with an intravenous device or with device-related infections such as catheter-associated urinary tract infections [161], it is obvious that catheters represent a serious threat to patients. So great is the risk they pose that the EPIC 2 [86] guidelines clearly state:

'Catheterising patients places them in significant danger of acquiring a urinary tract infection. The longer a catheter is in place, the greater the danger.'[86] (page S23). In other words, urinary catheters can kill.

THE PATHOGENESIS OF CATHETER-ASSOCIATED URINARY TRACT INFECTIONS

While the urethra is colonised with bacteria, urine proximal to the distal urethra is normally sterile. The urethra remains closed except when urine is being voided, and the bladder is protected from microbial invasion by the regular emptying and voiding of urine which flushes away micro-organisms. Urinary tract infections in uncatheterised individuals are particularly common in women because of the short female urethra and its close proximity to the perineum, which has a resident population comprised of faecal and genital flora, and this can result in endogenous infection. Bacteria can also be transiently displaced into the bladder during sexual intercourse, giving rise to cystitis.[156] In the catheterised state, the urethra remains open and the catheter forms a bridge between a naturally sterile organ and the external environment, effectively acting as a gateway for the ascending passage of bacteria. The catheter retention balloon prevents complete emptying of the bladder, allowing for a small residual volume of urine in the bladder below the volume of the catheter drainage holes [162], and any bacteria present will multiple within this stagnant pool. The retention balloon can also damage the lining of the bladder if it is under- or over-inflated, irritating the lining of the bladder and interfering with the correct positioning of the bladder tip by resting against the bladder mucosa in an area known as the delicate trigone, where it can cause the equivalent of a small pressure sore.[163,164]

Table 7.3 Routes of access to the bladder

Bacteria introduced into the bladder on insertion
Via the hands of staff – resident/transient flora
Via the jug used to empty the drainage bag
Via the sampling port
Via the catheter bag junction
At the meatal junction
Along the outside of the catheter
Inside the catheter lumen

Catheters and their associated drainage systems provide a wonderful environment for bacteria as they support the growth of bacterial biofilms [39,40,41] (see Chapter 2 Bacterial and Viral Classification, Structure and Function). Once they have made contact with the surface of the catheter they attach to it by secreting a polysaccharide matrix which consists of sugars and proteins. This encases them, affording protection from the effects of antibiotics and host immune defence mechanisms such as phagocytosis.[165] The presence of bacteria such as *proteus, pseudomonas* and *Klebsiella* encourage biofilm formation. *Proteus mirabilis*, which belongs to the family *Enterobacteriaceae,* is an opportunistic pathogen which inhabits the GI tract. On culture media, *P.mirabilis* swarms over the culture plate with a spreading growth that covers other organisms that may be present within the culture, and it does the same on catheters.[156] It produces a very potent urease (an enzyme that catalyzes the hydrolysis of urea, forming ammonia and carbon dioxide) which makes the urine more alkaline, leading to the formation of struvite crystals and encrustation which can block the catheter.[156,166] When the catheter is removed, biofilm may be visible around the catheter tip as a slimy coating. Encrustation is not always as easily spotted as it may be inside the catheter lumen.[166]

There are numerous ways in which bacteria can gain access to the bladder, and these are summarised in Table 7.3.

BACTERIAL CAUSES OF URINARY TRACT INFECTIONS

More than 95 % of UTIs are caused by a single bacterial species and uropathogenic strains of *E.coli* are the commonest bacterial cause of urinary tract infections, particularly in relation to community-acquired infections.[167,168] *E.coli* is part of the normal faecal flora and can be pathogenic if it is transferred to other body sites. It possesses fimbriae (see Chapter 2 Bacterial and Viral Classification, Structure and Function), which enables it to adhere to mucosal surfaces, such as the lining of the bladder. The commonest cause of UTIs in women is *Staphylococcus saprophyticus*, a coagulase negative staphylococci which forms part of the normal vaginal flora. *Serratia, Klebsiella* and *Pseudomonas aeruginosa*, like *Proteus*, belong to the bacterial genus *Enterobacteriaceae* and are normal inhabitants of the colon, predominantly causing infections among hospitalised patients.[168] They produce exotoxins which act on the host cells and posses fimbriae which facilitate adherence to invasion of the urinary epithelium.[156,167] *P.aeruginosa* is a particularly virulent organism which secretes an extra-polysaccharide slime (biofilm), facilitating adherence and evading host defences.

Some bacteria such as *Klebsiella* species and *E.coli* secrete an enzyme called lactamase which renders the bacteria resistant to antibiotics such as the cephalosporins. As discussed in Chapter 8 (The Problem of Antimicrobial Resistance), this has implications for the treatment of infections caused by antibiotic-resistant bacteria, and the potential risk of cross-infection with resistant organisms to other patients has to be avoided[169]. Extended-Spectrum Beta Lactamase- (ESBL) producing bacteria are not just confined to the hospital setting and have been found extensively in the community as well.

CLINICAL FEATURES OF UTIS

Detecting a urinary tract infection in an uncatheterised patient is relatively straightforward. In cases of cystitis, which has an abrupt onset, the symptoms are due to inflammation and irritation of the bladder mucosa as well as the mucosal surface of the urethra. This gives rise to frequency of urination (micturition) which is often accompanied by a feeling of urgency; dysuria (pain on urinating); suprapubic or loin pain/tenderness and a temperature. In severe cases the urine may be blood-stained (haematuria)[156] as well as cloudy and malodorous.

Pyelonephritis is a more severe infection affecting the kidney and the upper renal tract, which can lead to kidney damage and the onset of septic shock (see Chapter 5). Symptoms include flank pain, a temperature which exceeds 38 °C and rigors. As the infection progresses, the patient may develop diarrhoea and vomiting.

UTI is less apparent in patients who are cathterised as the key symptoms of frequency and pain on urinating are absent. While suprapubic tenderness and cloudy, malodorous urine may be present, these features are not reported in all cases and in elderly patients fever may be the first symptom, along with confusion/delirium.[170]

DIAGNOSIS

Unsurprisingly, urine specimens comprise the largest single category of specimens examined in most medical microbiology laboratories.[171]

Laboratory confirmation of a urinary tract infection is dependent upon the examination of a sample of normally sterile urine and the detection of bacteria and the accompanying inflammatory response which is evident by the number of white blood cells present in the sample.[156] The specimen should be obtained either as a 'clean catch', a mid-stream urine (MSU) or in catheterised patients taken from the sampling port on the catheter using an aseptic technique[86] in order to avoid contaminating the sample. Urine should never be taken directly from the drainage bag as bacteria may have multiplied within the urine, and the results could be misleading. Chapter 3 describes how a urine sample should be obtained. Isolation of $> 10^4$ bacteria/mL of urine is indicative of infection.[168]

The results need to be carefully interpreted alongside the clinical symptoms. As the prevalence of bacteriuria in catheterised patients is virtually 100 % if the catheter has been in situ for three to four weeks, the results are not clinically significant in the absence of clinical symptoms.[171] The routine collection of urine specimens from catheterised patients should be discouraged as it is of no proven value, and should only be sent from catheterised patients if there is evidence of sepsis.[172,173] Treatment of asymptomatic bacteriuria can lead to the emergence of drug-resistant bacteria, a significant problem particularly as it is known that catheter-associated UTIs comprise perhaps the largest institutional reservoir of antibiotic-resistant organisms.[172,174]

TREATMENT

A urine sample should be obtained before the patient commences antibiotics. Trimethoprim is typically the first drug of choice. Other suitable antimicrobial agents include cotrimoxazole, nitrofurantoin, cefixime and ciprofloxacin.

PREVENTION

The best method of prevention is to avoid catheterisation where at all possible and consider other methods such as the use of convenes for the management of urinary incontinence. For the management of urinary retention, intermittent catheterisation may be an option. In patients who do have an indwelling urinary catheter, the use of a flipflo valve as opposed to a drainable urine bag means that the closed circuit is not broken. The EPIC 2 guidelines[86] recommend the use of lubricant gels to facilitate the insertion of urinary catheters. Although these have been used for many years in male catheterisations to facilitate the passage of the catheter along the long male urethra, their use during female catheterisations has not been consistent, with the general consensus being that as the female urethra is shorter, the discomfort experienced on catheterisation is less.[175] The urethra in both men and women has a good blood and nerve supply and contains collagen which reduces its elasticity, making it susceptible to trauma during catheterisation. The use of a single-use lubricant gel that has both anaesthetic and antiseptic properties, inserted into the urethra approximately five minutes before the procedure takes place, reduces pain and discomfort, increases patient compliance, and reduces the risk of infection occurring as a result of a traumatic catheterisation.

THE USE OF SILVER CATHETERS

The broad-spectrum antibacterial properties of silver have long been recognised[176], and the use of silver-impregnated wound dressings and silver-coated central venous catheters have received favourable press in relation to reducing the incidence of infection.[86,177] Silver alloy with hydrogel and silver oxide urethral catheters have both been proven to reduce the **incidence** of catheter-associated UTIs by 32–69 %[178,179,180], although the literature suggests that silver alloy with hydrogel is more effective.[181,182] The Department of Health Rapid Review Panel gave the

Bardex IC silver alloy-coated hydrogel coated catheter (manufactured by CR Bard) a level one recommendation in 2004.[183] The catheter, which contains a layer of gold and palladium over a layer of silver, reduces microbial adherence to the catheter which minimises biofilm formation, and inhibits the migration of bacteria along the catheter surface and into the bladder.[184] The use of silver catheters however should not be viewed as a quick fix to solving the problems of catheter-associated UTIs. They are not a cure for existing infections, but they can be utilised as a preventive measure in conjunction with sound clinical practice.

The following guidelines for the management of urinary catheters were developed by East Kent Hospitals NHS Trust, based on recommendations within the Royal Marsden Manual of Clinical Nursing Procedures[62] and the EPIC 2 Guidelines[86] and are for illustrative purposes only. The reader should refer to their own local guidelines.

Table 7.4 Recommendations for practice in the management of urethral urinary catheters and drainage systems[62,86,163,164]

Action	Rationale
Hand hygiene Decontaminate hands (preferably using alcohol hand rub on visibly clean hands, or by using liquid soap and water) and wear a new pair of clean non-sterile gloves before manipulating a patient's catheter. Decontaminate hands after removing gloves.	To reduce the risk of cross-infection.
Catheter size Select the smallest gauge that will allow free urinary flow.	Smaller gauge catheters with a 10 ml balloon minimise urethral trauma, mucosal irritation and residual urine in the bladder (EPIC 2 recommendation).
Balloon size 10 ml balloon for routine drainage. It is essential to inflate the balloon with the correct amount of sterile water.	The weight of water in larger balloons may cause them to rest against the delicate trigone of the bladder, causing tissue damage and dragging of the bladder (and associated patient discomfort). Balloons that are under- or over-inflated become misshapen and increase the risk of irritating the bladder mucosa.
Catheter insertion Catheterisation is a skilled aseptic procedure and should only be carried out by staff who are competent to undertake the procedure. The Royal Marsden Manual of Clinical Nursing Procedures documents the correct technique.	

Table 7.4 (Continued)

Action	Rationale
Clean the urethral meatus with sterile normal saline prior to inserting the catheter.	
If a catheter is not introduced into the bladder with the first attempt, use a new sterile catheter for each subsequent attempt.	To reduce the risk of introducing infection on catheter insertion.
Record the residual volume of urine.	
Use an appropriate lubricant for both male and female catheterisation.	To facilitate insertion of the catheter, minimising urethral trauma and patient discomfort (EPIC 2 recommendation).
The urinary drainage system 2-litre catheter bags should always be used. A catheter valve, e.g. flipflo, should ideally be the first choice for patients unless clinical/patient indications prevent their use.	To avoid breaking the system.
Link system For those patients with leg bags or valves, a non-drainable overnight bag (without a tap) should be attached. Each morning the bag should be disconnected, emptied and disposed of.	Reduced infection rate through the maintenance of the closed system of drainage (EPIC 2 recommendation).
Urinary drainage bag stands/hangers All 2-litre drainage bags should be supported on a dedicated stand/hanger, which should be cleaned thoroughly in between patient use. The tap should never be in contact with the floor. The bag should be changed only when necessary (some hospitals may have local recommendations, e.g. weekly). This should be done using a non-touch technique.	To reduce the risk of cross-infection (EPIC 2 recommendation).
Bag emptying The bag should be emptied frequently to maintain urine flow and prevent reflux, using a separate and clean container for each patient. Contact between the urinary drainage tap and the container should be avoided (EPIC 2 recommendation).	To avoid breaking the system unnecessarily. Cross-infection can occur when urinary catheter bags are emptied.
Position of the drainage bag The drainage bag should be positioned below the level of the bladder on a stand that prevents contact of the bag with the floor (EPIC 2 recommendation).	

SURGICAL WOUND INFECTIONS

Wound infections are a common but potentially avoidable complication following any surgical procedure during which the skin is breached and opportunistic resident or transient micro-organisms gain entry to the wound, causing local or deep tissue infections. They are associated with significant distress to the patient and are often interpreted as a marker of poor standards of care, particularly in relation to standards and practices within the operating theatre. While most heal without complication, deep-seated infections can result in systemic illness and can be fatal.[185]

The main bacterial causes of surgical wound infections are shown in Table 7.5. There are three routes by which wounds can become infected:[186]

1. Direct contact via the hands of healthcare workers or from contaminated equipment.
2. Airborne – skin squames can be carried in dust on air currents and can settle on open wounds if wounds are dressed while activities such as bed making or ward cleaning are in progress. The use of electric fans in ward areas can also disseminate dust and skin squames and they should be used with caution.
3. Endogenous infection – caused by the patient's own skin flora, which may migrate from one site of the body to another.

RISK FACTORS FOR THE DEVELOPMENT OF SURGICAL WOUND INFECTION

Patient susceptibility

Age, underlying illness/disease or infection, malnutrition, obesity and medication (e.g. steroids which suppress the immune response, or antibiotics which can alter the body flora) are acknowledged risk factors for the development of any infection (see Chapter 5 Understanding the Immune System and the Nature and Pathogenesis of Infection). Associated co-morbidities at the time of surgery increase the risk

Table 7.5 Common bacterial causes of surgical wound infections

Staphylococcus aureus (including MRSA)
Pseudomonas aeruginosa
Klebsiella species
Proteus species
Clostridium perfringens
Bacteroides
Group A Streptococcus
Enterobacteriaceae
Anaerobes

of post-operative wound infection and the American Society of Anaesthiologists devised a pre-operative risk score (ASA score) to identify those patients most at risk.[187] Patients are given a score of 1–5, with 1 representing the lowest risk (a normal, healthy patient) and 5 the highest risk (patient not expected to survive 24 hours with or without surgery).

Wound classification

Wounds are classified into different categories according to their origin.[188,189,190]

- Clean wounds are surgical wounds which are created under controlled conditions using an aseptic technique. At the time of surgery, there is no inflammation present and sites such as the GI tract which contain their own flora are not breached.
- Clean-contaminated wounds are surgical wounds which extend into the GI, respiratory, genital or urinary tracts but without contamination of the wound occurring.
- Contaminated wounds include those that arise as a result of trauma; where there has been a major break in sterile technique; contamination as a result of spillage from the GI tract, or where inflamed tissue is encountered but without the presence of pus.
- Dirty or infected wounds are contaminated with foreign material (dirt/debris) or from the contents of perforated viscera. Infected wounds may contain necrotic devitalised tissue.

Duration of surgery

When tissues are exposed to the air during surgery, there is a risk that bacteria carried on airborne particles can settle in the wound, on surgical instruments or the hands of operating staff. The majority of micro-organisms are from the staff present in the theatre and the dispersal of micro-organisms increases with movement. It has been estimated that each person sheds approximately 10,000 micro-organisms per minute when they are at rest, increasing to 50,000 per minute during periods of activity[191], and so the number of staff present at the time of surgery should be limited to essential personnel only. In order to further reduce airborne transmission and contamination of the wound, operating theatres should have at least 20 air changes an hour, equating to one air change every three minutes, which will reduce airborne contamination to 37 % of its former level.[192] In orthopaedic surgery, the consequences of an infection occurring in a wound where a prosthetic implant has been inserted can be particularly devastating, and the use of laminar flow systems in conjunction with high-efficiency particulate air (HEPA) filters in orthopaedic theatres has been shown to significantly reduce infection rates.[188]

Surgical technique

Poor technique can lead to contamination of the site (e.g. perforation of the bowel will contaminate the operative site with anaerobic gut flora), prolong the duration of surgery and damage tissues and blood/oxygen supply to the area.[188]

Presence of foreign material

Prosthetic implants, sutures and drains have all been found to increase the risk of post-operative infection. Without a suture, 6.5 million bacteria would be required to initiate an infection, but in the presence of just one suture, only 100 bacteria are required.[193] Prosthetic implants including those used in orthopaedic and cardiac surgery 'attract' organisms such as coagulase negative staphylococci which produce biofilm and adhere to implanted material.

Length of hospital stay and time interval between admission and surgery

Many patients for routine elective surgery are now admitted on the day of operation, having had pre-operative investigations such as full blood count, ECG and x-rays carried out in the pre-assessment clinic. This has the benefit of reducing bed occupancy. Plus the less time the patient is in hospital before surgery, the less opportunity there is for the patient's normal body flora to be replaced by hospital pathogens.[194]

Pre-operative hair removal

Pre-operative shaving with a razor has been identified as a major contributing factor to wound infection.[195,196] Nicks and cuts on the skin's surface reduce its integrity, and liberate resident dermal bacteria into the operative field, making the skin environment more favourable to bacterial proliferation.[197] In order to reduce the risk of infection:

- Hair removal at the operative site should be avoided where possible unless it physically interferes with the correct anatomical approximation of the wound edges.[198]
- If hair has to be removed it should be done in a manner that preserves skin integrity, hair removal should be kept to a minimum, and it should only be removed with the use of a surgical clipper incorporating a single-use blade.
- Hair removal should be undertaken as near to the time of surgery as practical[198] and undertaken away from the sterile field to minimise contamination of the surgical site.

Antibiotic prophylaxis

The first three hours is considered to be the critical period during which bacterial contamination of the wound leading to infection can occur[191], and antibiotics may be administered perioperatively and during surgery to minimise the risk. The administration of antibiotic prophylaxis depends on: the patient's risk of developing a post-operative surgical wound infection; the severity of the consequences of an infection (in patients with an orthopaedic implant, the implant and possibly the joint may have to be removed); the effectiveness of the antibiotic and the potential consequences of administration, such as the risk of developing *Clostridium difficile* and pseudomembranous colitis.[199] The antibiotics used for surgical prophylaxis are chosen to target the pathogens that commonly cause infections in specific types/sites of wounds and are administered at induction, as near to the time of incision as possible, and during surgery. The timing of administration is important – the aim is to achieve the correct concentrations of the drug in the blood and in the tissues at the time surgery and to maintain them while the procedure is taking place.[193] Prophylaxis is indicated in the following types of surgical procedures although there may be exemptions based on local policy and this is not an exhaustive list[199]:

- cardiothoracic surgery – pacemaker insertion; open heart surgery
- head and neck surgery – contaminated/clean-contaminated wounds
- neurosurgery
- orthopaedic surgery – for prosthetic implant insertion and internal fixation of fractures
- general surgery – colorectal surgery; appendicectomy; open biliary tract surgery; endoscopic procedures; oesophageal surgery; small bowel surgery
- vascular surgery – abdominal and lower limb; lower limb amputation
- obstetrics and gynaecology – caesarean section, hysterectomy
- urology – transurethral resection of the prostate.

CLINICAL FEATURES OF SURGICAL WOUND INFECTION, DIAGNOSIS, AND MANAGEMENT

Inflammation and tenderness at the incision site are often the first signs of infection. The surrounding tissues are often oedematous and any discharge from the site can be purulent and malodorous, particularly if anaerobic bacteria are present. These signs are often accompanied by a pyrexia which indicates that an inflammatory response is taking place in response to the infection. If the infection is deep-seated, the pain is generally more severe (described as throbbing) and the wound can dehisce. Following abdominal surgery, complete wound dehiscence with visible loops of bowel appearing through the incision is a surgical emergency and the patient needs to be swiftly returned to the operating theatre. Discolouration at the wound margin and friable granulation tissue which bleeds easily are also indicators of infection.[193,200] Although an infection can be diagnosed based on clinical signs, the causative organism needs to be identified in order to ensure that the infection is treated with the appropriate antibiotic (see Chapter 3 The Collection and Transportation of Specimens), and in deep-seated infections, these will need to be administered intravenously. In some cases, further surgical intervention is required for incision and drainage in the event of abscess formation, debridement of necrotic tissue or removal of a prosthetic implant. Depending upon the extent of the infection and subsequent tissue damage, vacuum-assisted closure of the wound may be required. The patient may need to be referred to a tissue viability nurse for specialist wound care.

BLOODSTREAM INFECTIONS ASSOCIATED WITH IV DEVICES

While potentially life-threatening bloodstream infections can occur as a result of infection elsewhere in the body, the majority are associated with intravenous access devices such as peripheral IVs and central venous catheters (CVCs).[201] Approximately 6,000 patients in the UK develop a catheter-related bloodstream infection (CR BSI) each year and each case of septicaemia costs in the region of £6,000 to treat.[26] It is estimated that between 18–80 % of patients admitted to hospital will have an intravenous access device inserted at some point during their admission [202,203], and many devices are inserted unnecessarily.[203] The acquisition of a bloodstream infection associated with a CVC is acknowledged to be one of the most dangerous complications of healthcare that can occur.[86] In view of the risk to the patient, the use of IV devices needs to be justified and the device managed appropriately to reduce the risk of infection.

Peripheral insertion is usually in the arm for short-term therapy. Short-term central venous catheters (CVCs) are generally inserted into the subclavian, jugular or femoral veins.[204] Lines inserted into the subclavian vein are associated with lower rates of infection than the other two sites – lines in the jugular vein can become contaminated by endotracheal secretions if the patient requires suctioning, and lines in the femoral vein can become contaminated with faecal flora.[205]

THE PATHOGENESIS OF CATHETER-RELATED BLOODSTREAM INFECTIONS (CR BSIS)

Colonisation is an essential prerequisite in the pathogenesis of CR BSIs and results from contamination of the IV device during insertion and subsequent care.[206] The point at which colonisation changes to infection is unclear but is thought to relate to the number of inoculating organisms and the length of time that the device is in place. Catheter-related bloodstream infections can occur as a result of endogenous or exogenous means. Endogenous infections are caused by the patient's own skin flora, the majority of which are opportunistic, only causing infections if the patient is particularly susceptible and there is a suitable portal of entry for the organism to gain access to the tissues and/or the bloodstream. *S. aureus* and *S. epidermidis* are the common culprits implicated in these infections [86], and they are known as pathogens of plastic [207], readily colonising IV devices and producing biofilm.

Exogenous infections occur as a result of cross-infection, from organisms (particularly transient organisms) carried on the hands of healthcare staff or from contact with the environment or contaminated equipment. CR BSI is generally caused by skin micro-organisms at the insertion site that contaminate the catheter on insertion, impacting on the distal tip, or migration of micro-organisms along the cutaneous catheter track, or transferred on the hands of healthcare workers to contaminate and colonise the catheter hub.

THE MANAGEMENT OF PERIPHERAL VENOUS CANNULA

The following guidelines for the insertion and maintenance of peripheral venous cannula were developed within East Kent Hospitals NHS Trust, based on recommendations within the EPIC 2 [86] and the Royal College of Nursing Infusion Standards.[208] They are included here for illustrative purposes. Readers should also refer to their own local guidelines.

Table 7.6 The insertion and management of peripheral venous cannulae[86,208]

Insertion Procedure	Rationale
Identify the patient as per EKHT identification policy.	To ensure correct patient.
Explain the procedure to the patient; ask for preference regarding site and obtain verbal consent and co-operation.	To ensure patient understanding.
Discuss previous experiences and check for need of local anaesthetic.	To establish venous history.
Select the correct cannula size (visible through the pack) for patient/infusion needs.	To reduce unnecessary trauma to the vein.
Decontaminate hands using alcohol hand rub or handwashing with liquid soap.	To minimise risk of cross-infection.
Check integrity of packaging and expiry date. Open the pack onto clean trolley/surface.	To maintain asepsis.
Wash and dry patient's arm if visibly dirty.	To adequately clean skin.
Position the patient with arm supported with pillow or if required ensure assistance from a colleague. Place the drape under the patient's arm.	To ensure patient comfort and safety.
Choose site according to patient condition and apply tourniquet at least 10cms above the selected insertion site.	To dilate veins by obstructing venous return.
Find a suitable PALPABLE vein. Clip hairs using surgical clippers incorporating a single-use disposable head, if necessary.	To reduce trauma to the vein.
Decontaminate hands using alcohol hand rub and then apply examination gloves.	
Disinfect site with chlorhexidine and alcohol solution for 30-60 seconds (included in the pack). Use an alcoholic povidone-iodine solution for patients with a history of chlorhexidine sensitivity. Allow the antiseptic to dry before inserting the catheter. Allow to air-dry. Do not re-palpate the vein or touch the skin.	To minimise risk of infection.
Fold down wings of cannula and inspect for faults. **DO NOT WITHDRAW THE NEEDLE.**	To detect faulty equipment.

Anchor the vein by applying tension to skin below site and insert the needle/cannula bevel at an angle of 10-45 degrees depending on device.	To immobilise the vein and ensure a successful cannulation.
Level the device and advance the cannula a few mms into the vein and withdraw needle slightly, observing flashback of blood in shaft	To avoid the vein wall and to ensure cannula is in a patent vein.
Maintaining anchor tension with one hand and holding the flashback chamber or thumb plate with the other, advance the cannula forward over the needle.	To ensure the vein remains immobilised thereby reducing risk of through puncture.
Only one vascular access device should be used for each cannulation attempt.	To maintain asepsis.
Release tourniquet.	To decrease pressure in the vein.
Apply digital pressure above tip of cannula and remove needle. Discard directly into sharps bin. **NEVER REINSERT THE NEEDLE.**	To reduce risk of needlestick injury.
Attach an injection cap, needleless connector or pre-primed solution set.	To prevent air entry/protect against contamination.
Apply dedicated sterile, vapour permeable, IV cannula dressing supplied in the pack.	To minimise risk of infection and to secure the cannula.
Flush the cannula with 5–10 mls of sterile sodium chloride 0.9 % for injection then commence IV fluids if appropriate * **The normal saline (0.9 %) should be prescribed on the drug chart. Alternatively a Patient Group Direction (PGD) can be used by a trained and competent PGD user.**	To prevent occlusion.
Discard gloves and decontaminate hands.	
Remove waste into appropriate container.	To ensure safe disposal.
Document insertion time, date, site, size of cannula, batch number, and name of person inserting the device. Record the review/removal date (72 hours) (use sticky labels supplied in the pack).	To meet legal and patient care requirements.

NB A peripheral cannula inserted in an emergency situation where aseptic technique has been compromised should be replaced within 24 hours.

MANAGEMENT OF THE PERIPHERAL CANNULA WHILST IN SITU

Management of the Cannula	Rationale
The number of lines and ports will be kept to an absolute minimum consistent with clinical need.	To reduce the risk of cross infection (EPIC 2 recommendation).[86]
A needlefree system should be used for accessing an injection access site.	RCN recommendation.[208]
IV administration sets should be changed:	

– When the vascular device is replaced
– At 72 hour intervals
– At the end of the infusion or within 24 hours of initiating the infusion when administering lipid emulsions.

Table 7.6 (Continued)

Management of the Cannula	Rationale
Blood transfusion administration sets should be changed: – On completion of transfusion or after two units when multiple units of blood are administered.	EPIC 2 recommendation. [86]
Intermittent administration sets should be changed every 24 hours if remaining connected to the device. Discard after each use if disconnected e.g. metronidazole infusion bags.	To reduce the risk of infection.
The maximum expiry date for any infusion prepared in a clinical area is 24 hours or less in accordance with the manufacturer's specification of product characteristics.	To help avoid the risk of infection.
Bandages should be avoided wherever possible. However, if a bandage is used it should be removed at least daily in order to inspect the insertion site.	
Devices designed for splinting should be used to facilitate infusion delivery only when the device is placed in or around an area of flexion or it is at risk of dislodgement e.g. being used in a child.	RCN recommendation. [208]
Splints should be removed and the circulatory status of the patient's extremity should be assessed at regular intervals.	
When manipulating the line/cannula a non-touch technique should be applied. Ensure equipment in contact with the circuit is sterile e.g. syringes.	To prevent cross infection (RCN recommendation). [208]
Prior to accessing the system, disinfect access ports using an alcoholic chlorhexidine solution (spray or steret) unless contraindicated by manufacturer's recommendations.	Essential to prevent entry of microorganisms into the system via the portal.
The cannula should be flushed at least once daily and pre and post drug administration with 5–10mls normal saline (0.9 %) in a 10ml syringe. * **The normal saline (0.9 %) should be prescribed on the drug chart. Alternatively a Patient Group Direction (PGD) can be used by a trained and competent PGD user**.	To maintain patency.
The dressing should be changed when it becomes loose, damp or soiled.	To reduce the risk of cross infection.
An aseptic non-touch technique should be used when changing the dressing. The area should be cleaned with alcohol/chlorhexidine moving from the catheter site outwards, providing it is compatible with the device. The area should be allowed to **dry** and a sterile peripheral dressing applied (use an alcoholic povidone iodine for patients with a history of chlorhexidine sensitivity).	Skin cleansing/antisepsis of the insertion site is one of the most important measures for preventing catheter related infection.
A cannula that has migrated externally should not be readvanced prior to restablisation.	
The site should be examined to ensure the device has not become dislodged, for signs of infection and extravasation. The Visual Infusion Phlebitis (VIP) score should be recorded three times daily using the Vygon pack VIP scoring tool (sticky label).	To identify mechanical complications and signs of infection.

If the VIP is greater or equal to 2 the cannula should be removed.

If the site appears infected (VIP score of 2 or greater), a swab should be taken and sent with the tip of the cannula to Microbiology for culture and sensitivity.

The microbiology results may indicate which antibiotic is required should the patient develop signs of septicaemia.

Any incidence of phlebitis, along with intervention, treatment, and corrective action, should be documented in the patients' nursing notes.

To provide evidence of any actions taken and aid communication.
RCN recommendation. [208]

Peripheral cannula should not be used for routine blood sampling. However, if necessary the cannula can be used to draw blood using a large syringe (larger than 10mls) ONCE ONLY immediately following insertion. Reapply the tourniquet above the cannula, wait for vein engorgement and draw blood SLOWLY using minimal force. Excess force will both haemolyse the sample and cause thrombophlebitis of the vein.

If a peripheral venous cannula is not being used/required for access, it should be removed.

The longer a peripheral venous cannula remains insitu, the greater the risk of infection.

Removal of Peripheral Cannula	Rationale
Peripheral cannula should be re-sited every 72 hours wherever clinically possible.	EPIC 2 recommendation.[86]
Removal of the intravenous cannula should be an aseptic procedure.	To prevent cross infection as well as contamination of the catheter tip.
Explain procedure to the patient and gain consent.	To ensure patient understanding.
Decontaminate hands using alcohol hand rub or handwashing with liquid soap.	To reduce cross infection.
Apply clean examination gloves.	To maintain universal precautions.
Remove dressing.	To expose cannula site.
Gently withdraw cannula using a slow, steady movement and keeping hub parallel with skin.	To ease withdrawal and prevent damage to the vein.
Check integrity of cannula before disposing into sharps bin.	To ensure all removed.
Apply pressure for 2-3 minutes with gauze.	To prevent haematoma.
When bleeding has stopped apply gauze dressing.	To aid healing.
Document the date and time of removal in the patients notes including the name of the person removing the device.	To meet legal requirement.
If the site appears infected (VIP score of 2 or more) a swab should be taken and sent with the tip of the cannula to microbiology for culture and sensitivity. The infection control incident form should be completed.	The microbiology result may indicate which antibiotic is required should the patient develop signs of septicaemia.

Figure 7.1 shows 10 important points for the care of peripheral IV cannualae (East Kent Hospital NHS Trust) based on the EPIC 2 recommendations.[86]

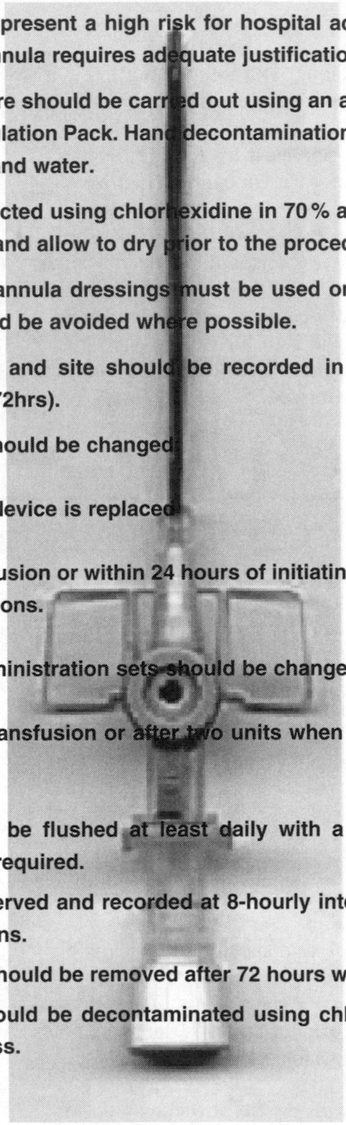

1. Intravenous cannulae present a high risk for hospital acquired infection; the need for an intravenous cannula requires adequate justification.

2. The insertion procedure should be carried out using an aseptic technique using the Vygon Biovalve Cannulation Pack. Hand decontamination is essential, using alcohol hand rub/liquid soap and water.

3. Skin should be disinfected using chlorhexidine in 70% alcohol. Gently rub over the skin for five seconds and allow to dry prior to the procedure.

4. Sterile dedicated IV cannula dressings must be used on all permanent IV cannula sites. Bandages should be avoided where possible.

5. The date of insertion and site should be recorded in the nursing notes with a review/removal date (72hrs).

6. Administration sets should be changed:

   - when the vascular device is replaced
   - at 72 hour intervals
   - at the end of the infusion or within 24 hours of initiating the infusion when administering lipid emulsions.

   Blood transfusion administration sets should be changed:

   - on completion of transfusion or after two units when multiple units of blood are administered.

7. The cannulae should be flushed at least daily with a normal saline solution or removed if no longer required.

8. The site must be observed and recorded at 8-hourly intervals according to the VIP score recommendations.

9. Peripheral cannulae should be removed after 72 hours whenever clinically possible.

10. The injection port should be decontaminated using chlorhexidine in 70% alcohol before and after access.

Figure 7.1 10 important points for the care of peripheral IV cannualae

CENTRAL VENOUS CATHETERS

As the potential consequences of catheter-related infections are so serious with CVCs, enhanced efforts are necessary in order to reduce the risk of infection to the absolute minimum. For this reason hand antisepsis and an aseptic technique are essential for CVC insertion, care of the site and accessing the system.

The following guidelines for the insertion, maintenance and removal of CVCs are those used by East Kent Hospitals NHS Trust, based upon the latest recommendations from EPIC 2 [86], and the Royal College of Nursing [208], and are included here for illustrative purposes. The reader should refer to their own local guidelines.

Table 7.7 The insertion, maintenance and removal of CVCs [86]

Insertion Procedure	Rationale
Healthcare personnel caring for a patient with a central venous catheter should be trained and assessed as competent in using and consistently adhering to infection prevention practices.	
It is strongly recommended that CVCs should be inserted in designated clean areas, e.g. treatment rooms, critical care units, operating theatres. **Insertion should be performed by trained and competent staff.**	To reduce the mechanical and infection risks associated with insertion.
Hands should be decontaminated using alcohol hand rub on visibly clean hands (apply one shot, cover all surfaces, rub hands together until dry). Alternatively, using an antimicrobial liquid soap e.g. Hibiscrub, povidone iodine, hands should be thoroughly washed, using a technique which aims to cover all surfaces of the hands. Hands should be rinsed in running water before and after applying the cleansing agent and dried well.	To reduce the risk of cross infection from the operator's hands during the procedure.
Use optimum aseptic technique, including a sterile gown, gloves and a large sterile drape (dedicated CVP insertion packs must be used).	Evidence has identified that using maximal barrier precautions reduces the risk of subsequent CVC-related infection (EPIC recommendation).
Effective skin preparation will remove bacteria from both hair and skin, avoiding the need for shaving, which can result in microscopic damage and thus microbial colonisation. If hair removal is considered necessary, **clipping** is the preferred option using a disposable clipper head.	Evidence suggests that shaving results in microscopic damage and thus microbial colonisation of the skin.
Using Chloraprep 2 % (two applicators of Chloraprep 3mls) applying gentle friction, disinfect the skin insertion site for 30 seconds. Allow to dry before inserting the catheter. Use an alcoholic povidone iodine solution for patients with a history of chlorhexidine sensitivity.	Skin cleansing/antisepsis of the insertion site is one of the most important measures for preventing catheter related infection. EPIC recommends an alcoholic solution of chlorhexidine 2 % as this combines the benefits of rapid action and excellent residual (ongoing) activity.

Table 7.7 (Continued)

Insertion Procedure	Rationale
The CVC should be firmly anchored to prevent movement.	CVCs readily become colonised and carry micro-organisms from the skin into the insertion tract.
Use a sterile, transparent, semi-permeable polyurethane CVC dressing i.e. IV 3000.	To allow for continuous inspection of the site (EPIC recommendation).
If total parenteral nutrition is being administered use one central venous catheter or lumen exclusively for that purpose.	EPIC recommendation.
The procedure must be documented in the nursing and medical records, stating the name of the person inserting the CVC, the date of insertion, site, catheter size and reason for insertion (insert product label into patient's notes).	To meet legal and patient care requirements/facilitate audit.
Radiological confirmation of the position of the catheter tip must be undertaken.	To confirm precise location of the catheter tip.
The number of access points should be kept to a minimum.	To reduce the risk of infection (EPIC recommendation).
IV administration sets should be changed:	EPIC 2 recommendation.
– When the vascular device is replaced – At 72 hour intervals *(unless disconnected)* – At the end of the infusion or within 24 hours of initiating the infusion when administering lipid emulsions. *If the solution only includes glucose and amino acids, administration sets in continuous use do not need to be replaced more frequently than every 72 hours.*	
Blood transfusion administration sets should be changed:	
– On completion of transfusion or after two units when multiple units of blood are administered.	
Intermittent administration sets should be changed every 24 hours, if remaining connected to the device or discarded after each use if disconnected e.g. flagyl bags.	To reduce the risk of infection.
The maximum expiry date for any infusion prepared in a clinical area is 24 hours or less in accordance with the manufacturer's specification of product characteristics.	To help avoid the risk of infection (EPIC 2 recommendation).
Administration sets should be labelled with the date of commencement and anticipated change.	To ensure that administration sets are changed according to policy.
The use of needleless connectors are recommended and should be used according to the manufacturers' instructions	Catheter hubs/ports are a potential source of entry for micro organisms (EPIC 2 recommendation).

(recommendations for the frequency of change of needleless components). When needleless devices are used, healthcare personnel should ensure that all components of the system are compatible and secured, to minimise leaks and breaks in the system.

When needleless devices are used, the risk of contamination should be minimised by decontaminating the access port with an alcoholic chlorhexidine gluconate solution unless contraindicated by the manufacturer's recommendations, in which case aqueous povidone iodine should be used.

The insertion site should be visually inspected at least daily for signs of local infection, e.g. heat, pain, tenderness, erythema, purulent discharge. The observation should be. recorded in the nursing notes. Signs of infection should be reported immediately to the medical team *who should consider removing the device.*

To detect signs of infection that are apparent at the insertion site.

Using a aseptic technique, the dressing should be changed when no longer intact, or when moisture collects at the site (must be changed at least every 7 days) (EPIC 2).

To reduce the risk of infection.

Hands should be decontaminated ideally using alcohol rub or washed using liquid soap and water.

To reduce the risk of cross infection from the operators hands.

Clean examination gloves may be used for undertaking dressings using a non-touch technique.

A sterile dressing pack must be used when changing the dressing. The area should be cleaned using 1 applicator of single use Chloraprep, moving from the catheter insertion site outwards. The area should be allowed to dry (use alcohol povidone iodine for patients with a history of chlorhexidine sensitivity. An aqueous solution of chlorhexidine gluconate should be used if the manufacturer's recommendations prohibit the use of alcohol with their product). A sterile CVC dressing should be applied.

Skin cleansing/antisepsis of the insertion site is one of the most important measures for preventing catheter related infection. EPIC 2 recommends an alcoholic solution of chlorhexidine 2 % as this combines the benefits of rapid action and excellent residual (ongoing) activity.

An aseptic technique should be applied for accessing the system. Decontaminate hands. Disinfect the external surfaces of the catheter hub before and after use with an alcoholic solution of chlorhexidine gluconate, unless contraindicated by the manufacturer's recommendations when an aqueous povidone iodine solution should be used.

Essential requirement to prevent cross-infection.

Table 7.7 (Continued)

Removal of the CVC	Rationale
Assess the need for continuing venous access on a regular basis and remove the CVC as soon as clinically possible.	Evidence suggests that the longer a CVC remains in situ, the greater the risk of infection.
Clean the skin with chlorhexidine in 70% alcohol and allow to dry fully prior to removing the device. Avoid accidental contamination of the tip, if culture is clinically indicated, i.e. signs of infection, pyrexia, high WCC etc. In this case, cut off 5cm of the distal catheter tip with sterile scissors and place in a sterile container and send for microscopy, culture and sensitivity (MC+S).	To ensure the catheter tip is obtained aseptically.
Apply a sterile occlusive dressing to the site.	To protect the insertion site whilst healing.
The date of catheter removal should be documented in the nursing and medical records.	To meet legal and patient care requirements.

Reproduced by permission of East Kent Hospitals NHS Trust

ADDITIONAL IMPORTANT POINTS[86]

Skin decontamination

The EPIC 2 guidelines recommend the use of 2% chlorhexidine gluconate 70% isopropyl alcohol for skin decontamination. Chloraprep[209] is effective against a wide range of micro-organisms within 30 seconds and has residual activity for up to 48 hours after application.

Number of catheter lumens

The EPIC 2 guidelines make the recommendation that single lumen catheters should be used rather than those with multiple ports, and that if the patient is receiving parenteral nutrition, it should be administered by either by a single-lumen catheter or a designated port on a multi-lumen catheters.

Tunnelled and totally implantable ports

EPIC 2 recommend that where long-term vascular access is anticipated (defined as longer than three–four weeks) tunnelled or implanted vascular devices are inserted.

Antimicrobial impregnated CVC

If the CVC is likely to remain in situ for longer than three–four weeks, the use of an antimicrobial impregnated vascular device should be considered.[86]

Selection of catheter insertion site

Identifying the most appropriate insertion site can be problematic and can influence the risk of infection. The subclavian vein should be used in preference to the jugular or femoral sites for non-tunnelled CVCs as it is associated with less risk of contamination. EPIC 2[86] recommends that the risk of infection is assessed against the risks of mechanical complications, such as bleeding, pneumothorax and thrombosis.

Replacement of CVCs

EPIC 2 recommends[86]:

- Non-tunnelled CVCs should not be routinely replaced to prevent infection.
- If the CVC needs to be removed because it is not functioning, or if the device needs to be replaced, a new catheter should be inserted over a guide wire as long as there is no evidence of infection.
- If a catheter-related infection is suspected, but there is no evidence of infection at the insertion site, the CVC can be removed and a new device can be inserted over a guide wire. If a catheter-related infection is confirmed, the newly inserted catheter should be removed and a new catheter inserted at a different site if it is still required.
- All fluid administration tubing and connectors should be replaced when the vascular device is replaced.
- When adherence to aseptic technique cannot be assured i.e. if the CVC is inserted during a medical emergency, it should be replaced as soon as possible (within 48 hours).

HOSPITAL-ACQUIRED PNEUMONIA

Pneumonia is the most severe and life-threatening of all respiratory tract infections, and the most commonly acquired infection in intensive care units where it is strongly associated with endotracheal intubation and mechanical ventilation. It has a case fatality rate approaching 70 %.[210,211,212] Hospital-acquired pneumonia is defined as pneumonia with an onset of at least 48–72 hours after admission to hospital, or in the case of ventilator-associated pneumonia, occurring within 48 hours of intubation.[213] Most cases of hospital-acquired pneumonia are caused by bacteria such as *Pseudomonas aeruginosa, Acinetobacter* species, *Staphylococcus aureus, Streptococcus pneumoniae* and *Haemophilus influenzae,* although viruses and fungi can also be implicated. It is not uncommon for more than one organism to be identified, as the longer the patient is in hospital the wider the exposure to potential pathogens, which are also more likely to be multi-drug resistant.[214] Risk factors for hospital-acquired, and in particular ventilator-associated, pneumonia are summarised in Table 7.8.

Table 7.8 Risk factors for hospital-acquired/ventilator-associated pneumonia[210,212]

Age
Malnutrition
Immunosupression
Underlying illness/disease
History of alcohol or substance misuse
Pre-existing chronic lung disease
Prolonged hospital stay
Admission to ITU
Administration of antibiotics (alteration of normal body flora; colonisation with
    drug-resistant bacteria)
Naso-gastric tube insertion
Endotracheal intubation
Aspiration
Surgery involving the head, neck, thorax or upper abdomen
Restricted mobility due to age/trauma/surgery or on prolonged bed rest
Prolonged mechanical ventilation
Exposure to contaminated respiratory devices
Transmission of pathogens on the hands of healthcare workers or from contaminated
    equipment

Table 7.9 Ways in which bacteria can access the lower airways[210,216,217,218,219,220]

Contaminated respiratory equipment – nebulisers, humidification circuit tubing, ventilator
    circuits.
Endotracheal suctioning.
Manipulation of endotracheal tubes and ventilator circuits.
Contaminated diagnostic equipment – bronchoscope/spirometer.
Routes of transmission can also occur from device to device, patient to patient,
    endogenously from a body site on the patient to the lower respiratory tract via the hands
    or a contaminated device.

THE PATHOGENESIS OF INFECTION

The most common cause of hospital-acquired pneumonia is the aspiration of
naso/oropharyngeal secretions. In mechanically ventilated patients, the endotracheal
tube bypasses the normal host defence mechanism, providing a direct route of entry
into the normally well-protected respiratory tract, and organisms colonising the
oropharynx may be carried into the trachea during intubation. Secretions pool above
the inflated cuff of the endotracheal tube [210] and often contain Gram-negative bacilli
and *S.aureus* which colonise the upper respiratory tract in patients who have been in
hospital for longer than five days. [210] Once the secretions have been aspirated into
the lower respiratory tract, they cause inflammation and infection in the terminal

Table 7.10 Prevention of hospital-acquired/ventilator-associated pneumonia[210,221,222,223]

General

Adequate post-operative pain relief to facilitate coughing/deep breathing.

Chest physiotherapy.

Early mobilisation.

Hand decontamination in between patients, after handling respiratory secretions or contact with medical equipment/devices.

Wear gloves when contact with respiratory secretions is anticipated; discard as clinical waste and either wash or decontaminate hands with alcohol hand rub after gloves have been removed.

Ensure that all respiratory therapy equipment is decontaminated appropriately in between patients according to manufacturer's instructions (used as single-use/single-patient use; cleaned, disinfected or sterilised).

Ventilated patients

Semi-recumbent positioning (if safe for the patient) with elevation of the head of the bed to 30–45 ° (decreases the risk of aspiration of gastro-intestinal contents/oropharyngeal or nasopharyngeal secretions).

Sedation holding – daily interruption of sedation reduces the duration of ventilation.

Airway humidification – use of heat and air moisture exchangers (HMEs) to prevent drying out of the respiratory mucosa. Use sterile water. Change the HME when it becomes visibly soiled.

Management of ventilator circuit – change when visibly soiled.[210]

Use a sterile technique for performing endotracheal suction to prevent contamination of the suction catheter before it is introduced into the trachea; use each suction catheter only once.

---

bronchioles and alveoli in the lung, filling the alveolar spaces with fluid instead of air, preventing gases exchange and resulting in consolidation.[215] There are other means by which bacteria can access the lower airways and these are summarised Table 7.9.

Table 7.10 summarises the methods for preventing pneumonia in hospitalised patients.

8 The Problem of Antimicrobial Resistance

INTRODUCTION

In spite of the number of antimicrobial agents available to treat infections, they still remain a serious cause of patient morbidity and mortality, and this has been compounded by the development of antimicrobial resistance among micro-organisms. It is hardly a new phenomenon, having been in existence now for at least 50 years, but it has become increasingly endemic and so prevalent that it is acknowledged to be a major public health threat and a global concern.[224,225] Many key documents have been published over the last nine years. In 1998, the House of Lords Select Committee on Science and Technology[226] published a report emphasising the need for resistance to be tackled on a global scale as '... resistance is not a short-term activity; it is a long-haul task requiring partnerships between government(s) and a wide range of organisations and individuals across many disciplines both in the UK and internationally' (page 7). Following the publication of this report, a health service circular was issued from the Department of Health in 1999[227], highlighting the need for the NHS to take action over antimicrobial prescribing and use, and calling for the prevention and control of infection in relation to resistant organisms to be strengthened. Then, in 2000, the Department of Health published the UK Antimicrobial Resistance Strategy and Action Plan[228] which outlined eight key areas which needed to be addressed in order to tackle the problem. This was followed in 2002 and 2003 by yet more Department of Health publications[3,142] which emphasised the need for the ongoing monitoring and surveillance of antimicrobial resistance, and identified the prudent use of antibiotics as an area requiring intensified control measures.

However, it is not just antibiotic resistance that is the only concern. Resistance to anti-viral and anti-fungal agents has been developing markedly[229,230], with serious implications for the treatment of patients with HIV, and other vulnerable patients at risk from opportunistic infections. Resistance is also now seen among fungi (e.g. *Candida albicans*) and protozoa (*Plasmodium falciparum*, or malaria).[231] Antimicrobial agents incorporated into household soaps, lotions and cleaning products are adding to the problem.[232]

Hospitals, particularly intensive care units, are an important breeding ground for the development and spread of antibiotic resistant bacteria, a consequence of exposing to heavy antibiotic use a high density population in frequent contact with healthcare staff and the attendant risk of cross-infection.[233] The National Audit Office Report in 2004[36] acknowledged that the problem of multi-drug resistant bacteria increases the complexity of patient care. Within the healthcare setting antimicrobial resistance, particularly among bacteria, limits treatment options by reducing the number of therapeutic agents available for use which in turn puts constraints on those that can be used. This sometimes leads to the use of more expensive, more toxic or less efficacious agents for the treatment of infections. Overall, this means that patient treatment options can be limited and as a result patient morbidity and mortality increased.[234]

It should be noted here that antimicrobial therapy and antimicrobial resistance are vast and complex topics which are beyond the scope of this book. The aim of this chapter is to provide the reader with a basic understanding of how antimicrobial agents work and the mechanisms of resistance, primarily focusing on antibiotics for the treatment of bacterial infections. The chapter begins by briefly looking at the development of antibiotics, and moves on to describe the principles of antibiotic therapy. The mechanisms of resistance among bacteria are explained, followed by problems with specific resistant organisms, such as *Acinetobacter, Klebsiella* and glycopeptide resistant enterococci (GRE). Controlling antimicrobial resistance is also discussed. The infection control precautions to be taken when caring for patients with resistant organisms are summarised in a Table 8.5 at the end of the chapter.

LEARNING OUTCOMES

After reading this chapter the reader will be able to:

- Understand the principles of antibiotic therapy
- Understand why antimicrobial resistance has occurred and how micro-organisms become resistant
- Understand the infection control precautions that need to be taken when caring for patients with resistant organisms.

THE HISTORY OF ANTIMICROBIAL CHEMOTHERAPY

The term 'antibiotic' was originally applied to naturally occurring compounds such as penicillin, which attacked the infecting bacteria without harming the host. Alexander Fleming discovered the antibacterial effect of penicillin in 1928, when he noticed that a fungal mould (*Penicillium notatum*) growing as a contaminant on an agar plate containing *Staphylococcus aureus*, caused the bacteria to lyse.[235] The term 'antimicrobial' is now applied to both natural and synthetic compounds, and 'antibiotic' is commonly used to describe the agents (mostly antibacterial agents) used to treat systemic infections.[236] The sulphonamides were the first group of broad-spectrum antibacterial agents to be introduced into clinical practice in 1935, and although their discovery marked the beginning of the effective treatment of infections with antibacterial therapy, they also marked the beginning of antimicrobial resistance.[237] Sulphonamide-resistant strains of previously sensitive bacteria soon became common. For example, in 1938 almost all strains of *Neisseria gonorrhoea* were sensitive to sulphonamides. However, by 1948, less than 20 % of clinical isolates were still sensitive and sulphonamides were no longer regularly used in the treatment of gonorrhoea.[238] Sulphonamide resistance was subsequently identified in many other bacteria including meningococci, haemolytic streptococci, pneumococci and coliforms.[237]

Penicillin wasn't commercially available until the 1940s, when it was mass produced for widespread use, and it was hailed as 'the wonder drug'. It was seen as the 'magic bullet', with the ability to kill bacteria without harming the host, and there was great optimism that it would completely revolutionise the treatment of infections and infectious diseases. However, the bubble began to burst in 1950, when penicillinase-producing resistant strains of *Staphylococcus aureus* began to emerge as a major cause of serious infection in hospital patients.[239] The penicillins and the cephalosporins are closely related families of compounds which share the structural features of a beta-lactam ring. Such compounds are known as beta-lactam antibiotics. Many bacteria, however, produce enzymes known as beta-lacatamase or penicillinase, which is capable of breaking open the beta-lactam ring, rendering the antibiotic ineffective. During the 1960s, the aerobic enteric Gram-negative bacilli (*Escherichia coli* and other species) emerged as important pathogens. Antibiotics effective against these Gram-negative species were introduced, including modified penicillins such as ampicillin, carbenicillin, the early cephalosporins and aminoglycosides. However, resistance developed and multi-drug resistant Gram-negative bacteria became the main therapeutic problem of hospital acquired infections during the 1970s and 1980s.[239] By the mid 1990s, it was acknowledged that there was a potential resistance mechanism among micro-organisms for every antimicrobial drug, including vancomycin, an antibiotic to which resistance was thought to be impossible.[239,240]

Since the 1960s a wide range of antimicrobial agents have been available for the treatment of infections caused by Gram-positive bacteria (staphylococci and streptococci), including the penicillins, cephalosporins, aminoglycosides, glycopeptides, tetracylines, macrolides and sulphonamides. However, due to this wide range of effective antimicrobial agents, there was very little research into the development of new drugs for the treatment of these organisms, and the last decade has seen an emergence of opportunistic Gram-positive bacteria resistant to some or all of these agents. This is possibly because the widespread use of cephalosporins, aminoglycosides and quinolones for Gram-negative infections has selected Gram-positive species that are inherently resistant to these antimicrobial agents, and their capacity for acquiring antibiotic resistant determinants.[241]

Infections caused by Gram-positive cocci have become predominant over the last two decades, notably MRSA which first emerged in the 1960s and increased in frequency as an important hospital pathogen during the 1980s and 1990s, and to date (see Chapter 9). Enterococci are also rising in prominence as hospital pathogens; not only do they have a natural resistance to most commonly used antibiotics, they also have the capacity to acquire resistance to those antibiotics to which they are sensitive, for example, amoxicillin.[241] Multiple antibiotic resistance to useful classes of antibiotics, including the penicillins, cephalosporins, aminoglycosides and fluroquinolones, has gradually increased among a number of Gram-negative hospital pathogens, notably *Klebsiella pneumoniae,* Enterobacter species, and *Pseudomonas aeruginosa.*[241,242]

Community acquired resistance to antibiotics is also increasing, particularly amongst *Streptococcus pneumoniae* and *Mycobacterium tuberculosis*, where resistance to seven antitubercular drugs has been reported.[243,244] Tuberculosis, with particular reference to multi-drug resistant disease, is discussed in detail in Chapter 10. Reports of resistance to trimethoprim in urinary tract infections caused by *E.coli* is increasing in the community, along with urinary tract infections caused by extended spectrum beta-lacatamase (ESBL) producing strains of *Klebsiella.*

THE PRINCIPLES OF ANTIBIOTIC THERAPY

Antibiotics are generally highly effective at treating infections caused by bacteria because of their selective toxicity. This means that they are able to kill bacteria (bactericidal action) or prevent their growth and replication (bacteriostatic action) without actually harming the host.[245] The choice of the appropriate antibiotic is multi-factorial and is dependent upon the organism (or likely organism), the site of infection (not all antibiotics are able to penetrate bone, joints or cerebral spinal fluid), likely antibiotic susceptibilities (see Chapter 4 The Microbiology Laboratory), the severity of the infection, and whether or not the patient has a past medical history of allergy to any antibiotics (penicillin allergy being the most common).

They can be administered topically, orally, rectally and by intra-muscular (IM) and intra-venous (IV) injection. The IM/IV route is commonly used to treat infections where it is particularly important to ensure that adequate concentrations of the antibiotic have been achieved, or in situations where the oral route cannot be tolerated. In these instances, the concentration of the antibiotic in the blood stream has to be monitored to ensure that the correct therapeutic dose is being achieved and to detect toxicity. For example, when IV vancomycin is prescribed, blood is taken pre-dose and one–two hours post-dose every three days and the dose adjusted where appropriate (either increased or decreased) to ensure that it is within the therapeutic range. Antibiotics can also be prescribed in combination, as certain antibiotics have a synergistic effect. Combination therapy can be used in the initial treatment of potentially life-threatening infections before microbiology results are available, if the causative organism can't be isolated or if the infection is poly-microbial, with more than one organism implicated. Combination therapy can also help combat or delay the emergence of antibiotic resistance.

Antibiotics are classified according to their mode of action; interference with bacterial cell wall synthesis, disruption of the cell membrane, inhibition of protein synthesis, and inhibition of nucleic acid synthesis. Groups of antibiotics that interfere with bacterial cell wall synthesis, either by preventing the cell wall from forming, or weakening it so that osmotic pressure exerted outside the cell causes it to swell and burst, include the beta-lactam antibiotics such as the penicillins and the cephalosporins.[245] Penicillin, for example, targets the enzyme transpeptidase, which is necessary for the cross-linking of the peptide-sugar chains which build the peptidoglycan wall. Polymixins, such as colistin, disrupt the bacterial cell membrane, which causes the cell to break open.[246] Aminoglycosides inhibit protein synthesis in aerobic bacteria[245] and quinolones are among groups of antibiotics that act directly or indirectly on DNA or RNA synthesis, either preventing DNA being transcribed into RNA, or disrupting the coiling/uncoiling of DNA.[236]

Antibiotics are also described according to their spectrum of activity, which may be narrow or broad. Antibiotics with a narrow spectrum have restricted activity and are only effective against certain organisms, whereas broad-spectrum agents are effective against a wide range of bacteria.

Table 8.1 lists some of the most commonly prescribed antibiotics according to their mode of action, antibiotic class or group and spectrum of activity. This list does not include all antibiotic groups.

All antibiotics have side effects, the most common being gastro-intestinal disturbances following disruption of the normal bowel flora (see Chapter 11 *Clostridium difficile*). Other side effects include skin rashes, ranging from mild urticaria to **Stevens-Johnson Syndrome**, and renal and hepatic toxicity. The most serious allergic reaction is anaphylaxis, which is a medical emergency characterised by laryngeal oedema, bronchospasm and hypotension. It can carry a high mortality rate unless treated promptly with adrenaline, oxygen therapy and antihistamines (See Chapter 5 Understanding the Immune System and the Nature and Pathogenesis of Infection).

ANTIMICROBIAL RESISTANCE

Resistance is acknowledged to be a complex phenomenon, involving the organism, the antimicrobial drug, the environment and the patient, both separately and in their interaction.[240] An organism can be classed as resistant if it is not inhibited or killed by one or more classes of antibiotic at concentrations achievable after normal dosage. From a microbiology laboratory perspective, this essentially means that a sensitive organism is one that is likely to respond to therapy with the antimicrobial agent tested, and a resistant isolate is one that will not.[239]

Resistance among micro-organisms can be inherent or acquired. Inherent, or natural resistance, is part of the organism's genetic make-up, and it is encoded on

Table 8.1 Some commonly used antimicrobial agents

Mode of action	Class	Agents	Comments
Inhibitors of bacterial cell wall synthesis	Beta-lactam	Penicillins (Flucloxacillin, Ampicillin, Amoxicillin, Benzylpenicillin, Piperacillin)	Early agents have a limited spectrum of activity due to susceptibility to beta-lactamases, but are used to treat staphylococcal, streptococcal and meningococcal infections. Respiratory and urinary tract infections; effective against pseudomonas and proteus species.
		Co-Amoxiclav, Tazobactam (Piperacillin with Tazocin) and Ticarcillin (Timentin) – extended spectrum penicillins by virtue of combination with a beta-lactamase inhibitors	
		Cephalosporins (1st generation – Cefalexin, Cephradine; 2nd generation – Cefuroxime; 3rd generation – Cefotaxime, Ceftriaxone, Ceftazidime)	1st generation agents had limited spectrum of activity and were available orally; later 3rd generation agents have broad-spectrum activity against most Gram-positive and Gram-negative organisms except Enterococci and anaerobes.
	Carbapenems	Imipenem, Meropenem, Ertapenem	Broad-spectrum Gram-positive/Gram-negative aerobic/anaerobic bacteria. (Ertapenem is not effective against Enterococci, Pseudomonas or Acinetobacter).
	Glycopeptides	Vancomycin, Teicoplanin	Aerobic and anaerobic Gram-positive cocci, including multi-resistant staphylococci.
Inhibitors of bacterial protein synthesis	Tetracyclines	Tetracycline, Minocyline, Doxycycline	Broad-spectrum antibiotics but use is limited due to bacterial resistance; often used in the treatment of acne and periodontal disease.

Aminoglycosides	Streptomycin, Gentamicin and Amikacin	Streptomycin may be used in the treatment of MDR-TB in combination with other agents; Gentamicin is commonly used in the treatment of septicaemia, biliary tract infections and endocarditis; Amikacin is used for the treatment of serious infections caused by Gram-negative bacilli that are Gentamicin-resistant.
Macrolides	Erythromycin, azithromycin, Clarithromycin	Respiratory tract infections, otitis media, skin and soft tissue infections; Legionnaires' disease, campylobacter.
Quinolones	Ciprofloxacin	Effective against Gram-positive and Gram-negative bacteria (Gram-negative in particular) but should be used with caution as frequently implicated in cases of pseudomembranous colitis.
Inhibitors of nucleic acid synthesis	Moxifloxacin	Second-line treatment of community-acquired pneumonia.
Other agents	Linezolid	Virtually all infections caused by Gram-positive bacteria, including MRSA and VRE; particularly effective against MRSA pneumonia.
	Metronidazole	Infections caused by anaerobes (i.e. *Clostridium difficile*, and in the treatment of polymicrobial necrotising fasciitis) and protozoa.
	Daptomycin	A completely new class of antibiotic (cyclic lipopeptide). Perforates the bacterial cell membrane; effective against most Gram-positive bacteria (including MRSA) but not Gram-negatives; cannot be used in the treatment of respiratory tract infections as it is partially inactivated by surfactant.
	Tigecycline	First of the glycylcline antibiotics; derived from the Tetracyclines; acts on inhibiting bacterial cell synthesis; wide spectrum of activity including most medically important bacteria, including MRSA, VRE and multi-resistant Gram-negatives.

the bacterial chromosome, meaning that the organism is naturally not susceptible to a certain antibiotic. Resistance that is acquired, however, is the most worrying, with spontaneous genetic mutation and/or genetic recombinations leading to the emergence of an antibiotic-resistant organism. Organisms can acquire resistance through the transfer of genetic material from one organism to another by plasmids or transposons. Plasmids are self-replicating circular pieces of DNA, which exist outside of the chromosome, and they can be encoded for multi-drug resistance. Transposons are mobile DNA segments that often carry genes for resistance and virulence which migrate between unrelated plasmids and/or the bacterial chromosome.[64] The transfer of plasmids or transposons is acquired by conjugation, transduction or transformation.

Conjugation is the major mechanism for the transfer of antibiotic resistance, and the exchange of genetic material can occur between unrelated species of bacteria.[247] It is the process by which DNA is transferred from a donor cell to a recipient cell, requiring direct cell-to-cell contact. One cell has to posses a self-transmissible plasmid (F plasmid) which contains a specialised structure known as the sex pilus, which attaches to the recipient cell and penetrates the cell membrane, allowing the transfer of DNA from one cell to another.[247,248] Transduction involves the transfer of DNA between cells by bacteriophages, viruses which infect bacteria, carrying DNA from one bacteria to another.[248] Some bacteria are able to take up DNA from another organism that has been released by lysis of the cell, incorporating it into their own chromosome through recombination. This process is known as transformation, and can occur between closely related species of bacteria.[64]

There are many other mechanisms of resistance. Some bacterial species may produce an enzyme capable of destroying the antibiotic, as seen with *Staphylococcus aureus* and penicillin. The bacterial cell wall may be naturally impermeable to certain antibiotics, or the bacteria may acquire an inner membrane protein which acts as an efflux pump and pumps the antibiotic out of the cell.[249] Bacteria can also alter the target site of the antibiotic; the antibiotic can enter the cell but is unable to inhibit the activity of the cell because of structural changes within it that prevent the antibiotic from binding and attaching to it.[250] They can also develop an alternative metabolic pathway, so that the antibiotic bypasses the site at which it would normally be effective.

FACTORS LEADING TO THE EMERGENCE OF ANTIMICROBIAL RESISTANCE AND PROBLEMS WITHIN THE HEALTHCARE SETTING

Resistance often occurs among normal bacterial flora in patients receiving antibiotics. If a further infection requiring treatment subsequently develops, that bacterial population is more likely to become resistant than in patients who have not received treatment. Darwin's theory of the 'survival of the fittest' favours selection systems.[251] Within the microbial population there is variation amongst microorganisms and selection occurs, which favours those organisms with traits that are most advantageous in the prevailing environment. Antibiotics therefore 'select' for resistance by targeting the susceptible or antibiotic sensitive organisms, 'allowing' the resistant ones to survive, so if there is a resistant mutant present, it has a competitive advantage over other bacteria, with natural selection always ensuring that dominant organisms survive.

The driving force behind the whole 'resistance problem' has been the widespread use of antibacterial drugs, and the misuse and overuse of antibiotics worldwide in the treatment of humans and animals. Antimicrobial agents are used to treat infections in animals, but in those animals bred for human consumption they are often administered prophylatically to protect whole herds from disease, and also for growth promotion.[252,3]

They are administered continuously at sub-therapeutic levels, often in feed. Resistant bacteria can either be transferred to humans via the food chain, or resistant pathogens in animals can transfer resistance genes to human pathogens.

Within the UK, 50 % of all antibiotics prescribed are used to treat infections in humans (the other 50 % are used in the animal industry), 80 % of which are prescribed in the community, predominantly for the treatment of upper respiratory and urinary tract infections.[252] Historically there has been huge pressure on general practitioners to prescribe antibiotics for the treatment of minor coughs and colds and other illness because of the level of patient expectation and demand for treatment. This has lead to the prescription and administration of antibiotics in situations where their use is not justified and the emergence of resistant organisms within the community, partly through poor prescribing, with the dose prescribed at sub-therapeutic levels, and partly due to poor patient compliance.[231]

Table 8.2 lists some of the factors in relation to antimicrobial prescribing which have exacerbated the development of resistance.

Pressures on healthcare systems for greater efficiency, with greater bed occupancy rates and stretched nursing and medical care, along with heavy antimicrobial use, increase the risk of infection to patients.[253] Resistant strains can spread among patients, with selection of resistance in infected or colonised patients enhanced by various patient factors. These include immunosupression, use of indwelling invasive devices, alteration of the patient's own flora during antibiotic therapy, length

Table 8.2 Factors contributing to the development of antibiotic resistance

Treatment of conditions where antibiotics are not indicated (e.g. coughs/colds due to viral infections).
Prophylactic administration where there is no proven value, or duration of prophylaxis too long.
Inadequate dose/duration.
Monotherapy, when treatment with combination antibiotic therapy would be clinically indicated.
Poor patient compliance – course of antibiotics not completed (e.g. lack of understanding; side effects; patient starts to feel better and so doesn't complete the course).

Table 8.3 Factors exacerbating the spread of resistant organisms

Travel to other countries with higher rates of resistant organisms – resistant organisms can
be imported.
Indiscriminate use/prescribing and over-the-counter availability of antibiotics in countries
where there are insufficient control measures.
Overcrowding in hospitals/high bed occupancy rates and mixing of patient populations.
Poor standards of infection control practice – failure to decontaminate hands, change
gloves/aprons, decontaminate equipment, poor standards of cleanliness.

of hospital stay, intensity and duration of exposure to broad-spectrum antibiotics,
severity of illness and other associated co-morbidities, and contact via the contaminated hands of healthcare staff. The hospital environment can harbour resistant
organisms, and healthcare staff need to work together to reduce reservoirs of infection within the hospital environment.[3]

Table 8.3 summarises the factors that exacerbate the spread of resistant organisms.

RESISTANCE AMONG SPECIFIC ORGANISMS – ANTIBIOTIC RESISTANT 'COLIFORMS'

Antibiotic resistant 'coliforms' include organisms such as members of the family
Enterobacteriaceae, for example *E.coli, Klebsiella* and *Proteus*, and *Acinetobacter*.
They are a normal inhabitant of the gastro-intestinal tract but can become opportunistic pathogens when transferred to other body sites. As well as causing endogenous infection in their host, they can also be spread to other patients via the
contaminated hands of healthcare workers, and via contaminated equipment such
as humidifiers, nebulisers, wash bowls or any equipment that is shared between
patients. They are killed relatively easily by heat, e.g. 80 °C for one minute as with
bedpan washers, but they multiply readily at room temperature, particularly in moist
conditions, and humidifiers and nebulisers act as potential sources for the spread
of infection, particularly in areas where their usage may be high, such as intensive
care units and respiratory wards, therefore in equipment, resistant coliforms may
already be present in the gastro-intestinal tract at the time of the patient's admission
to hospital. These organisms may already be present in the gastro-intestinal tract,
colonising the patient's bowel on admission to hospital. This section briefly looks at
antibiotic-resistant *Acinetobacter* and *Klebsiella* as important causes of healthcare
associated infection, and concludes with the specific problems caused by another
resistant pathogen – glycopeptide-resistant Enterococci (GRE).

Acinetobacter

Acinetobacter species not only colonise the bowel and skin of humans and animals,
they are also widespread within the environment, occurring naturally within drinking
and surface waters, soils and sewage. Compared to many other organisms, they lack

the virulence factors that would class them as major pathogens, but they can cause opportunistic infections, particularly in patients who are immunocompromised, and they can affect any body site. Isolation of *Acinetobacter* in a clinical specimen is not always of clinical significance; the patient's general condition and the antibiotic susceptibilities of the organism need to be taken into account in order to determine whether or not the patient is colonised or infected.

Acinetobacter bumannii is the most commonly reported species of *Acinetobacter*, accounting for approximately 80 % of reported infections such as pneumonia, bacteraemia, wound and urinary tract infections.[254,255] These infections tend to occur in already ill hospitalised patients, and can be spread by direct/indirect contact, contaminated equipment and environmental exposure. It can be multi-antibiotic resistant, which is defined as resistance to any aminoglycoside, such as gentamicin, as well as resistant to any third generation cephalosporin, such as cefuroxime and cefotaxime. Some isolates are now also resistant to the carbapenems such as imipenem and meropenem, which has implications for the treatment of infections. In view of this, and because this organism is now causing so many problems nationally, guidelines on the control and management of multi-resistant *Acinetobacter* which incorporate recommendations on isolation, antibiotic prescribing, environmental cleanliness and decontamination were published in 2005.[255] They can be accessed via the Health Protection Agency website.[256]

Klebsiella species

Klebsiella are opportunistic pathogens implicated in many healthcare associated infections, with *Klebsiella pneumoniae* a common cause of pneumonia and urinary tract infections. Infection is preceded by colonisation, and is associated with length of stay, the severity of the patient's illness and the manipulation of any invasive indwelling devices.[257] Widespread environmental contamination can occur and one documented outbreak of *Klebsiella pneumoniae* involved nearly 300 patients over a period of three-and-a-half years.[258] They are often referred to as ESBLs, or extended beta-lacatamase producers, meaning that they produce enzymes rendering them resistant to the cephalosporins such as cefuroxime, cefotaxime and ceftazidime, as well as aminoglycosides and fluroquinolones, making treatment of infections difficult.[259]

Glycopeptide-Resistant Enterococci (GRE)

Enterococci are inhabitants of the gastro-intestinal tract and the female genital tract, existing as part of the normal faecal flora. They are a common cause of healthcare associated infections, and *Enterococcus faecalis* and *Enterococcus faecium* are implicated the most in infections, with *E.faecalis* responsible for approximately 90 % of clinical infections.[260] While some infections can be attributed to endogenous sources, outbreaks of patient-to-patient spread can occur, with transmission via direct or indirect contact, and the reservoir of infection is usually the bowel. Common sites of infection are the urinary tract, wounds (especially following abdominal and biliary tract surgery, where they can be found mixed with other faecal flora) and the bloodstream.[261]

Acquired resistance to glycopeptides (vancomycin) by resistance encoded plasmids has emerged in enterococci, and particularly in *E.faecalis* and *E.faecium*, reducing the treatment options in cases of severe infection.[231] This has been a mounting concern since 1992, when it was first discovered that the gene that codes for vancomycin resistance, *vanA*, could be transferred from enterococci to meticillin-resistant *Staphylococcus aureus*[262]; in 1997, the first strain of *S.aureus* with reduced susceptibility to vancomycin and teicoplanin was reported in Japan.[263]

Risk factors for colonisation with GRE depend on first of all being exposed to other patients with GRE, especially those with diarrhoea and who will be carrying or shedding high numbers of the organism, as the environment is likely to be heavily contaminated.[264,265,266,267] Other risk factors include prolonged hospital stay, admission to intensive care units, and renal, liver and oncology units, and prior antibiotic therapy, especially with glycopeptides and cephalosporins.[260]

As colonisation with GRE is more common than infection, the need for antibiotic therapy needs to be carefully reviewed. If the patient has an indwelling invasive device in situ, such as a urinary catheter, removal may be sufficient enough in itself to resolve the problem of colonisation/infection. Some individuals may be long-term carriers of GRE, with stool carriage persisting for months or years. These patients can represent a potential source of cross-infection, especially in high risk clinical areas.[260] As GRE has also been isolated from frozen meat and animal carcasses and in the bowels of animals who are administered food supplements containing a glycopeptide called avoparcin, it is highly likely that GRE enters the food chain, leading to colonisation of the bowel in humans and exacerbating the problem of intermittent or long-term carriage.[268,269]

Table 8.4 details the risk factors for colonisation with resistant organisms.

Table 8.5 details the infection control precautions to be taken when caring for patients who are colonised or infected with multi-antibiotic resistant organisms.

Table 8.4 Patient risk factors for colonisation/infection with resistant organisms

Prolonged hospital stay – including time spent in the Intensive Care Unit.
Treatment with multiple antibiotics, especially broad-spectrum agents.
Surgery.
Invasive indwelling devices.
Severity of illness.
Underlying co-morbidities.
Exposure to other colonised/infected patients.

Table 8.5 Infection control precautions for patients colonised/infected with resistant organisms[86,260]

Isolation	Patients who are colonised/infected with resistant organisms, especially those which are multi-antibiotic resistant, should be isolated in a single room where possible to reduce the risk of cross-infection to other patients. Sometimes a risk assessment is required, taking into account the patient's overall medical condition (isolation could compromise the patient's safety), the site of colonisation/infection, the isolation facilities available (general lack of facilities or patients with other infections who also require a side room), the nature/speciality of the ward, and the susceptibility of other patients. If the patient is colonised/infected with GRE and they have diarrhoea, isolation of the patient is particularly important because of the need to reduce environmental contamination. The infection prevention and control team will normally advise when patients can be de-isolated. In cases of infection/colonisation with GRE, stool samples/rectal swabs and wound swabs (if applicable) may be required for clearance according to local policy.
Hand hygiene	Hands should be decontaminated with alcohol hand rub in between each episode of patient contact, or washed with liquid soap and water if they are visibly contaminated with dirt, blood or body fluids.
Personal protective equipment and clothing	Disposable gloves and aprons should be worn for any episode of direct contact with the patient or with equipment within the immediate patient environment. They should be changed in between each episode of patient contact and disposed of as clinical waste according to local policy and national guidance.
Decontamination of equipment	As equipment can harbour micro-organisms, equipment should be designated single-patient use wherever possible to reduce the risk of cross-infection to other patients. If this is not possible, *any* equipment that is shared between patients such as commodes, monitors, sphygmomanometers (dynamaps) for example should be decontaminated before it is used on another patient, either with detergent wipes or cleaned according to the manufacturer's instructions. Stocks of equipment/supplies within the patient's isolation room, such as dressings and boxes of gloves, should be kept to the minimum; anything extraneous which is unused on patient discharge will need to be discarded, as the outer packaging will be contaminated.
Environmental cleanliness	Antibiotic-resistant organisms can survive for hours – days on hard surfaces and ledges, material (bed clothes, curtains) and dust-traps within the ward environment. Thorough cleaning of the patient's bed area and the ward in general is absolutely crucial in preventing the establishment of environmental reservoirs. For GRE, there is no evidence that one cleaning regimen is preferable to another, and the method of cleaning will depend on local policy. To reduce environmental reservoirs of Acinetobacter, chlorine based agents (e.g. sodium dichlorisocyanurate 1000 ppm available chlorine with a compatible anionic agent) are recommended. On patient discharge, the bed frame, mattress and pillows should be decontaminated.

Table 8.5 (Continued)

	Dynamic Airwave Mattresses or either specialist beds/mattresses should be decontaminated according to local policy/manufacturer's instructions. Bedside curtains should be changed when the patient is discharged, and bedside audio-visual equipment decontaminated, along with any other equipment remaining at the bedside.
Restricting patient movement	The transfer of colonised/infected patients with antibiotic-resistant organisms to other wards should be avoided where possible to reduce the risk of spread to other areas, but patient care should not be compromised, particularly if the patient requires specialist care on another ward or has to undergo investigations. The receiving ward/department/hospital should be informed so that they can ensure that the appropriate infection control precautions are put in place.

Extracts in this chapter are reproduced with permission from the British Journal of Infection Control. Vol 2 Issue 1; The Problem of Antimicrobial Resistance (2000)

Part II

9 Meticillin-resistant *Staphylococcus aureus* (MRSA)

INTRODUCTION

No organism has had such an extraordinary media profile in recent years as Meticillin-resistant *Staphylococcus aureus*. Extensive media coverage has increased the profile of MRSA, caused considerable public anxiety and forced the issue of antibiotic-resistant organisms, dirty hospitals and poor compliance with infection control to the top of the political agenda. Yet it is by no means a new problem – it has been in existence for nearly 50 years. It was first reported in 1961, with the first hospital outbreaks of MRSA following in 1963.[270,271] Epidemic strains of MRSA began to emerge throughout the 1960s, causing huge problems in Australia during the 1970s, and then exploding into the healthcare arena during the late1980s/early 1990s, with the emergence of epidemic strains EMRSA15 and −16. An outbreak at Kettering Hospital in Northamptonshire during 1991–1992 affected 400 patients and cost more than £400,000, seeding the spread of MRSA across the country.[26,3] National guidelines on the control of MRSA were first issued in 1986[272] and reviewed again in 1990, 1998 and 2006[273,274,275] but MRSA had become so endemic that many experts were of the opinion that the window of opportunity to control MRSA had passed, and that its presence in UK hospitals should be accepted as inevitable. Screening to detect colonised individuals was viewed as a considerable financial burden to the cash-strapped NHS, diverting attention from other important infection control activities and other organisms; its clinical impact was considered to be less than that of ordinary Meticillin-resistant strains of *Staphylococcus aureus*, and it was considered by many to be an organism of low virulence in the light of little convincing evidence that it caused significant morbidity.[276,277] Indeed, MRSA is just one of a number of potentially problematic organisms, and infection prevention and control teams have long been concerned about other organisms such as *Clostridium difficile* (see Chapter 11) which have greater pathogenic potential. However, it is dangerous to under-estimate the clinical importance of MRSA. The true extent of the MRSA 'problem' is not known, and while it would appear that asymptomatic carriage/colonisation with MRSA is more common than infection, colonised individuals are susceptible to developing an invasive infection if they undergo 'high risk' surgery or clinical interventions, and infection is associated with increased morbidity and mortality. It is also likely that there is a huge reservoir of colonised patients, both in hospital wards and out in the community who, while they may never progress to developing clinical disease themselves, pose a considerable threat to other more vulnerable patients. MRSA now has the distinction of being the most commonly reported antibiotic-resistant pathogen in the world and it is a global healthcare problem and a major cause of both community acquired and hospital acquired infections. Although the prevalence of MRSA varies among countries, the UK has the highest prevalence of MRSA infections in Europe, particularly in relation to bloodstream infections, which have increased from 2 % to more than 40 % in the last 10 years.[3,36]

This chapter looks at the management and control of MRSA. The organism, *Staphylococcus aureus,* and the pathogenesis of infection are discussed, along with the clinical significance of MRSA infection, and the patient risk factors for acquisition. The problems with community acquired strains of *S.aureus,* reported in the UK press during the latter part of 2006, the MRSA bacteraemia mandatory surveillance scheme and the Department of Health's national MRSA target are also explored, along with detection, prevention and control measures such as screening, decolonisation of colonised individuals, isolation and the principles of infection control. Reference is also made to other Department of Health initiatives to drive down MRSA rates.[30]

LEARNING OUTCOMES

After reading this chapter the reader will:

• Understand the clinical significance of Staphylococcal/MRSA infection
• Be able to list the patient risk factors for MRSA infection/colonisation, common body sites for MRSA carriage/colonisation and understand the importance of patient screening
• Understand how to administer topical decolonisation protocol
• Understand the significance of MRSA bloodstream infections
• Be able to describe the infection control precautions that need to be taken in order to reduce the risk of transmission to other patients

STAPHYLOCOCCUS AUREUS AND MRSA

Staphylococci are Gram-positive, catalase-positive, facultative anaerobes, measuring 0.5–1.5 micro-metres in diameter. Cultured on agar or in broth for 12–24 hours at 37 °C, they produce golden-yellow colonies ('golden staph') with a smooth shiny surface and grow in grape-like clusters (*Staphyle* – Greek – 'bunch of grapes'), or in pairs, chains or singly.[278,279,280] Staphylococci are characterised by the ability to clot plasma and the catalase test is carried out to distinguish the organism from Streptococci (See Chapter 4 The Microbiology Laboratory).

Although there are more than 30 species of Staphylococci, only three are considered to be pathogenic in humans:

- *Staphylococcus aureus* (including MRSA) – discussed in detail in this chapter.
- *Staphylococcus epidermidis* – which forms part of the normal skin flora in large numbers and is frequently associated with infections involving invasive indwelling devices such as IV cannualae, urinary catheters and prosthetic implants (see Chapter 7 Types of Healthcare Associated Infection).
- *Staphylococcus saprophyticus* – a common cause of cystitis in women.

STAPHYLOCOCCUS AUREUS

S.aureus causes a wide range of infections, ranging from mild to potentially life-threatening.

Table 9.1 Infections caused by *Staphylococcus aureus*

Localised skin infections – boils, styes, abscesses
Deep-seated infections – osteomylitis, septic arthritis
Acute endocarditis
Septicaemia
Meningitis
Pneumonia
Hospital associated infections – post-operative wounds/invasive devices
Toxin mediated infections – toxic shock syndrome and food poisoning

It is carried by 20–30 % of the population, either as part of the resident skin flora or intermittently, colonising the skin (including skin folds, hairline, perineum and umbilicus), the anterior nares and chronic wounds such as varicose and decubitus ulcers. It can be shed or dispersed in large quantities, particularly from patients with chronic skin conditions such as eczema or psoriasis, and disseminated into the environment, resulting in environmental contamination and potential cross-infection. *S.aureus* is most notorious for being a major cause of healthcare associated infections involving post-operative wounds and invasive indwelling devices, and it has been causing problems in hospitals since 1955. In 1957, a large outbreak of post-operative wound infections among patients, and skin sepsis among both patients and staff, at the Royal Devon and Exeter Hospital led to the appointment of the first infection control sister in the UK.[1]

PATHOGENESIS OF S.AUREUS INFECTION

S.Aureus possesses many virulence factors.[278,279,280] Surface proteins facilitate colonisation of the host tissues and invasions (leukocidin, kinases and hyaluronidase) assist the spread of the organism through the tissue. The bacterial capsule, together with a surface protein called protein A, protects the bacteria against phagocytosis, along with other components which assist it in evading host immune defences (see Chapter 5 Understanding the Immune System and the Nature and Pathogenesis of Infection). It also produces potent toxins, commonly referred to as super-antigens, which are potent activators of the immune system and trigger an immune response by the host that is actually responsible for many of the signs and symptoms of *S.aureus* infections. Enteroxins A, B, C, E and G are produced by approximately half of all *S.aureus* isolates[278] and are the principle cause of vomiting and diarrhoea in cases of staphylococcal food poisoning. If contaminated food is ingested, the enterotoxins bind to receptors in the upper gastro-intestinal tract, stimulating the vomiting centre in the brain and inducing nausea, vomiting and diarrhoea within six hours of eating. Toxic shock syndrome toxin (TSST-1) causes toxic shock manifesting as a high fever; a widespread rash resembling sunburn which leads to skin desquamation, vomiting and diarrhoea; hypotension; and multi-organ failure. It has been particularly associated with tampon use, and is believed to have accounted for at least 22 deaths in the UK between 1990–2000.[281] Epidermolytic toxins (A and B) cause blistering skin diseases, the most dramatic of which is scalded skin syndrome, sometimes seen in small children where parts of the skin blister and slough away.[280]

METICILLIN-RESISTANT *STAPHYLOCOCCUS AUREUS* (MRSA)

Although *S.aureus* is inherently sensitive to many antibiotics, approximately 90 % of the strains seen in hospital are resistant. Meticillin-resistant *Staphylococcus aureus* is a strain of the organism that is resistant to many of the antibiotics that are used to treat infections. *S.aureus* developed resistance to penicillin soon after penicillin was introduced into clinical practice, producing an enzyme called penicillinase which rendered the antibiotic ineffective. The development of antibiotic resistance and the mechanisms by which bacteria develop resistance are examined in Chapter 8 The Problem of Antimicrobial Resistance. Antibiotics that were stable against penicillinase were developed during the 1950s and 1960s. The first of these was Meticillin, a semi-synthetic derivative of penicillin which was introduced in 1959, but the first reported cases of Meticillin resistance were made in 1961, followed in 1963 by the first hospital outbreak and an increase in Meticillin-resistant *S.aureus* across England.[270,282] Although Meticillin is no longer used to treat infections, it is used in the laboratory to test *S.aureus* for susceptibility to flucloxacillin. Resistant strains of *S.aureus* are still referred to as Meticillin-resistant, which means the same as flucloxacillin-resistant. Ordinary strains of *S.aureus* that are not Meticillin-resistant are referred to as MSSA (Meticillin-sensitive *Staphylococcus aureus*).

There are now 17 strains of MRSA[283], some of which have more epidemic potential than others, distinguishable by molecular typing and antibiotic sensitivity. Strains 1, 3, 15 and 16 have historically caused the most problems in the UK.

THE CLINICAL IMPORTANCE OF MRSA INFECTION AND RISK FACTORS ASSOCIATED WITH MRSA COLONISATION/INFECTION

Although MRSA is no more virulent than MSSA, the fact that the organism is antibiotic-resistant can mean that treatment for an MRSA infection is more difficult and more prolonged, and the number of MRSA strains in existence means that it has more epidemic potential. As well as the effects on the patient – distress, fear and anxiety, the psychological effects of isolation, delayed discharge, potential loss of earnings, the risk of additional surgery if the patient acquires an infection (limb amputation, wound debridement or removal of a prosthetic orthopaedic implant), and additional antibiotic therapy – the financial burden on the health service is considerable. Delayed discharges equate to lost bed days for the Trust and loss of revenue, along with money spent on litigation, empirical antibiotic therapy, extra equipment, protective clothing and hotel services. Public confidence in the Trust is also dented as a result of adverse publicity, and under the new payments by results tariff[28], patients may choose to receive their treatment elsewhere if a hospital is perceived to have problems with MRSA or indeed any other healthcare associated infection. With healthcare associated infections estimated to cost the health service in excess of £1 billion per annum, and the cost of treating a single healthcare associated infection estimated to be between £4,000 –£10,000, MRSA cannot be ignored.[29]

MRSA colonisation can predispose patients to developing invasive disease, particularly if the patient is in a high-risk patient group. As colonisation is generally asymptomatic, particularly if just the anterior nares and/or skin folds are colonised, patients are often upset when they are told that they have MRSA, often equating MRSA carriage/colonisation with infection. It is important that healthcare workers are able to make the distinction clear between carriage/colonisation and infection. Carriage/colonisation refers to the presence of MRSA at or on a body site in the absence of any symptoms. People can be carriers of MRSA intermittently or for prolonged periods of time but without any adverse effects to themselves. If an infection is present the patient will display systemic signs which can include a raised temperature, pain or discomfort at the affected site, an inflamed oozing wound which may have broken down or be slow to heal post-operatively, or tenderness and inflammation at the insertion site of an invasive indwelling device. Not all infections are severe, and not all patients require treatment with antibiotics.

COMMUNITY ACQUIRED MRSA

Although the acquisition of MRSA has always been linked to hospitals, and it is commonly unhelpfully referred to in the media as the 'hospital superbug', there has been an increase in recent years in the number of people acquiring serious life-threatening MRSA and MSSA infections who have no prior history of exposure to the healthcare setting.[284] Resistant and sensitive strains of *S.aureus* have started to emerge worldwide that produce a toxin called Panton-Valentine Leukocidin (PVL) which destroys white bloodcells, and community strains of MRSA have been found to be more likely to produce PVL than the strains which are commonly found in hospitals.[285] PVL producing strains can cause severe invasive infections, the most lethal of which is necrotising pneumonia, which presents as a rapidly progressive, haemorrhagic, necrotising, community-acquired pneumonia in previously young, fit and healthy individuals, and is rapidly fatal.[286,287,288,289] Patients with invasive PVL infections require aggressive management in an intensive care unit and combination antibiotic therapy.

There is always a risk that PVL-MSSA/MRSA could become endemic within hospitals, and in April 2006 the Health Protection Agency (HPA) produced interim guidance on diagnosis and management of PVL-associated Staphylococcal infections in the UK.[285]

SURVEILLANCE OF MRSA BLOODSTREAM INFECTIONS AND THE NATIONAL TARGET TO REDUCE BACTERAEMIA RATES

Attributable mortality due to MRSA may be difficult to ascertain, but there is evidence to suggest that MRSA bacteraemia carries twice the attributable mortality of MSSA bacteraemia[290], and colonisation with MRSA is a recognised risk factor for the development of an MRSA bloodstream infection. In April 2001, the Department of Health introduced mandatory surveillance and reporting of MRSA bacteraemias. Under this scheme, hospitals are categorised as specialist, acute or single speciality Trusts, and the bacteraemia rate for each Trust is expressed as the number of bloodstream infections per 1,000 bed days, based on bed occupancy data provided by each NHS Trust to the Department of Health. During the first three years of the scheme, the results were published annually as league tables, with each Trust awarded a national ranking according to their Trust category, bacteraemia rate per 1,000 bed days and the number of positive blood cultures reported. Since 2005, they have been published six-monthly. This data is available from the Health Protection Agency website.[291] This information can easily be misinterpreted by the general public, and is sometimes misrepresented by the media, which reports on MRSA rates rather than differentiating between MRSA in general and bloodstream infections. Bacteraemias reported under this scheme are not necessarily acquired within the Trust that reports them, as MRSA can be imported from one Trust to another with the transfer of colonised patients. Patients may have a blood culture taken on attending the A&E Department which, if positive, indicates that they were bacteraemic on admission; they may have no previous history of healthcare exposure or may have received care previously in another Trust, but under the surveillance programme the Trust that takes the blood culture records and reports the bacteraemia. This is why bacteraemia rates can be higher in some Trusts than others. The specialist nature of the Trust can also affect bacteraemia rates, as the more vulnerable the patient group along with the specialist interventions and procedures being undertaken, the greater the risk to the patient of acquiring an infection.

Results from the fourth year of the surveillance scheme (2004–2005) showed a slight downward trend but this was not a convincing enough picture. In November 2004 the then Health Secretary, John Reid, announced that the Department of Health was setting each acute NHS Trust in England the target of reducing its MRSA bacteraemia rate by 60% based on its 2004 baseline, to be achieved by March 2008.[31] Each Trust has been given a trajectory which sets out the number of MRSA bacteraemias 'allowed' each year, demonstrating a year-on-year reduction in order to reach the target. This target has, perhaps more than any other Department of Health report or initiative, pushed infection control right to the top of every Trust's agenda, requiring engagement from senior managers and the appointment of nominated infection control leads among nursing and medical staff in every service area/clinical directorate. Some will find achieving their 60% reduction relatively easy, particularly if they are starting from a high baseline. Trusts already starting from a low baseline will find it more of a challenge.

In order to achieve this reduction Trusts are having to look at a number of issues such as the screening of high-risk patients, isolation of colonised patients (often compounded by a lack of isolation facilities and infections caused by other organisms which place an added demand on isolation facilities), hand hygiene programmes, the decontamination of equipment, environmental cleanliness, and the use and management of invasive indwelling devices. Healthcare workers are personally accountable for their own practice and in order to provide the best care for patients and prevent healthcare associated infections such as MRSA, they must adhere to infection prevention and control policies and guidelines. Undertaking a root cause analysis[32] each time a bacteraemia is confirmed will assist in identifying where poor practice, such as failure to screen patients in accordance with local policy or manage invasive devices appropriately, may have contributed to the infection. These areas of poor practice can then be addressed and managed through the development of a ward/directorate-based action plan to improve compliance and manage risk, reducing the risk of a bloodstream infection occurring in another patient.

In 2004, the Department of Health published *Towards cleaner hospitals and lower rates of infection: A summary of action.*[19] This document emphasised the importance of controlling healthcare associated infections through actions such as the implementation of the *Matrons' Charter*[141], which includes recommendations on how to ensure that high standards of hospital cleanliness are achieved and maintained, the importance of patient involvement, the implementation of the national *cleanyourhands* campaign (see Chapter 6 The Principles of Infection Prevention and Control), and independent inspection and audit by the Healthcare Commission.

In June 2005, *Saving lives: a delivery programme to reduce healthcare associated infection including MRSA*[30], was published by the Department of Health, providing a framework which would assist Trusts in meeting the MRSA bacteraemia target. The programme consists of a number of initiatives. Trusts are required to complete a balanced score card, which illustrates the Trust's overall infection control activities according to nine key challenge areas. Completion of the score card highlights where improvements need to be made and compliance heightened, with red boxes within the score card highlighting high priority areas, amber indicating areas that require review and green showing the areas in which the Trust is compliant. Based on these results, each Trust completes a self-assessment and action planning tool, against which compliance can be measured. The programme also consists of a series of high impact interventions, which are simple evidence-based audit tools that reinforce the actions that should be taken by staff in order to significantly reduce the risk of the patient acquiring a healthcare associated infection each time a key procedure is performed.

CONTROL OF MRSA

The latest national evidence-based guidelines[275] provide detailed advice on all aspects of the management and control of MRSA including screening, decolonisation, antibiotic usage, isolation, patient management, cleaning and decontamination and surveillance, and many infection prevention and control teams have based their local MRSA policy on this guidance.

Screening

The purpose of screening for MRSA is to detect those individuals with asymptomatic MRSA carriage/colonisation, as they represent the most important reservoir of MRSA in healthcare facilities.[292] Some countries, most notably The Netherlands and Denmark, adopted rigorous 'search and destroy' policies during 1980 and the prevalence of Meticillin-resistant isolates amongst *S.aureus* is low.[293] 'Search and destroy' policies centre on early identification, detection and containment of MRSA and are labour-intensive and resource-dependent. Historically, screening programmes within the UK have been variable, although the recommendation has been that screening should be targeted at those patients who are considered to be at high risk of MRSA carriage or colonisation (see Table 9.3), and as identified within the national guidelines. While the universal screening of all patients admitted to hospital has often been debated, and would perhaps appear to be the most logical step towards reducing the risk of MRSA colonisation/infection, it is labour-intensive for staff, extremely costly and would require far greater resources than those which are currently available. These include laboratory support and the national availability and implementation of the PCR rapid test, currently only licensed for the detection of MRSA in nasal swabs.[294]

In November 2006, further guidance on screening was issued by the Department of Health[294] to assist acute NHS Trusts to further reduce the risk of MRSA colonisation and the incidence of MRSA bacteraemias. Categories of high-risk patients who should be screened for MRSA on admission, and in whom decolonisation should be considered are recommended as follows.[294]

- Pre-operative patients in certain surgical specialities where the clinical impact of MRSA infection can have serious consequences. This category includes those patients undergoing elective orthopaedic surgery, cardiothoracic surgery and neurosurgery. It is recommended that decolonisation of these patients is undertaken prior to surgery as although they themselves may be categorised as low risk, the nature of their operative procedure means that an MRSA infection could have devastating consequences.
- Emergency orthopaedic and trauma patients. This encompasses many elderly patients from residential and nursing home environments where there are often undiagnosed cohorts of MRSA colonised patients. Elderly patients often have multiple hospital admissions or healthcare contact, and as such are at an increased risk of being colonised with MRSA.
- Patients in critical/intensive care units, who have undergone major surgery/high risk procedures and who have multiple indwelling invasive devices in situ, are at an increased risk of acquiring MRSA and developing a significant infection, including bloodstream infections.
- Patients from renal units who undergo dialysis are at risk of developing MRSA bloodstream infections.
- Patients admitted from other high risk settings, such as those transferred from other hospitals or admitted from nursing/residential homes, should also be screened.
- Consideration should be given to screening all emergency admissions[295], all patients previously known to be MRSA-positive, all elective surgical patients and oncology patients, particularly those undergoing chemotherapy and who will therefore be immunosupressed.

The majority of patients who are admission screened will only have swabs taken from the nose and groin/perineum, although some Trusts may also include throat swabs in their screening programme. The national guidelines[275] also recommend the regular screening of known MRSA-positive inpatients at a frequency to be determined by local policy, and these patients too may require screening of multiple body sites. Table 9.2 summarises the risk factors for MRSA colonisation and Table 9.3 summarises the body sites that should be screened.

Table 9.2 Risk factors for MRSA colonisation/infection

Previous healthcare contact, particularly overnight stay/multiple hospital admissions/transfer from another healthcare facility, including recent stay in a hospital abroad and residence in a nursing or residential home.
MRSA colonisation.
Surgery – particularly surgery involving the insertion of prosthetic implants such as hip prosthesis.
The presence of invasive indwelling devices – peripheral/central venous cannulae and other lines, urinary catheters, wound drains.
The elderly – immune system less able to fight off infections.
Individuals who are immunocompromised or who have associated co-morbidities.

Table 9.3 Body sites to be screened for MRSA[275]

Anterior nares
Groin/perineum
Skin lesions/skin breaks
Wounds
Sites of indwelling invasive devices such as lines and drains
Sputum if expectorating
Tracheostomy sites
PEG sites
Urine if catheterised
Umbilicus in neonates

Staff screening

The routine screening of healthcare staff for MRSA carriage is no longer undertaken routinely, and is only required if there is evidence of cross-infection occurring to patients. It is recognised that staff can acquire MRSA transiently during the course of their duties (i.e. transient nasal carriage) but this is generally lost very quickly, and nasal carriage among staff carries little risk in terms of transmission to patients. However, staff with skin lesions may be colonised with MRSA, and any skin breaks should be included in the screen. The implementation of staff screening needs to be carefully planned, with staff screened at the beginning of a shift and not halfway through or at the end, in order to minimise the possibility of detecting transient carriage, and may be undertaken in conjunction with both the occupational health department and the infection prevention and control team. The number of screens required for clearance and the amount of time required off work is again dependent upon local policy.

TREATMENT OF MRSA COLONISATION/INFECTION

Topical agents such as an antibiotic nasal cream (e.g. Bactroban or Naseptin) and disinfectant body wash (e.g. Aquasept) are recommended to eradicate or reduce nasal and/or skin carriage. While there is no evidence to suggest that it is always possible to completely eradicate MRSA, and patients can recolonise either with the same strain or through acquisition of a new one, the use of these topical agents can decrease MRSA carriage in the short term, reducing the risk of transmission to other patients within the healthcare environment, as well as reducing the risk to the patient of developing an infection. How effective the decolonisation regimen is depends in part on the presence of 'foreign bodies' such as clips or sutures and invasive indwelling devices, and wounds or skin lesions.[275] Table 9.4 describes how topical decolonisation agents should be applied.

Table 9.4 Topical decolonisation protocol[275]

Nasal decolonisation

Mupirocin (Bactroban) nasal cream in a 2 % paraffin base – applied to the inner nostrils (anterior nares) three times a day for five days (repeated courses are not recommended because of the risk of mupirocin resistance developing). The patient should be able to taste the mupirocin cream at the back of the throat. If possible, encourage the patient to pinch the nostrils together and then sniff once the cream has been applied. If the patient has a naso-gastric tube in situ, the efficacy of the mupirocin may be affected but it should still be administered.

Skin decolonisation

Either 4 % Chlorhexidine gluconate aqueous solution or 2 % Triclosan are prescribed as a body wash for eradicating or reducing skin colonisation. The patient should wash or bathe (or be bed-bathed) daily for five days, applying the body wash neat to the skin, like a liquid soap; it should not poured into a bowl of water or into a bath. All areas of the skin should be treated and attention paid to common skin carriage sites such as skin folds, the groin/perineum and axilla. Hair should be washed on the first day of treatment to reduce staphylococcal carriage. If the patient has a skin condition, the underlying skin condition should be treated where possible, and dermatology advice may be required. Oilatum or Oilatum plus may be prescribed (Oilatum plus contains Triclosan 2 %).

Patients with an infection will be treated with the appropriate antibiotic, depending upon the antibiotic susceptibilities of the MRSA strain involved. Deep-seated or severe infections are treated with vancomycin, which has long been the antibiotic of choice.[270] The dose is adjusted in the elderly and/or those patients with renal impairment. Too much vancomycin can be potentially toxic, and too little can be sub-therapeutic, so serum blood levels are recorded pre dose and one–two hours post dose every three days, and the dose decreased or increased as required. There are increasing concerns about bacterial resistance to vancomycin among entero-cocci and staphylococci, with resistance to vancomycin recorded in both sensitive and resistant strains of *S.aureus*, which obviously has implications not only for the treatment of MRSA, but also other infections.[296,297] Teicoplanin is also effective against severe Gram-positive infections, penetrating tissues including skin, fat and bone. Teicoplanin blood assays are only performed where there is severe deep-seated infection and/or renal impairment. Linezolid is a newer antibiotic which is increasingly being prescribed for the treatment of severe infections. The exact modes of actions of these antibiotics, and the problem with vancomycin-resistance, are discussed in Chapter 8 The Problem of Antimicrobial Resistance.

INFECTION CONTROL PRECAUTIONS

The basic principles of infection control should be applied to minimise the transmission of MRSA to other patients, including minimising environmental contamination, and these are summarised in Table 9.5.

Table 9.5 Infection control precautions to be taken when caring for MRSA colonised/infected patients[86,275]

Isolation	Wherever possible, patients colonised/infected with MRSA should be nursed in a single room with the door kept closed. Sometimes a risk assessment is required, taking into account the patient's overall medical condition (isolation could compromise the patient's safety), the site of the MRSA colonisation/infection, the isolation facilities available (general lack of facilities, or competing organisms that are more high-risk in terms of spread than MRSA, such as tuberculosis or *C.difficile*), the nature/speciality of the ward, and the susceptibility of other patients on the ward. Where it is not possible to care for patients in single rooms, they should be cohort-nursed along with other MRSA-positive patients, either in a separate bay or another defined area within the ward. Care should be taken to ensure that the patient's recovery/rehabilitation is not affected if the patient is nursed in a single room, and physiotherapy and occupational therapy-based interventions should continue. The infection prevention and control team will generally advise when patients can be 'de-isolated', again according to local policy. In some areas, particularly those which are designated high risk, this may be after the patient has received three consecutive sets of negative swabs.
Visitors	Patients with MRSA can receive visitors. No special precautions are required – visitors do not need to wear protective clothing for example – but they should be asked to decontaminate their hands with alcohol hand rub on leaving the isolation room/ward. The patient and their relatives should be provided with written information on MRSA in the form of a patient information leaflet and be given the opportunity to speak with a member of the infection prevention and control team if they have any anxieties.
Administration of MRSA decolonisation protocol and follow-up screening	Topical decolonisation protocol should be administered as prescribed according to local policy in order to reduce carriage. Patients should be screened for clearance at intervals determined according to local policy.
The management of invasive indwelling devices and wounds	Intravascular cannulae (peripheral and central), other lines, urinary catheters and drains present a risk factor for the development of MRSA infection, and should be removed as soon as possible. Insertion sites should be examined at least daily for signs of infection and managed according to local policy. Wounds should be covered until healed to prevent inoculation of the wound with MRSA.
Hand hygiene	All staff should ensure that they decontaminate their hands with alcohol hand rub on entering and leaving isolation rooms/cohort bays, and in between each episode of patient contact, particularly when handling indwelling invasive devices. If visibly soiled with dirt and/or body fluids (and if the patient is co-infected with *Clostridium difficile*) hands should be washed with liquid soap and water. Visitors should also be asked to decontaminate their hands.

Personal protective equipment and clothing	Disposable aprons and gloves should be worn if there is any episode of direct contact with the patient or with equipment within the immediate patient environment. They should be removed and disposed of as clinical waste immediately after each activity. Masks are generally not required but the national guidelines recommend that they are worn in the event of procedures being undertaken which may generate staphylococcal aerosols (e.g. sputum induction).
Linen	All linen should be treated as contaminated/infected and disposed of in red linen bags and according to local policy/national guidance.
Waste	Clinical waste should be disposed of according to local policy and national guidance.
Decontamination of equipment	Equipment can harbour bacteria, potentially increasing the risk of the spread of infection. Where possible, patients with MRSA should be allocated equipment that is single-patient use and disposable, or equipment that can remain with the patient during their time in hospital and either be disposed of or decontaminated appropriately when the patient has been discharged home. Any equipment which is multi-patient use, such as wheelchairs, commodes, monitors, sphygmomanometers etc must be decontaminated in between each patient use, either using detergent wipes or cleaned according to the manufacturer's instructions.
Environmental cleanliness	MRSA can survive for long periods in the environment, particularly in dust, and the patient environment should be kept clean and free from dust and dirt, reducing environmental reservoirs of MRSA contamination and decreasing the risk of the spread of MRSA to others. This is particularly important if the patient is cared for in the open ward. When the patient is de-isolated, discharged or if the patient is transferred to another ward, the immediate bed area must be thoroughly cleaned according to local policy, bedside curtains changed and equipment decontaminated. This should include the cleaning of bedside audio-visual equipment.
Restricting patient movement	The transfer of colonised patients to other wards should be avoided where possible to minimise the risk of spread, but patient care should not be compromised, particularly if the patient requires specialist care on another ward or has to undergo investigations. The receiving ward/department/hospital should be informed of the patient's MRSA status so that they can ensure that they take the appropriate precautions.
Patients who require surgery	Patients who require surgery and who are colonised/infected with MRSA may be placed last on the theatre list, although this may not always be possible or appropriate. Antibiotic prophylaxis may not be indicated but if so, it should be administered as prescribed. Extraneous equipment within the operating theatre should be removed, and all surfaces and equipment within the theatre decontaminated before the next patient is operated upon.

Table 9.5 (Continued)

	Most Trusts, as well as having a general policy for the management and control of MRSA, will also have a local theatre policy in relation to infection control.
Discharge arrangements	Patients can be discharged when they are medically fit, regardless of whether or not they are still MRSA-positive. The patients general practitioner should be notified of the patient's MRSA status. Follow-up screens for MRSA carriage are rarely required but there may be individual circumstances where this is clinically indicated. If travelling by hospital transport, such as ambulance or authorised car, no special precautions are required but any open lesions/wounds should be covered, and high-risk susceptible patients should not be transported in the same ambulance as a known MRSA-positive patient. Ambulance staff should decontaminate their hands with alcohol hand rub after patient contact. No special cleaning of the vehicle is required, but any spillages of blood or body fluids should be attended to according to local policy. No special precautions are required once the patient is at home beyond 'normal' hygiene measures.
Last offices	No special precautions are required for deceased patients beyond those which are undertaken routinely when caring for MRSA colonised/infected patients in life. Skin lesions/wounds should be covered with an impermeable occlusive dressing. The use of body bags is not required unless blood and body fluids are leaking from wounds/orifices. Relatives are able to view and touch the body.

More information on the management and control of MRSA for healthcare workers, patients and members of public is available from the Royal College of Nursing and the Department of Health.[298,299]

10 Tuberculosis

INTRODUCTION

In 1993, the World Health Organization (WHO) declared tuberculosis (TB) a global emergency.[300,301] This age-old disease, which has been identified in the skeletal remains of prehistoric humans and the spines of Egyptian mummies,[302] has historically had many names – 'consumption', 'white plague', 'phthisis' and 'scrofula' to name but a few – and it is now the second most common infectious cause of death in the world after HIV/AIDS. It can affect virtually any area of the body, although pulmonary tuberculosis is the most clinically important disease. According to WHO[301], one third of the world's population (approximately two billion people) is currently infected, with someone in the world newly infected with tuberculosis every second; left untreated, each person with active disease will go on to infect on average 10–15 people a year. Although TB is a curable disease and it can be controlled, around two million people die from it every year (5,000 people every day), particularly in countries within sub-Saharan Africa, where there are 1.6 million new cases and 6,000 deaths a year. Although the epidemiology of tuberculosis has changed over the years, more than 8,000 people in England, Wales and Northern Ireland were diagnosed with TB in 2006[303] and 350 people in England die from it each year.[304] Inner cities have a significant TB problem, particularly London, which has a highly mobile population, the highest proportion of HIV-related cases, and the highest rates of drug-resistant strains. The emergence of drug resistance in the 1990s continues to pose a threat to the worldwide control of TB[305] by limiting treatment options and shortening life expectancy. Outbreaks of sensitive and drug-resistant strains have occurred in hospitals and prisons throughout the world, principally affecting patients with HIV but posing a threat to any individual who is exposed.

Prompt recognition of symptoms, confirmation of cases and the appropriate infection control precautions to minimise spread are key to preventing and controlling tuberculosis, and this chapter focuses on the prevention and control of tuberculosis in the UK, with reference to the 'national guidelines'.[306] These were written by the National Collaborating Centre for Chronic Conditions and published in 2006; they were funded by the National Institute for Clinical Excellence (NICE) and are referred to here as the 'NICE guidelines'. This chapter examines the organism, *Mycobacterium tuberculosis*, with particular emphasis on the pathogenesis, diagnosis and treatment of infectious pulmonary tuberculosis. Infection with environmental opportunistic mycobacteria and extra-pulmonary tuberculosis is discussed briefly, and specific problems associated with multi-drug resistant disease and the link between TB and HIV are examined in detail.

LEARNING OUTCOMES

After reading this chapter, the reader will:

- Be able to describe the process of infection with pulmonary tuberculosis
- Understand the difference between, and the clinical significance of, infection with *M.tuberculosis* and environmental opportunistic mycobacteria
- Be able to describe the risk factors for multi-drug resistant TB
- Understand the drug treatments

THE ORGANISM

There are more than 80 species of mycobacteria[307], and those which are human pathogens belong to a group of organisms known as the *Mycobacterium tuberculosis* Complex (MTC), consisting of *M. tuberculosis, M.bovis, M. africanis* and *M.microti*.[308] *M.tuberculosis* is the principle cause of infectious tuberculosis in humans, with pulmonary disease the most clinically significant illness. Mycobacteria are slender Gram-positive rods (bacilli). They are obligate aerobes, with no capsule. They are motile and non-spore forming and compared to most other bacterial pathogens which divide every hour, mycobacteria are slow growers, dividing once every 16–24 hours and forming visible colonies on solid agar at three–six weeks.[309,310] The bacterial cell wall consists of 60 % lipids, and this high lipid content means that the organism cannot be identified by the traditional method of Gram-staining; the ZN stain technique used to identify the waxy bacterial cell wall is described in Chapter 4 The Microbiology Laboratory.

Some species of mycobacteria are environmental opportunists (see Table 10.1) isolated from water, soil, dust, milk, animals and birds.[307] Although they are of low virulence and low grade pathogenicity, they can cause a wide range of opportunistic infections in immunocompromised individuals, particularly those with HIV infection or pre-existing chronic pulmonary disease. Human to human transmission is very rare, and even if an environmental mycobacteria is isolated from the sputum, the normal notification and contact tracing procedures that would be initiated in the event of infection with *M.tuberculosis* do not apply. Environmental mycobacteria such as *M.chelonae* have been isolated from bronchoscopes, where the water supply feeding into the endoscopy washer-disinfector has contaminated the rinse water, and also isolated from clinical specimens such as bronchial washings.[150,151]

Mycobacterium kansasii is the most common opportunistic mycobacterial pathogen isolated in England and Wales, and along with *M. exenopi*, and

Table 10.1 Environmental opportunistic mycobacteria

M.aviaum complex
M.exenopi
M.chelonae
M.kansasii
M.fortuitum
M.malmonense
M.scrofulaceum
M.marinum
M.ulcerans
M.abscessus

M.avium complex (MAC), often causes lung disease which clinically is very similar to pulmonary disease caused by *M.tuberculosis*.[311] These organisms cause pulmonary disease, lymphadenitis, and disseminated disease, as well as infections at other body sites involving soft tissues, bones and joints and the genitourinary tract. The detection of environmental mycobacteria is not always clinically significant, and only those who are immunocompromised through HIV infection or with underlying pulmonary disorders require treatment for opportunistic mycobacterial infections.

EXTRA-PULMONARY TUBERCULOSIS

Tuberculosis can affect almost any area of the body, commonly affecting the central nervous system (TB meningitis), the abdomen, renal/genital tract, bones and joints (including the spine), lymph nodes and the skin. It gives rise to general non-specific symptoms such as fatigue, weight loss, fever and night sweats, together with clinical features specific to the site of infection. Individuals with extra-pulmonary tuberculosis are generally considered to be non-infectious and do not require isolation, but pulmonary involvement must be investigated and excluded. In the case of tuberculosis affecting the lymph nodes or skin where there may be open discharging lesions or cavities which require irrigating, aerosol-generating procedures should be avoided in open ward areas. Treatment of extra-pulmonary tuberculosis includes the standard six-month four-drug regimen with anti-tuberculosis drugs as discussed later in this chapter.

THE PATHOGENESIS OF TUBERCULOSIS INFECTION

The initial site of TB infection is usually the lung, and takes place through the inhalation of TB bacilli, which are expelled in small droplets of moisture from infected individuals through coughing, talking and sneezing. These airborne droplets contain just a few viable bacilli but as they are released into the air, water evaporates from the surface of the droplets and they become much smaller, forming droplet nuclei with a more concentrated bacterial count. Droplet nuclei can float in room air for several hours and it has been estimated that a single cough can generate as many as 3,000 infected droplet nuclei, with inhalation of less than 10 bacilli sufficient to initiate pulmonary infection in a susceptible individual.[309] The inhaled droplet nuclei implant into alveoli in the middle and lower lung fields, areas of the lung that receive the highest air flow[312] where they are attacked and engulfed by non-specific alveolar macrophages (see Chapter 5 Understanding the Immune System and the Nature and Pathogenesis of Infection). While phagocytosis will destroy some of the TB bacilli, others will survive and replicate within the macrophages but without harming the host. Most of the infected macrophages will die, releasing a new generation of bacilli and cell debris and initiating a cycle of infection, bacterial replication and host cell death. Bacilli may be transported within the macrophages through the lymphatic system to the lymph nodes draining the affected site, where they may be disseminated via blood and lymph tissue to other sites such as the liver, spleen, bone, brain and kidneys, giving rise to clinical disease affecting any of these organs[309], known as extra-pulmonary tuberculosis. Secondary foci may develop in the lymph nodes in the hilum of the lung.

THE PATHOGENESIS OF PULMONARY TUBERCULOSIS

In pulmonary TB, a local inflammatory lesion called the Ghon focus develops in the middle or lower lung field. This develops into a granuloma, a feature of chronic infection consisting of infected macrophages, lymphocytes and fibroblasts, which walls off and isolates the site of infection within the lung. As the macrophages within the granuloma are metabolically active they consume oxygen, and the centre of the granuloma becomes necrotic, producing a hostile environment in which the majority of the bacilli will die. Bacterial replication subsequently becomes inhibited, infection is arrested and over time the granuloma may become calcified. The 'infected' individual has no idea that they have TB, and in most people an efficient and effective immune response can contain the infection. In fact, 90–95 % of initial infections do not progress to clinical disease, with the individual in the asymptomatic or dormant (latent) phase. However, not all of the bacilli contained in the alveolar macrophages within the granuloma are destroyed; 'persisters' may survive for months or years, and clinical disease can subsequently develop later in life. The predisposing factors leading from primary infection to active disease are not always evident but are thought to be related to the number of infecting bacilli inhaled, and the efficiency of the host's immune response, which may become compromised by an underlying illness or disease, increasing age, alcoholism, malnutrition or stress.[309]

In individuals who are immunocompromised as a result of HIV infection or following transplant surgery, the interval between infection and the development of

Table 10.2 Clinical features of pulmonary tuberculosis

Non-specific symptoms
Generally unwell – fatigue and lethargy
Anorexia and weight loss
Fever and drenching night sweats
Enlarged lymph glands

Pulmonary symptoms
A chronic cough – which may have been unresponsive to a course of antibiotics – becoming more productive
Shortness of breath.
Chest pain
Haemoptysis

---

active disease is considerably shorter.[307] Active clinical disease occurring after the initial primary infection is known as post primary, or reactivation, TB. Here, the granuloma becomes more necrotic and takes on a tumour-like appearance, called a tuberculoma, which eventually erodes into the bronchi, leading to the formation of pulmonary cavities in the lung. Although the interior of the tuberculoma is not very conducive to the replication of the bacilli, the oxygen-rich environment of the pulmonary cavity supports the growth of the bacilli, which can be found in huge numbers in the cavity walls.[313] From there, the bacilli gain access to the sputum and the patient becomes infectious. The clinical features of pulmonary tuberculosis are presented in Table 10.2.

DIAGNOSING TUBERCULOSIS

MICROSCOPY AND CULTURE

Healthcare workers should assume a high index of suspicion of any patient presenting with the above symptoms, even if another presumptive diagnosis has been made. Tuberculosis is known as one of the 'great imitators'[312] and mis-diagnosis can put other patients at risk and obviously delay the onset of treatment for the patient. As discussed in Chapter 4, the definitive method of confirming TB infection is through the detection of acid-fast bacilli in a clinical specimen, and the laboratory techniques used are described within that chapter. A diagnosis of infectious pulmonary tuberculosis is generally based upon a combination of a positive sputum smear, clinical features and chest x-ray findings. Table 10.3 identifies the different types of clinical specimens that may be obtained depending on the suspected site of infection.

The number of bacilli present in a clinical specimen can vary by the hour so generally the more specimens collected, the higher the chance of detection.

Table 10.3 Types of clinical specimens for the diagnosis of tuberculosis

---

Sputum
Urine
Cerebral-spinal fluid (CSF)
Pleural fluid
Bronchial washings/aspirate
Tissue biopsy – taken at surgery/during investigative procedure/during post mortem
Lymph node biopsy
Pus
Gastric aspirate

A diagnosis of infectious pulmonary tuberculosis is made if 5,000–10,000 acid-fast bacilli are detected in 1 ml of sputum.[308,314] Three sputum specimens should be obtained on three consecutive occasions and at least one of the specimens should be an early morning sample. Ideally, specimens should be obtained prior to the commencement of anti-tuberculosis therapy, but where there is clear clinical evidence of pulmonary disease, a decision may be made to initiate treatment before any specimens have been obtained or the microbiology results are available. Attempts should still be made to obtain a specimen, which can be sent for microscopy and culture within seven days of treatment starting. In situations where it is difficult to obtain a specimen, either because the patient is physically unable to produce a specimen, or if there is no productive cough, sputum production can be produced by the administration of nebulised saline, or by bronchoscopy and lavage. The generation of sputum via nebuliser is an aerosol-generating procedure and should only be carried out with the implementation of the appropriate infection control precautions, which are discussed later on in this chapter. Patients with bacilli detected in the sputum are said to have infectious or 'open' tuberculosis. If no bacilli are detected on sputum smear, this does not exclude pulmonary TB; the patient may still be treated as positive based on the clinical features and also chest x-ray findings, but they are considered to be less infectious.

RADIOLOGY

All patients with a presumptive diagnosis of TB affecting any body site should have a chest x-ray to exclude or confirm co-existing pulmonary disease. Lesions, shadows, calcifications and cavities will be evident on chest x-ray. As lesions and shadows are also indicative of a diagnosis of lung cancer, a more detailed image of the lung fields can be provided by CT/MRI scanning.

PCR

Identification and typing of TB bacilli can be achieved by Polymerase Chain Reaction (PCR), which amplifies the bacterial DNA. This technique is described in Chapter 4 The Microbiology Laboratory.

SKIN TESTING AND INTERFERON-GAMMA TESTING

The Mantoux test is predominantly used as a screening test to detect latent TB, and recent TB infection (shown by conversion of the Mantoux from negative to positive) but it can also be used as an aid to diagnosis in the presence of clinical symptoms. A 0.1 ml solution of tuberculin purified protein derivative (PPD) is injected intradermally into the forearm, and the transverse diameter of the induration that arises at the injection site is read 48–72 hours later. The Department of Health 'Green Book'[52] describes the exact technique required for administering the Mantoux. The test measures the degree of hypersensitivity to tuberculin, *not* immunity to TB, and the results need to be interpreted with care. An induration diameter of 15 mm or more *suggests* TB infection or disease, and the result should be viewed in the light of any clinical features that are suggestive of active disease. A reaction of 6 mm or greater indicates an immune response which *may* be due to TB infection, infection with environmental mycobacteria, or previous BCG vaccination. A skin reaction of 6 mm or less is reported as negative, indicating that the individual has no significant hypersensitivity to tuberculin protein; in this situation BCG vaccination may be given to unvaccinated individuals. The result of the Mantoux may be affected, and the skin reaction suppressed, if the individual being tested has glandular fever, any viral infection, is immunocompromised as a result of other disease or treatment, on corticosteroid therapy, has had a live vaccine (viral) within the previous four weeks, or suffers from **sarcoidosis**.[52]

Two blood-based immunological tests are now commercially available in the UK – QuantiFERON-TB Gold, and TSPOT-TB.[306,315] These detect tuberculosis antigens known as 'early secretion antigen target 6' (ESAT–6) and 'culture filtrate protein 10' (CFP-10), interferon gamma produced by T-cells in specific response to *Mycobacterium tuberculosis*, which are not present in the BCG vaccine and are only found in a few strains of environmental mycobacteria. NICE guidance recommends that individuals with a positive Mantoux test, or those in whom Mantoux testing may be unreliable, should be considered for interferon-gamma testing if it is available.[306]

MULTI-DRUG RESISTANT TUBERCULOSIS (MDR-TB) – THE THREAT, THE EXTENT OF THE PROBLEM AND CONTROL MEASURES

Drug-resistant TB is becoming an increasing problem around the world, posing a major public health threat, for while it is no more virulent than 'ordinary' drug-sensitive disease, infection with a resistant strain prolongs the amount of time that the individual is infectious, compromises the effectiveness of treatment and increases the mortality rate. In addition, complex treatment regimens are required with more toxic, more expensive but less effective drugs, and each case costs in the region of £60,000–£70,000 to treat.[316] Patients may initially be infected with a drug-resistant strain, or an initially drug 'sensitive' strain may become drug-resistant as a result of inadequate treatment and poor patient compliance with therapy.

A resistant organism can be defined as one whose growth is not inhibited by clinically achievable concentrations of an antimicrobial agent.[246] Two types of drug resistance have emerged in TB. Multi-drug resistant tuberculosis (MDR-TB) is defined by WHO as resistance to at least rifampicin (the main killing, or bactericidal, drug) and isoniazid (the 'sterilising' drug).[317,318] WHO estimates that there are at least 4,500,000 cases of MDR-TB worldwide in 109 countries, accounting for 4.3 % of all TB.[319] More than 40,000 of these are in African countries which have the highest prevalence of HIV. The former Soviet Union has a huge prison population, and of the 300,000 prisoners released each year who are infected with TB, 100,000 have a drug-resistant strain.[320]

Rather worryingly, WHO has identified another form of drug-resistant TB known as extensively drug resistant, or XDR-TB. XDR-TB is defined as MDR-TB *plus* resistance to (i) any fluroquinolones and (ii) at least one of three injectable second line drugs – capreomycin, kanomycin and amikacin, and 27 countries have now confirmed that they have cases of XDR-TB.[321,322,323] While XDR-TB is still relatively rare, it poses a big risk to patients who are HIV positive, and there is always the possibility of community or hospital acquired XDR-TB outbreaks.

The driving factor behind the emergence of drug-resistant TB in general has been the inadequate treatment of drug-sensitive strains through poor prescribing practice and poor patient compliance with therapy. Inadequate dosage together with inadequate duration of therapy will, as with any infection, result in an illness which has not been fully treated or eradicated; similarly, if patients do not complete the course of medication exactly as prescribed/recommended, the end result will be a partially and insufficiently treated infection. Patient compliance issues are often due to poor communication on the part of the healthcare worker and lack of understanding on the part of the patient, together with poor supervision of drug therapy.

The treatment of drug-resistant disease continues for at least 18 months, often longer, and involves the use of multiple drugs, including antibiotics such as amikacin and capreomycin. Risk factors for the acquisition of drug-resistant tuberculosis are summarised in Table 10.4.

Table 10.4 Risk factors for MDR-TB

Previous drug treatment for tuberculosis
HIV infected
Contact with a known case of MDR-TB
Failure of clinical response to treatment
Prolonged sputum smear (at four months) or culture positive (at five months) while on
    treatment

INFECTION CONTROL PRECAUTIONS FOR MDR-TB

Patient isolation

There are certain infection control precautions that need to be taken when caring for patients with drug-resistant tuberculosis that differ from those required when dealing with drug-sensitive disease. While patients with suspected or confirmed smear-positive pulmonary tuberculosis must be isolated in a single room, patients with suspected or confirmed drug-resistant pulmonary tuberculosis require isolation in negative pressure isolation facilities which conform to the standards described by the Interdepartmental Working Group on Tuberculosis.[324] This is because air currents can transport bacteria and viruses within buildings and rooms, increasing the risk of infection to other patients and staff, and ventilation in buildings, whether natural or mechanically induced, dilutes airborne droplet nuclei by removing contaminated air from within the room and replacing it with 'clean' air. An ordinary standard ventilated hospital single room will usually have six air changes an hour. The air changes within the room by passing under the door, or whenever the door or a window in the room is opened, mixing with the air in the corridor or within the ward area. With multi-drug resistant tuberculosis, it is important to prevent air contaminated with infectious bacilli from mixing with 'clean' air, and so the ventilation system must expel the air *away* from other areas, venting it to the outside so that it is not sucked back into the building. Where there is no existing negative pressure ventilation system, a suitable single room can be adapted to negative pressure through the installation of a Vent-Axia exhaust fan, which will discharge air from the room to the outside. Ideally, negative pressure rooms should be purpose built, with air pressure that is automatically controlled and monitored so that if the system fails, an alarm sounds, alerting the staff when the pressure falls. In order to maintain the negative pressure within the room, there should be no gaps underneath or around the doors through which air can enter into and escape from the room, and it should not be possible to open the windows. Negative pressure rooms should have an en-suite toilet and bathroom, and also be equipped with a telephone and a television – some patients may require isolation for many months, either until they are no longer considered to be infectious, or until they have had three consecutive negative sputum cultures.[306]

Respiratory protection

The NICE guidance does not recommend the routine use of respiratory protection by healthcare workers when caring for patients with tuberculosis except in the event of suspected or confirmed drug-resistant disease.[306] This recommendation has been the subject of recent debate and there have been requests for NICE to revisit and clarify this advice further.[325,326]

For MDR-TB, disposable FFP3 respirators which conform to European Standard EN149:2001 should be worn during patient contact. While conventional surgical face masks provide a generally adequate level of protection, helping to prevent droplets being expelled into the environment by the person wearing them and also protecting the wearer against splashes of blood or body fluids, they are not designed to effectively filter air as it is breathed in.

EN149 is the European respiratory protection standard for disposable filtering respirators which filter particulates including bacteria and viruses, worn as face masks and covering the nose, mouth and chin. The FFP3 respirator provides 99 % particle filtration efficiency, and affords the highest level of protection under the EN standard for disposable respirators. So that the FFP3 respirator can provide the optimum filtration efficiency and protection against airborne particles, it is absolutely essential that the respirator fits the face snugly, and healthcare workers will have to be fit-tested to ensure that there is a tight seal and that no air can enter from the sides. Facial hair such as beards and moustaches, and also stubble, can prevent a tight seal against the skin and so the skin should be clean-shaven. Each time a new respirator is worn, the fit will need to be checked. Although the respirators can be worn for eight hours at a time, they must not be re-used and must be disposed of as clinical waste.

Public health legislation

If a patient with infectious pulmonary tuberculosis, particularly one with MDR-TB, refuses to comply with treatment, that individual may pose a risk to public health. For health protection purposes, the consultant in communicable disease control (CCDC) at the local health protection unit (HPU) may consider it necessary to seek a magistrate's order for admission to hospital and detention under sections 37 and 38 of the Public Health (Control of Disease) Act 1984. Compulsory treatment of the patient, however, is not allowed.

TB AND HIV

The HIV epidemic has been a major contributing factor in the dramatic resurgence of tuberculosis, which is one of the leading causes of death in those living with HIV (see Chapter 16 Blood-borne Viruses). HIV positive individuals are 50 times more likely to develop tuberculosis in a given year than those who are HIV negative[327] and approximately 90 % die within months of contacting tuberculosis, as the suppression of the immune system with HIV rapidly accelerates the progression of tuberculosis from latent infection to active disease. Tuberculosis is harder to diagnose in someone who is HIV positive as it can present in a non-specific, or atypical way, leading to mis-diagnosis and a delay in treatment with rapidly fatal consequences. Extra-pulmonary disease and disseminated tuberculosis are more commonly seen in HIV positive patients compared to other patient groups, and may co-exist alongside other opportunistic infections. TB can be acquired through healthcare contact[243,244] and hospital outbreaks of TB have occurred where as many as 40 % of HIV positive patients have developed active TB within two months of exposure to the index case[328], and in the 1990s two separate outbreaks of MDR-TB occurred in HIV units in two London teaching hospitals. One of the outbreaks, which occurred at St Thomas' Hospital, resulted in the death of seven HIV positive patients from MDR-TB.[329] HIV and tuberculosis patients should not be cared for together in the same ward environment.[306,324] Where patients may be infected with HIV or immunocompromised due to other illness, patients with suspected pulmonary disease should be viewed as potentially infectious and isolated until the diagnosis is excluded.

THE TREATMENT OF TUBERCULOSIS

Prior to the discovery of the antibiotic streptomycin during the 1940s which became the mainstay of treatment of TB, patients were cared for in TB sanatoria which were often located in remote areas in the countryside. Fresh air, in all weathers, and bed rest were considered to be the 'cure' for tuberculosis but where that failed, the diseased lung, or part of the lung, was often removed.[330] The effectiveness of streptomycin against tuberculosis brought new hope, but the emergence of drug resistance has meant that it can only be used in combination with other antimicrobial agents, and for the last 15 years, the evidence-based gold standard for the treatment of tuberculosis, both pulmonary and extra-pulmonary disease, has been a six-month four-drug regimen with isoniazid, rifampicin, pyrazinamide and either streptomycin or ethambutol.[306] The treatment of drug-sensitive tuberculosis is given in two phases; the initial phase, lasting two months, involves the use of isoniazid and rifampicin, supplemented by pyrazinamide and either ethambutol or streptomycin, followed by a continuation phase with rifampicin and isoniazid for a further four months. These drugs have three modes of action; they prevent the replication of the bacilli, they destroy the bacilli, and they sterilise the pulmonary cavities.

The aim of treatment during the initial phase is to reduce the bacterial population as much as possible so that the patient becomes non-infectious as quickly as possible, and to prevent the emergence of drug-resistance.[331] Streptomycin may be prescribed during the initial phase of treatment as part of combination therapy where resistance to isoniazid has been identified. During the first few weeks of treatment, isoniazid is the principle 'killing' drug, destroying all of the rapidly replicating bacilli within the pulmonary cavity, assisted in its work by ethambutol and rifampicin. This combination is so effective that patients with sputum smear-positive drug-sensitive disease are not infectious once they have had two full weeks of treatment[306,311], and if they are in hospital they can then be moved out of isolation, although bacilli will continue to be visible in sputum specimens for several weeks. Rifampicin and pyrazinamide continue the killing process by targeting the less active bacilli lurking within the macrophages and the inflammatory lesions, where they also sterilise the pulmonary cavities. After the initial phase of treatment has been completed, isoniazid and rifampicin are continued for the remaining four months; rifampicin kills any dormant bacilli, and isoniazid targets any that are rifampicin-resistant.[331]

The side effects of these drugs can adversely affect patient compliance with therapy, and this is a potential problem area as poor compliance with treatment is a known risk factor for the development of drug-resistant disease. A side effect of isoniazid is peripheral neuropathy, which commonly affects patients with pre-existing illnesses such as HIV and diabetes, and other risk factors including malnutrition, alcohol dependence and chronic renal failure. Rifampicin can cause transient disturbances in liver function and in patients with pre-existing liver disease treatment may have to be changed; it can also affect the action of oral contraceptive pills, an important point to note when prescribing rifampicin for women of reproductive age. While pyrazinamide is a powerful, rapidly bactericidal drug, it can induce liver toxicity and for this reason its use has to be discontinued after two months treatment. Ethambutol can induce visual disturbances such as loss of visual acuity and colour blindness and patients require eye examinations prior to starting therapy.

DIRECTLY OBSERVED THERAPY (DOT)

Within the UK patients who are unlikely to comply with taking anti-tuberculosis therapy unsupervised may be given their treatment under supervision, where they are directly observed to swallow their medication. While directly observed therapy is not necessary for all patients with TB, the NICE guidance[306] recommends that it is considered in particular patient groups with risk factors for poor compliance, such as street homeless people, patients with a history of poor compliance, patients with multiple drug resistances, and those with serious mental illness.

BCG (BACILLUS CALMETTE-GUERIN) VACCINATION

The BCG vaccine, first used in 1921, contains live organisms modified from *M.bovis*. It was discovered by two scientists working at the Pasteur Institute in Paris, who isolated the organism from a cow with bovine tuberculosis, and over a period of several years the organism underwent numerous genetic changes which altered the original strain of *M.bovis*, producing what is now known as BCG.[332] The BCG vaccine was introduced into the UK in 1953, and until the autumn of 2005 it was administered to schoolchildren between the ages of 10–14 as part of the schools vaccination programme to prevent the acquisition of pulmonary disease. However, the epidemiology of tuberculosis in the UK has changed significantly over the years and in 2005 the Department of Health announced changes to the BCG vaccination programme.[333] Within the UK, tuberculosis has changed from being a disease that affects the general population, to one that mostly affects high risk groups, and under the new vaccination programme, only those falling into 'at risk' groups will be vaccinated. Children who would have been vaccinated through the old schools vaccination programme will be screened for risk factors, skin tested and offered vaccination if appropriate.

Table 10.5 BCG vaccination 'at risk' groups[52]

All infants (aged 0–12 months) living in areas of the UK where the incidence of tuberculosis is 40/100,000 population or greater.

Infants with a parent or grandparent born in a country with a TB incidence of 40/100,000 population or greater.

Previously unvaccinated tuberculin-negative new entrants to the UK, under the age of 16 who were born in, or who lived for at least three months in, a country with an annual incidence of TB of at least 40/100,000 population.

Previously unvaccinated, tuberculin-negative children aged 0–16 years, with a parent or grandparent who was born in a country where the annual incidence of TB is 40/100,000 population or greater.

Individuals at risk through occupational exposure.

The aim of the vaccination programme in the UK is to protect those individuals who are at increased risk of developing tuberculosis through exposure to the disease. It does not offer protection against latent (reactivation) disease, or prevent primary disease from occurring.[52] As it is a live vaccine (although it does not contain any bovine material), BCG should not be administered to any individual who is immunocompromised as a result of any underlying illness/disease or treatment, as it could induce a severe reaction or, in some cases, disseminated disease. The vaccine is administered in a single dose (0.05 ml in infants under the age of 12 months, or 0.1 ml for infants over the age of 12 months, children and adults) and injected intradermally into the lateral aspect of the left upper arm.[52] Induration at the injection site is followed by a small lesion which may ulcerate initially but will subside over several weeks or months, leaving a small flat scar.

CONTACT TRACING AND SCREENING[306]

The principle aim of contact tracing is to identify any associated cases of tuberculosis, detect people with latent infection, and identify those who are not infected and offer vaccination in order to prevent infection where appropriate. It may also be a useful aid in detecting the source of infection in an outbreak situation where the index case is not obviously recognisable, and is of particular importance in cases of infectious pulmonary tuberculosis. Close contacts are defined as those from the same household, sharing a bedroom, kitchen, bathroom or sitting room with the index case. They may also include very close associates of the index case such as a partner or frequent visitors to the home. Most occupational contacts come under the heading of 'casual contacts' and follow-up would usually only be necessary if the index case is sputum smear-positive and any of the contacts are felt to be unusually susceptible, or if the index case is considered to be highly infectious, or in the event of an outbreak. In each case, the lifestyle of the index case needs to be carefully considered since other places of close contact may be revealed; for example, the index case may have recently been on a long-haul air flight, or may be living in a homeless shelter.

INPATIENT CONTACT TRACING[306]

Within the hospital inpatient setting, there is always the possibility of a patient with active TB being mis-diagnosed, or just not detected, and being placed in the middle of an open ward. Although the risk of infectivity to other patients is considered to be small, each patient needs to be individually risk assessed, and decisions around the appropriate action to be taken should centre around the degree of infectivity of the index case, the length of time which other patients were 'exposed' to the index case, the proximity of the contact, and whether any of the contacts were immunocompromised. Patients in the same bay as the patient, as opposed to all patients on the ward, should be regarded as being at risk only if the index case was found to be sputum smear-positive with a productive cough and was in the bay for more than eight hours. In the event of susceptible patients being on the same ward, but not necessarily in the same bay, as the index case, and the length of stay of the index case of that patient exceeding more than two days, individual patients should be risk assessed.

CONTACT TRACING/SCREENING OF HEALTHCARE WORKERS[306]

Although it is generally accepted that the incidence of tuberculosis in healthcare workers is no higher than in other members of the population at large, there is evidence to suggest that healthcare workers are at risk, particularly as staff have been recruited for employment within the NHS from countries where the burden of tuberculosis is high.[334] New employees who will either be having patient contact or who will be working with clinical specimens should undergo a health screen before they commence work, and the NICE guidance and new guidance from the Department of Health[335] published in 2007 details the processes that should be followed.

It is not recommended that the routine screening of healthcare workers following exposure to a patient with sputum smear-positive disease is undertaken unless the staff member concerned is considered to be at any significant risk. The NICE guidance recommends that after a 'TB incident' on a ward, staff are sent a 'one-off' reminder by the occupational health department, which details the signs and symptoms to look out for, and the importance of reporting any symptoms promptly. Any healthcare worker who is concerned about having been exposed to tuberculosis would generally be advised to seek assurance from their own occupational health department. In the event of a healthcare worker being diagnosed with tuberculosis, either from occupational exposure or a community source, liaison between the treating physician, the occupational health department, the Health Protection Agency and the infection prevention and control team is important. If that member of staff has been working while they have been infectious, patients and colleagues who have had significant contact will need to be identified. It will not always be known how long the index case has been infectious for, so it is recommended that contacts be reviewed for the period of time that the index case has had a cough. In the event of this not being known, contacts should be traced back from the first three months preceding the first sputum smear or culture-positive results.

SCREENING OF NEW ENTRANTS TO THE UK[306]

New entrants pose a risk to others if they arrive from a country where there is a high prevalence of tuberculosis, or if they have latent or active disease. The UK has had a policy of screening new entrants from high risk countries, with a TB incidence of 40/100,000 population, via the port of arrival scheme, and new entrants who are proposing to remain in the UK for longer than six months are identified by immigration staff and referred to the local port health control unit for assessment and screening.

The NICE recommendations are that new entrants should be identified for TB screening from port of arrival reports, new registrations with primary care, entry to education (including universities) and links with statutory and voluntary groups working with new entrants. The TB assessment should include a chest x-ray where one has not recently been done, and a clinical risk assessment in the event of an abnormal chest x-ray, a risk assessment for HIV infection, and a Mantoux and interferon-gamma test where clinically appropriate. BCG vaccination may be appropriate for unvaccinated individuals who have a negative Mantoux test.

INFECTION CONTROL PRECAUTIONS – DRUG-SENSITIVE/ DRUG-RESISTANT TB

These are summarised in Table 10.6. The reader is advised to consult their local infection control manual and familiarise themselves with their own local policy.

Further information on the control, prevention and management of TB can be found on the web.[336,337,338]

Table 10.6 Infection control precautions for patients with pulmonary tuberculosis

Isolation	Patients with suspected or confirmed (sputum smear-positive) pulmonary tuberculosis should be isolated in a single room until they have had two full weeks of anti-tuberculosis therapy; patients with extra-pulmonary tuberculosis do not require isolation if pulmonary disease has been excluded. If the patient is sputum smear-negative, isolation is not required and the patient can be moved to an open ward, provided that there are no HIV positive or other immunocompromised on the ward.

Table 10.6 (Continued)

	A risk assessment should be undertaken for multi-drug resistant disease, and if confirmed the patient should be moved into a negative pressure isolation room; this may necessitate the patient being moved to another hospital.
Personal protective equipment	Respiratory face protection is not generally required by healthcare workers unless aerosol-generating procedures such as bronchoscopy, sputum induction or nebuliser treatment are undertaken. Disposable FFP3 respirators should be worn for suspected or confirmed MDR-TB until drug-resistant disease is excluded, or the patient is no longer considered to be infectious. Masks should be removed *after* exiting the isolation room and disposed of as clinical waste. Patients with smear-positive pulmonary tuberculosis should be asked to wear a surgical face mask if they have any occasion to leave their isolation room. Disposable gloves and gowns are not required. However, some Trusts may have their own local policy for the use of PPE and the reader should refer to their infection control manual.
Visitors	Visitors should be restricted to those who have previously had close contact with the patient; they will be followed up for contact tracing.
Linen	Linen should be disposed of according to local policy.
Waste	Clinical and household waste should be segregated and disposed of according to local policy and national guidance.
Discharge arrangements	Patients may be discharged when they are clinically well and have shown a response to treatment; in some cases patients may be discharged prior to completing two full weeks of anti-tuberculosis treatment depending upon their clinical response, degree of infectivity and individual circumstances. If the discharge is complicated because the patient has complex social needs, or they require supervision with regard to taking their medication, a discharge planning meeting may be required.
Last offices	Deceased patients with tuberculosis should be placed into a body bag and the mortuary notified of the patient's infectious state so that the appropriate precautions can be taken.

11 Clostridium difficile

INTRODUCTION

Clostridium difficile was first described in 1935 as 'the difficult Clostridium'[339], a reference to the difficulties experienced in isolating and then culturing the organism under laboratory conditions, but its association with antibiotic administration and pseudomembranous colitis was not recognised until the 1970s.[340] *Clostridium difficile* is now notorious for being the most important cause of hospital acquired diarrhoea in adults and a significant cause of patient morbidity and mortality, causing a spectrum of illness which ranges from asymptomatic colonisation of the bowel to trivial diarrhoea to life-threatening illness. It also places a significant financial burden on the NHS, where costs due to increased length of stay have been estimated to be in excess of £4,000 per patient.[341] Although infection prevention and control teams have long been concerned about *C.difficile*, its importance as a hospital pathogen has been grossly underestimated by many other healthcare professionals and the media, but now major changes are being seen in relation to its epidemiology and pathogenicity with the emergence of the new 027 strain. The outbreak at Stoke Mandeville Hospital, in which 33 patients died[21], and the more recent outbreaks at Maidstone and Tunbridge Wells NHS Trust, have heightened media and public awareness and the prevention and control of *C.difficile* infection is proving to be as much of a problem and a challenge as MRSA, if not more.

This chapter looks at *C.difficile* in detail, discussing the organism; the pathogenesis of infection, including risk factors for acquisition; clinical features and diagnosis; antibiotic management and novel treatments such as the use of probiotics and immunoglobulin; infection control precautions and the UK mandatory surveillance scheme. It concludes by examining the Stoke Mandeville outbreak.

LEARNING OUTCOMES

After reading this chapter the reader will:

- understand and be able to describe the pathogenesis of infection and the risk factors for acquisition

- recognise and be able to describe the clinical features of *C.difficile* infection
- be able to discuss the infection control precautions that need to be taken when caring for a symptomatic patient and understand the importance of strict compliance
- understand the management of *C.difficile*, including the role of novel treatments

CLOSTRIDIA

Clostridia are the most clinically important of the Gram-positive anaerobic rods (the other significant Gram-positive rods being aerobes). As obligate anaerobes, they colonise oxygen-deficient areas of the body where they co-exist alongside the normal resident flora but if displaced into a sterile body site they can result in potentially life-threatening conditions.[342,343] Out of the 160 species[21] of Clostridia which occur naturally in the environment in soil, water, sewage and also within the human and animal gastrointestinal tract, only a very small minority are pathogenic to humans, such as *Clostridium tetani, Clostridium botulinum, Clostridium perfringens* and *Clostridium difficile*. They tend to cause opportunistic infections, and their potent exotoxins (see Chapter 2 Bacterial and Viral Classification, Structure and Function) can result in invasive and destructive damage to the host. Their ability to form endospores, which render them resistant to heat, disinfection and desiccation, facilitates their survival in extreme environmental conditions for months or years. They have the ability to return to their vegetative state when the environmental conditions are favourable.

Healthy adults carry at least 500 species of bacteria in the colon, of which 90 % are anaerobes.[344] This normal colonic flora inhibits the growth of other bacteria which could proliferate within the bowel if the normal balance of bacterial flora is disrupted. *C.difficile* are part of the normal bowel flora in 2–5 % of the population, with rates of carriage seen in hospitalised patients ranging from 13–50 % depending on their length of stay.[345,346] Within long-term care facilities such as nursing and residential homes, carriage rates of 7 % have been reported[347], and studies have reported hospital carriage rates of 14–21 % in patients on medical wards.[348] Carriage rates of *C.difficile* in healthy neonates (probably acquired from the mother during delivery) are much higher, between 35–65 %.[349] Signs of symptomatic infection tend to be absent in neonates and this is thought to be due to the immature nature of the intestinal flora and the lack of toxin receptors in the intestine, although children become increasingly susceptible to *C.difficile*-associated disease after the age of two years.[349]

THE PATHOGENESIS OF *CLOSTRIDIUM DIFFICILE* INFECTION

The main route of acquisition is via the faecal-oral route. The organism is ingested either in its vegetative form or as metabolically inactive spores. As they are not affected by stomach acid, spores are able to pass through the stomach, germinating

Table 11.1 Risk factors for *Clostridium difficile* infection

Age >65 years
Underlying disease
Immunocompromised
Intensive care
Prolonged hospital stay
Antibiotic treatment, including multiple antibiotic therapy/prolonged courses
Proton pump inhibitors

into the vegetative form (from which they replicate and produce toxins) in the small intestine where they are exposed to bile acids before reaching the colon, which they can then colonise. In the normal healthy adult, the flora of the colon is generally resistant to colonisation by *C.difficile*, and even if the organism is acquired, the risk of the individual progressing to clinical illness is negligible.[350,351] There are suggestions that 70 % of the adult population have antibodies to the toxins produced by the bacteria, which would indicate that exposure is common and linked to environmental factors, and that high antibody responses develop within days of acquiring the organism, which suggests previous exposure.[352,353] However, if the normal flora of the large intestine has been disrupted by the administration of antibiotic therapy, it can be readily colonised by *C.difficile* which does not have to compete with other bacteria for nutrients, and this can predispose the patient to developing diarrhoea.

The patient population, the use of antibiotics and the presence of colonised or symptomatic patients within the ward environment all influence acquisition rates.[349] While the risk of *C.difficile* infection depends in part on the virulence factors of the particular strain and the individual's immune response[345,354,355], there are numerous other factors which increase individual susceptibility to symptomatic infection, and these are summarised in Table 11.1.

Symptomatic disease will only develop if the strain of *C.difficile* possesses the gene for toxin production, producing toxins A and/or B. Enterotoxin A binds to receptors in the bowel wall and causes extensive tissue damage with injury to the mucosa, along with inflammation and oedema. The exact role cytotoxin B has to play is undefined, but it has a cytotoxic potency that is 1,000 times greater than that of toxin A, and is thought to play a major role in activating the inflammatory response.[349]

The resulting inflammation leads to the development of pseudomembranes, whereby the inflamed mucosa is studded with raised white and yellow plaques, consisting of neutrophils, fibrin, mucin and cellular debris[345], although there may be intervening patches of 'normal' mucosa.

THE ROLE OF ANTIBIOTICS AND PROTON PUMP INHIBITORS IN *C.DIFFICILE* INFECTION

The disruption and subsequent alteration of the bowel flora through the administration of antibiotics is the main precipitating factor for symptomatic *C.difficile* infection. Overgrowth of *C.difficile* has increasingly been linked to broad spectrum agents such as clindamycin, the cephalosporins (cefotaxime in particular has been implicated in the onset of symptomatic cases[356]) and penicillins, although any antibiotic with anti-bacterial activity can induce diarrhoea. The risk is partly dependant upon the antibiotic used and the duration of treatment.[346,357]

The natural acidity of the stomach serves as a 'disinfectant' for the gastrointestinal tract. Proton pump inhibitors and histamine H_2 antagonists, used to prevent the development of gastric and duodenal ulcers and reduce the secretion of gastric acid, have been implicated as possible contributing factors in *C.difficile* infection.[358,359] As gastric acid secretion is suppressed, the natural acidity of the stomach declines and the vegetative forms of *C.difficile*, including the spores, are less likely to be destroyed.

CLINICAL FEATURES AND DIAGNOSIS

Sudden onset of diarrhoea can occur during a course of antibiotics or up to two months after exposure. It has a characteristic 'farmyard' or 'manure' type smell and may be accompanied by mucous. Patients may pass unformed, or watery diarrhoea more than twice a day and in severe cases the diarrhoea is often profuse and watery, with the patient passing more than 20 stools a day, often accompanied by abdominal pain.[360] Abdominal distension, fever, and dehydration may also be present. Sigmoidoscopy in mild cases is generally of no value and will reveal a normal colon unless performed during severe cases where a characteristically inflamed colon with adherent yellow plaques will be seen. These plaques are usually confined to the distal colon although they can occur in the proximal colon, where they may be missed unless a colonoscopy is performed.[361] An endoscopy performed on a symptomatic but *neutropenic* patient may give a false negative result as pseudomembranes do not form because of the lack of neutrophils.[349] If symptoms progress, patients are at increased risk of developing paralytic ileus and toxic megacolon, which may result in perforation.[362] X-rays will reveal dilated colon and oedema of the mucosa; invasive investigations such as sigmoidoscopy and colonoscopy are contra-indicated here as they can induce perforation. The mortality rate ranges from 6–30 % in patients with pseudomembranous colitis.[352,363]

The definitive method and the 'gold standard' for diagnosing *C.difficile* infection is the detection of cytotoxin in tissue culture[344] and a single specimen of unformed stool, taken at the onset of symptoms, will generally be sufficient to establish the diagnosis.

MANAGEMENT OF INITIAL AND RECURRENT SYMPTOMATIC *C.DIFFICILE* INFECTION

Treatment is only indicated in patients who are symptomatic, and management therefore depends on the clinical presentation and the inciting agent. The most important first step in treating *C.difficile* infection is to stop the inciting antibiotic if it is medically appropriate to do so. In mild cases this in itself may lead to full recovery within two to three days without the need for any other intervention[364], although a delay in initiating treatment could result in a clinical deterioration in the patient's condition.

Metronidazole and vancomycin are the antibiotics of choice for the treatment of symptomatic *C.difficile* infection.[365] Although they are considered to be equally effective, oral metronidazole 400 mgs eight hourly for seven to ten days is the first line of treatment as most *C.difficile* isolates are highly susceptible to it and it is less expensive than vancomycin. It is contra-indicated in women who are pregnant or who are breastfeeding. Vancomycin is generally not the first drug of choice as it is known to contribute to the spread of vancomycin-resistant bacteria[260,261,262], particularly vancomycin or glycapeptide resistant enterococci (VRE) which colonise the bowel. It should only be given if treatment with metronidazole fails to respond or if the disease is severe.

A recurrence of symptomatic disease occurs in 5–20 % of cases, with 12–24 % developing a second case of *C.difficile* within two months of the initial infection.[361,366] Although there are a number of factors which can influence the possibility of recurrent disease re-occurring, there is disagreement in the literature when it comes to distinguishing whether or not recurrent disease in a previously symptomatic patient is a relapse or re-infection. A relapse has been defined as a recurrence of symptoms within two months of the initial diagnosis whereby treatment has failed to eradicate the organism; re-infection is a recurrence of symptoms after two months due to infection either by a new strain or cross-infection arising from environmental contamination.[366,367] Patient risk factors for recurrence include increased age, recent abdominal surgery, and the survival of *C.difficile* spores in the colon, in spite of high intraluminal levels of vancomycin.[368,369]

Treatment of recurrent disease can be problematic, although patients usually respond to prolonged courses of either metronidazole or vancomycin.[363] There have been some successes with tapering courses of vancomycin over a period of six weeks, and vancomycin combined with rifampicin for seven days.[370,371] There are also case reports of successful treatment with intravenous immunoglobulin which contains significant levels of antibodies to *C.difficile* toxins.[372,373] This is a particularly interesting development as one study demonstrated a 48-fold risk of recurrent disease in patients with a failed antibody response.[374]

Much has been written about the value of probiotics, commonly referred to as 'good bacteria', which are live organisms that improve the microbial balance of the host by fighting infections that affect the GI tract and mucosal surfaces. It is thought the administration of bacteria such as *bifidiobacterium* and *lactobacilius*, along with *Saccharomyces boulardii*, which is a yeast, have a role to play in restoring the equilibrium of the flora within the bowel after antibiotic administration. Although there have been some successes, particularly with the use of *Saccharomyces*[375,376,], it appears that the evidence to support their use generally is not very convincing and that the jury is still out as far as their effectiveness in the prevention and treatment of *C.difficile* is concerned.[377,378]

The administration of antiperistaltic drugs such as loperamide are contra-indicated in symptomatic *C.difficile* infection as they slow the faecal transit time, which is thought to result in the retention of toxins in the colon and extended toxin-associated damage.[343]

C.DIFFICILE RIBOTYPE 027

In March 2003, a virulent strain of *C.difficile* was detected at several hospitals in Quebec, Canada.[379] A prospective study at 12 hospitals during six months in 2004 revealed 1,703 patients who met the case definition for hospital acquired diarrhoea; 422 patients died within 30 days of the onset of diarrhoea, and *C.difficile* was the attributable cause of death in 117. The results of the study showed that there was a single predominant strain in circulation associated with high morbidity and mortality, increased virulence and antibiotic resistance. Between 2003 and 2005, outbreaks occurred at Stoke Mandeville hospital in the UK[21], in which relapse rates were noted to be on the increase, and deaths occurred from toxic megacolon and colonic perforation. The strain responsible for the Stoke Mandeville outbreak was identified as the 027 strain, very similar to the virulent strains that have caused outbreaks in North America and the Netherlands since 1999.

The most striking feature of 027 is hypertoxin production.[380] It produces 10–20 times more toxin than other strains as it lacks a gene that regulates how much toxin is produced.[381,382] It is resistant to ciprofloxacin and the new generation of fluroquinolones such as levofloxacin and moxifloxacin, and exposure to the fluroquinolones and cephalosporins are a recognised risk factor.[379] This is a significant development as the fluroquinolones have previously been regarded as 'safe' antibiotics and not linked to *C.difficile* infection. It is now the second most common strain identified by the Health Protection Agency's national sampling surveillance programme.[21] Patients infected with the 027 strain tend to have a more acute illness and increased severity of symptoms [379,381,382,383] (although diarrhoea may not always be present), together with important diagnostic markers – a raised white cell count and elevated *C-reactive protein* (CRP). They may fail to respond to metronidazole and have a higher rate of progression towards developing pseudomembranous colitis. Table 11.2 summarises the main features of *C.difficile* Ribotype 027.

Table 11.2 Clinical features of *C.difficile Ribotype 027*

Increased severity of illness – increased abdominal pain and frequency of diarrhoea.
   (*NB Diarrhoea may not always be present*)
Failure to respond to antibiotics.
Abdominal distension, raised CRP and rising WCC particularly in patients who may
   have appeared to respond to antibiotics.
Deterioration in condition.

INFECTION CONTROL PRECAUTIONS

Preventing the spread of *C.difficile* can present quite a challenge as hospitals tend to have an increasing population of elderly, debilitated and susceptible patients which naturally increases the number of susceptible hosts within the environment. Keeping the environment and equipment clean is another challenge altogether but one which must be met head on if environmental reservoirs are to be reduced and cross-infection prevented. It is important that the reader is familiar with the information and advice available from their own infection prevention and control team and they adhere to their local policy or guidelines for the prevention and control of *C.difficile* infection.

PATIENT ISOLATION

Given the explosive nature of diarrhoea, and the fact that patients with *C.difficile* may secrete up to 10^9 organisms per gram of faeces[346], there is a real risk of patient-to-patient transmission via the faecal-oral route if the environment becomes heavily contaminated. Department of Health and PHLS Guidelines[365] state that symptomatic patients should be isolated until formed stools have been obtained, although isolation tends to be discontinued when the patient has been asymptomatic for 48 hours. The pressure on available side rooms, and in many cases a lack of isolation facilities, together with competing infections and various patient factors all combine to make patient isolation difficult. However, the Healthcare Commission Report into the Stoke Mandeville Outbreak[21] recommends the prompt isolation of patients with diarrhoea in order to prevent outbreaks of *C.difficile*, and states that failure to isolate patients poses a significant clinical risk. A comprehensive risk assessment needs to be taken and if isolation facilities are not available for whatever reason, that reason should be documented and reviewed daily where appropriate. The infection prevention and control team should be informed that the patient cannot be isolated. If there is more than one symptomatic patient on the ward, they should be 'cohorted' or nursed in the same bay where possible. Where symptomatic patients are nursed in open areas of the ward, particular care and attention must be made to reducing environmental contamination and enhanced cleaning of equipment and the ward environment will be required.

HAND HYGIENE (SEE CHAPTER 6)

Hands of healthcare workers contaminated with *C.difficile* spores will transmit the organism onto equipment and from patient to patient. Although the introduction of alcohol hand rubs has increased compliance with hand hygiene within healthcare settings, they do not remove dirt and organic material and are ineffective against spores, so hands must be washed with liquid soap in between each episode of patient contact, or contact with contaminated equipment.[86,384]

Disposable gloves and aprons should be worn for each episode of direct contact with the patient and/or contaminated equipment. They should be disposed of as clinical waste and hands washed with liquid soap and water after the protective clothing has been removed. Linen should be treated as infected and disposed of in a red linen bag and clinical waste disposed of into the appropriate clinical waste bag. Care must be taken when disposing of linen and waste in order to ensure that local requirements in relation to the handling and disposal of infected linen and waste are followed.

DECONTAMINATION OF EQUIPMENT

Ideally, patients in isolation with any healthcare associated infection should have equipment dedicated for their own use. The reality is that equipment more often than not has to be shared among patients and this increases the risk of cross-infection. Research indicates that high levels of micro-organisms are present on a wide range of healthcare equipment such as bed frames, mattresses, patient call bells, blood pressure cuffs, telephones and numerous other objects [384,385,386], and that up to one third of healthcare associated infections can be prevented by cleaning equipment thoroughly. Some Trusts use single-use disposable equipment such as blood pressure cuffs to reduce the risk of cross-infection, and if these are available they should be used. Commodes have been implicated as vehicles of cross-infection in *C.difficile* outbreaks as they will become heavily contaminated with spores [385] and one report states that a commode contaminated with *C.difficile* was the source of cross-infection to eight patients within the space of one week.[348] Where possible symptomatic patients should be allocated their own commode, or have designated toilet facilities. In circumstances where this cannot be met, enhanced cleaning of toilet and bathroom facilities is required, and commodes must be thoroughly cleaned in between patient use ensuring that any physical soiling is removed, and decontaminated once a day using a solution of hypochlorite 1,000 ppm. Bedpan washers are potential problem areas if they are not reaching and holding their optimum temperature for heat disinfection at 80 °C for one minute. Inadequate decontamination of both a bedpan and a bed washer has been reported, with both testing positive for *C.difficile* before and after the disinfection cycle.[387] Most clinical areas have now replaced traditional bedpan washers with macerators. As alcohol is ineffective in the presence of organic material and bacterial spores, detergent wipes are generally sufficient for the routine cleaning of equipment. Note should be taken though of any specific manufacturer's instructions, as some cleaning materials may cause damage to equipment.

DECONTAMINATION OF THE ENVIRONMENT

Heavy environmental contamination with spores from colonised or infected patients are recognised as significant risk factors in terms of cross-infection, and close proximity to a symptomatic patient has been given an attributable risk of 12 %.[388] In addition, the level of contamination on healthcare workers' hands has been found to be proportional to the level of environmental contamination.[389] Studies have shown that environmental cleaning with a hypochlorite based solution rather than neutral detergent can significantly reduce the incidence of *C.difficile* infection and environmental contamination.[390,391] Special attention should be paid to the cleaning of bedside equipment such as telephones and television sets.

STOOL SPECIMENS FOR CLEARANCE

Once symptoms resolve, there is no need to send stool specimens for clearance as asymptomatic carriage of *C.difficile* may persist for up to three months after the initial infection[390], and a positive result in an asymptomatic patient is indicative only of colonisation, not infection. If symptoms return, the infection prevention and control team should be contacted for advice.

The infection control precautions are summarised in Table 11.3.

Table 11.3 Infection control precautions for patients with symptomatic *C.difficile* infection

Isolation	Patients with **symptomatic** *Clostridium difficile* infection should be isolated in a single room with the door kept closed. Sometimes a risk assessment is required, taking into account the patient's overall medical condition (isolation could compromise the patient's safety), the frequency/severity of diarrhoea, and the isolation facilities available. It may be necessary for the patient to remain in the open ward and if this is the case, it should be documented in the medical/nursing notes that isolation is not possible, the infection prevention and control team should be informed, and the patient's isolation status reviewed daily. If there is more than one symptomatic patient on the ward, cohort nursing may be considered. Patients generally remain in isolation until they have been asymptomatic ('normal' formed stool, depending on what is normal for the patient) for 48 hours.
Hand hygiene	Alcohol hand rub is ineffective against *C.difficile* spores; therefore, hands should be washed with liquid soap and water in order to physically wash the spores off the hands. Hand washing should take place immediately after each episode of direct contact with the patient, after removing protective clothing, after contact with the patient's faeces and before contact with another patient.
Personal protective equipment and clothing	Gloves and aprons should be worn for episodes of direct contact with the patient/faeces/contaminated equipment; they should be removed immediately after contact and disposed of as clinical waste, and hands should be washed with liquid soap and water.
Visitors	Patients can receive visitors; they do not need to wear protective clothing unless they are assisting the patient with bathroom/toilet needs and there is the possibility of direct contact with faeces. Visitors should be asked to wash their hands with liquid soap and water on leaving the patient's room/ward.

Table 11.3 (Continued)

Linen	All linen should be managed according to local policy/national guidance.
Waste	Clinical waste should be disposed of according to local policy/national guidance.
Decontamination	Where possible, patients with *C.difficile* should be allocated equipment that is single-patient use and disposable, or equipment that can remain with the patient during their time in hospital/isolation and either be disposed of or decontaminated accordingly when the patient has been discharged/de-isolated. Any equipment which is multi-patient use must be decontaminated in between each patient use. Patients should be allocated their own commode or own toilet if there are no en-suite facilities available. Commodes should be cleaned in between patient use with detergent wipes after any visible soiling has been removed with a solution of neutral detergent and water. They should be decontaminated daily using a solution of hypochlorite 1000 ppm.
Environmental cleanliness	It is essential that environmental reservoirs of infection are reduced, and ward based cleaning should be undertaken using a hypochlorite solution. Particular attention should be paid to cleaning toilets/bathrooms.
Restricting patient movement	The transfer of symptomatic patients to other wards should be avoided where possible to minimise the risk of spread, but may be necessary if the patient requires specialist care on another ward or has to undergo investigations. The receiving ward/department/hospital should be informed so that they can take the appropriate precautions.
Discharge arrangements	Patients should not be discharged/transferred to nursing/residential home accommodation while they are still symptomatic; the home should be informed that the patient has received treatment for symptomatic *C.difficile* infection when the patient is ready for discharge. Patients may be discharged home with symptomatic infection on the appropriate antibiotics at the discretion of the medical team if they are medically fit for discharge, but they should be made aware of the importance of completing the prescribed course of metronidazole/vancomycin, and of informing their general practitioner if their symptoms worsen, or if the diarrhoea returns.
Care of the deceased patient	Deceased patients do not need to be placed into a body bag.

MANDATORY SURVEILLANCE OF *C.DIFFICILE* IN THE UK

Voluntary reporting of positive *C.difficile* isolates was introduced in 1990 and became mandatory in January 2004, with acute Trusts in England required to report all cases of *C.difficile* infection in patients over the age of 65 to the Department of Health as part of their programme of mandatory surveillance of healthcare associated infections. The purpose of the surveillance programme is to detect and interpret trends in the incidence, distribution and severity of *C.difficile* by the collation of robust data which reports cases, outbreaks and hyperendemic situations. Trusts are also required to report outbreaks, defined as 'occurrence of two or more related cases over a defined period agreed locally taking account of the background rate'[344] to their strategic health authority and local health protection unit as serious untoward incidents (SUIs) associated with infection.[392]

In 2005, the Health Protection Agency and the Healthcare Commission distributed a survey to the directors of infection prevention and control at all 173 acute NHS Trusts in England, which focused on the management, prevention, laboratory investigation and surveillance of *C.difficile* infection. Of those responding, 67 % reported that they had seen an increase in the incidence of reported infections at their Trusts over the last three years, and 56 % had experienced consistently high background rates, as well as an increased frequency in the number of outbreaks. The survey revealed that 40 % of trusts did not routinely isolate symptomatic patients, Trusts generally were not working to an agreed definition of what constituted an outbreak of infection, there was variation in the techniques used for culture and typing between laboratories, the reporting of positive specimens under the mandatory surveillance scheme was inconsistent, and there was a need to review antibiotic policies and rigorously monitor compliance with antibiotic prescribing.[392]

The final report, published by the HPA in July 2006[393], stated that: 'The increased incidence of *Clostridium difficile* infection, possible changes in this infection's average severity and population distribution, and the emergence of new and possibly hyper-virulent strains of *C.difficile* highlight the need to review currently recommended procedures for prevention and control of *C.difficile*, particularly as regards adherence to recommendations on isolating cases and implementation of robust antimicrobial policies'.

THE STOKE MANDEVILLE OUTBREAK[21]

In July 2006, the Healthcare Commission published its report into the *C.difficile* outbreaks at Stoke Mandeville Hospital, part of Buckinghamshire Hospitals NHS Trust, in which 334 patients contacted *C.difficile* and at least 33 died in outbreaks which took place between October 2003 and June 2005. The outbreaks attracted national publicity and the patient deaths, which were due to the hyper-virulent 027 strain, were described as 'an awful tragedy' by the chairman of the Healthcare Commission. The enquiry was undertaken at the request of the Secretary of State to look at the systems and procedures that the Trust had in place for the control of infection. There had been several small outbreaks during 2003 prior to the main outbreak and the infection control team was concerned at the time that patients were not being isolated appropriately, which exposed other patients to the risk of cross-infection. The HCC found that there were numerous issues which contributed to the outbreak relating to the management of the Trust as whole, the hospital environment and the lack of facilities and resources, staffing shortages, and clinical practice issues. Failure to isolate symptomatic patients was seen as a significant contributing factor, as were the extreme nursing shortages on the ward, which meant that shortcuts in clinical practice were taken; staff were failing to wash their hands, change protective clothing in between patients, and decontaminate equipment. Hand washing facilities were lacking and in some cases access to them was obstructed. Sluice rooms contained antiquated bedpan washers and were cluttered with linen and waste bags which obstructed access to hand wash basins. There were also many issues in relation to hospital cleanliness. All of these factors and many more contributed to the spread of *C.difficile* infection. The report was damning, although the efforts of the hospital staff working under such extreme conditions were recognised, and the infection control team in particular was highly praised for its work in trying to contain the outbreak.

The Healthcare Commission has made a series of recommendations which have implications for NHS Trusts. It acknowledges the pressure that Trusts face in meeting government targets, stating that '. . . there is no doubt that the potential conflict between these targets and the control of infection is an issue that faces all Trusts'. However, the approach taken by the Trust 'compromised the control of infection and hence the safety of patients . . . we would reiterate that the safety of patients is not to be compromised under any circumstances'.[21]

In relation to the management of *C.difficile* outbreaks the report recommends:

- rapid isolation of patients with diarrhoea
- restricting the movement of patients between wards
- rapid identification and notification of outbreaks to the HPA and the strategic health authority
- the establishment of a multi-disciplinary outbreak committee which meets on a regular basis
- the rapid implementation of all recommended changes
- close monitoring of all aspects of the management of outbreaks and particularly those concerned with cleanliness of the environment, decontamination, the ward environment and antibiotic prescribing
- effective channels of communication with patients, hospital staff and outside agencies.

The Health Act[22] and *Saving Lives*[30] emphasise the importance of each Trust ensuring that it has a robust policy in place that encompasses surveillance, isolation/cohort nursing, environmental decontamination and antibiotic prescribing, and that prescribing with infection control practice is audited.

Further information on the prevention, control and management of *Clostridium difficile* can be found on the web[394,395,396].

12 Invasive Group A Streptococcal Disease

INTRODUCTION

Lancefield group A streptococcus (*Streptococcus pyogenes*) is one of the most prevalent human pathogens, responsible for a wide range of suppurative infections in the upper respiratory tract and skin, and invasive life-threatening soft tissue infections. The two most potentially devastating and lethal infections are discussed in this chapter – necrotising fasciitis and streptococcal toxic shock syndrome (STSS). The chapter begins by looking at the microbiology of streptococcus and *Streptococcus pyogenes*, before moving on to examine necrotising fasciitis (which has been the subject of sensationalist and alarmist newspaper headlines and is often referred to as 'the flesh-eating bug') and streptococcal toxic shock syndrome in detail. The risk factors, clinical presentation and pathogenesis of each infection are discussed, along with diagnosis, management and infection control precautions. The chapter concludes with a discussion of the UK Guidelines for the management of close contacts of invasive group A streptococcal disease.[397]

LEARNING OUTCOMES

After reading this chapter the reader will:

- Be able to relate the virulence factors of streptococci to the infective process
- Recognise the risk factors for, and clinical presentation of, necrotising fasciitis and streptococcal toxic shock syndrome
- Understand the management of invasive group A streptococcal disease, with particular reference to necrotising fasciitis and the infection control precautions
- Be familiar with the treatment of close contacts based on the UK guidelines

STREPTOCOCCUS

There are 40 species of streptococci which are anerobic, Gram-positive, catalase-negative cocci occurring either in pairs or chains. They are clinically important pathogens, existing as commensal flora in the mucous membranes of the upper respiratory tract and also colonising the bowel (enterococci), but they can cause invasive infections if they gain access into the bloodstream from the oral cavity or the gastro-intestinal tract.[398,399,400,401]

Streptococci are traditionally classified according to their ability to cause haemolysis of red bloodcells in blood agar and their antigenic type, both of which are used as markers for distinguishing between clinical species. B-haemolytic streptococci cause complete lysis of red cells, resulting in a clear ring around the colony on blood agar; A-haemolytic streptococci cause a partial lysis of red cells and a green ring, or halo effect, is apparent around the colony.[401] The antigenic characteristics of streptococci are based upon the C carbohydrate which is found in the bacterial cell wall. They are known as Lancefield antigens, and there are 18 of them, of which B-haemolytic streptococci groups A and B are the most clinically important.[398] Group A B-haemolytic streptococcus – *Streptococcus pyogenes* – is the most virulent of the species, with the ability to colonise, multiply quickly and spread within the host, invading seemingly intact skin and mucous membranes. Historically, *S.pyogenes* has been an important cause of sepsis following childbirth[402] (known as puerperal fever, puerperal sepsis or childbed fever), and streptococcal pharyngitis or tonsillitis, where scarlet fever was a severe complication of streptococcal pharyngitis before the advent of antibiotics. It also causes skin infections such as impetigo and cellulitis, and auto-immune conditions such as acute rheumatic fever and acute glomerulonephritis which can arise following streptococcal pharyngeal or soft tissue infections. Most devastatingly, it can cause invasive, immensely destructive, spreading soft tissue infections.

VIRULENCE FACTORS

S.pyogenes has a whole array of weapons at its disposal, which aid its invasion of the host and its destructive journey through the soft tissues.[398,399,400,401] The bacterial cell wall accounts for much of the organism's virulence factors, particularly those concerned with colonisation and evasion of phagocytosis and the host immune responses. Hair-like projections called fimbriae facilitate adherence to host cells and contain M proteins, which are the major virulence factor of *S.pyogenes*. There are 80 types of M protein, and individuals may experience several episodes of *S.pyogenes* infection during their lifetime if they encounter new M proteins which they have no antibodies against.[398] The bacterial capsule is composed of hyaluronic acid, which is chemically identical to the hyaluronic acid which is found in host connective tissue. This effectively disguises or hides the organism from the effects of the immune system, as it is not recognised as antigenic. In order to facilitate adherence to host tissues and mucous membranes, *S.pyogenes* produces a variety of acids and proteins which act as adhesions and allow it to establish itself at a portal of entry where it can colonise or invade the site. Its spreading ability is due to the secretion of additional proteins which aid invasiveness and spread to other areas of the body. These proteins kill host cells, initiating an inflammatory response which in turn stimulates the immune response to release cytokines, causing shock and tissue injury. Hyaluronidase, known as the original 'spreading factor', facilitates the spread of infection along fascial planes[45], and haemolysins (streptolysins O and S) damage cell membranes. Enzymes (hyaluronidase, deoxyribonucleases and streptokinase) facilitate the rapid spread of the organism through the tissues.[45]

INVASIVE DISEASE

Invasive group A streptococcal disease is defined as any infection associated with the isolation of group A streptococcus from a sterile body site, resulting in potentially lethal infections such as necrotising fasciitis and streptococcal toxic shock syndrome (STSS). The incidence of invasive disease, although relatively low at 3.8 cases per 100,000 population, carries a high mortality rate, with 20 % of cases dying within the first seven days of diagnosis.[397] Outbreaks of invasive disease have occurred in closed environments such as hospitals and nursing homes, and transmission to family members, other close contacts and healthcare workers has been documented.[403,404,405]

During the 1980s and the early 1990s there were increased reports of severe disease associated with *Streptococcus pyogenes,* predominantly from the United States, Norway, Sweden and Denmark.[406] A cluster of cases of necrotising fasciitis in Gloucestershire in 1994[407] was the trigger for the enhanced surveillance of invasive group A streptococcal disease both within the UK and Europe, determining trends of the disease in order to enhance understanding of its epidemiology.

NECROTISING FASCIITIS

Necrotising fasciitis is a potentially fatal, devastating and rapidly progressive bacterial infection involving the superficial fascia and deeper subcutaneous tissue (which contain vascular structures and nerves), characterised by rapidly spreading necrosis and gangrene of the skin and underlying structures.[401] It initially spares muscle, although muscles and other tissues will eventually become affected as a result of secondary infection if left undebrided.[408,409] The earliest records date back to Hippocrates in the 5th century BC.[410] It was described in 1924 as haemolytic streptococcal gangrene[411] and wasn't described as necrotising fasciitis until 1952.[412,413] It appears to be a relatively rare infection in the UK, with fewer than 500 cases reported each year.[410] In the initial stages of infection, it may be mistaken for cellulitis or a wound infection. Delay in diagnosis, late or inadequate surgical debridement, the extent of soft tissue involvement, advancing age and necrotising fasciitis involving the trunk or the chest all significantly increase the mortality rate, which is between 50–76 %.[414,415,416] Although *S.pyogenes* is the most common single pathogen isolated in 15 % of cases of necrotising fasciitis[417], the cause may be polymicrobial[418], with the number and type of organisms being dependent on the site of infection. A mixture of aerobic and anerobic bacteria are commonly isolated, such as *S.aureus*, clostridia, pseudomonas and bacteriodes[418], and it is believed that the combination of bacteria exerts a synergistic effect, although polymicrobial disease is more slowly evolving and there are fewer systemic complications.[419] Reports of an increased incidence of cases of necrotising fasciitis in America have been linked to a community acquired strain of MRSA.[420]

Risk factors

Individuals with underlying pre-existing medical conditions are most at risk from necrotising fasciitis as their immune defences are impaired; increasing age, renal disease, peripheral vascular disease, diabetes, malnutrition, obesity, and underlying malignancy[406,421] all increase patient susceptibility. Any area of the body can be affected and generally there is a history of trauma and damage to the skin[422,423] although this may be unknown in approximately 20 % of cases. It can also occur on the extremities secondary to trauma, including burns and lacerations, IV drug abuse and animal and insect bites, and cases have been reported following incidences of blunt trauma, varicella infection and incarcerated hernias.[421,422] There is also some evidence to suggest that the use of non-steroidal anti-inflammatory pain killers may mask the early signs and symptoms of streptococcal infections and could possibly predispose the individual to developing either necrotising fasciitis or streptococcal toxic shock syndrome.[423] However, necrotising fasciitis commonly occurs in the abdominal wall as a post-operative complication following abdominal surgery or in the perineum secondary to a pilonidal abscess, neglected perineal or ischiorectal abscess, or affecting the male genitalia and known as Fournier's gangrene.[410,416] The risk factors for developing necrotising fasciitis are summarised in Table 12.1.

Table 12.1 Risk factors for necrotising fasciitis

Underlying medical condition
Increasing age
Renal disease
Peripheral vascular disease
Underlying malignancy
Malnutrition
Obesity
Varicella infection
Anti-inflammatory non-steroidal drugs
Abdominal or perineal surgery
Incarcerated hernia
Trauma to the extremities – burns, lacerations, IV drug abuse, animal and insect bites
Blunt trauma

Clinical presentation

Symptoms may develop over a period of hours to several days, and the clinical presentation may vary between patients.[410] In the initial stages of infection, skin changes will be noticeable within 2–4 days of the inciting event. The patient may present with a mild area of erythema, or a more obvious tender, swollen hot area of erythema and cellulitis at the site of injury. The patient may also complain of a flu-like illness, with a headache, temperature and muscular aches and pains. This is generally the point at which necrotising fasciitis may be missed and treatment subsequently delayed, as the flu-like syndrome is often mistaken for the onset of influenza or a viral infection, and the skin changes diagnosed as a wound infection or cellulites.[416,424] One of the defining symptoms which should immediately trigger a high index of suspicion is that there is local severe pain at the site which is often disproportionate to the clinical findings on examination.[408,410] In the 50 % of patients without a defined portal of entry, the infection begins deep within the skin and is frequently at the site of a traumatic joint injury, muscular strain or haematoma.[401] As the condition progresses nerves within the fascia are destroyed and the severe pain will eventually be replaced by numbness.[425] The infection evolves rapidly over the next 24–72 hours, and even if the patient has been started on antibiotics, the erythema continues to spread, and the skin becomes smooth, shiny and intensely swollen.[409] This spreading erythema can progress by as much as 3–5 cm an hour[404,426] and failure of antibiotic therapy to halt its progression should be interpreted as a warning sign.[418] The skin begins to darken and takes on a patchy dusky blue hue with blistering, and as necrosis of the superficial fascia and fat takes place, 'dishwater' pus leaks from the skin which begins to take on a gangrenous appearance and starts to slough. By this stage, a large area of the skin/body may be affected. As organisms and toxins are released into the bloodstream, the patient displays signs of extreme systemic toxicity, and the cause of death is often from multi-organ failure as a result of overwhelming sepsis. The clinical presentation is summarised in Table 12.2.

Table 12.2 Clinical features of necrotising fasciitis

Erythema at the site of infection
Prodromal flu-like illness at the onset
Local severe pain which does not reflect the clinical finding
Spreading diffuse erythema
Skin begins to darken within the area of erythema – dusky blue with blistering
Skin becomes gangrenous – starts to slough

Diagnosis and management

Necrotising fasciitis is a surgical emergency and early diagnosis together with aggressive surgical debridement, empirical antibiotic therapy and supportive treatment in an intensive care unit are essential for a successful outcome.[416,427]

Although imaging techniques such as x-rays, computed tomography (CT) and magnetic resonance imaging (MRI) may show localised swelling of the deep structures, and infection spreading along tissue planes along with gas in the soft tissues[428], the patient's condition may have deteriorated to such an extent that the use of imaging techniques will not be an option. In some cases no abnormalities will be detected and any delay in initiating surgery can increase the mortality rate.[416,421,429] Surgical exploration is the only satisfactory way to confirm the diagnosis, and any patient presenting with atypical cellulitis should be referred for an urgent surgical opinion.[410] Tissue damage is often much more extensive than is apparent from an examination of the skin's surface, with the spread of infection internally out-pacing the apparent spread externally, and consequently the amount of debridement required is often grossly underestimated.[430,431] The involvement of specialist surgical teams may be required depending on the extent of the infection and the body site involved.[416,432] In order to ensure that all non-viable tissue is removed, surgical debridement has to be aggressive and extensive, and further exploration and debridement is required 24–48 hours later to check that the infection has been halted. This may be required on a daily basis for several days.[410,433] If the infection involves the perineum, the formation of a defunctioning colostomy may be required. In cases of necrotising fasciitis involving a limb, amputation of the extremity may be the only surgical option. Once surgical exploration and debridement is no longer necessary, patients may still have to return to theatre daily so that the wound dressings can be changed under general anaesthetic. Skin grafting is often required so the wound can be covered, and vacuum-assisted closure therapy (VAC) may be needed to promote healing and aid closure of the wound. Reconstructive surgery may be required at a later date.[410,416] Patients will be cared for in the intensive care unit in order to provide the intravenous fluid resuscitation, mechanical ventilation and inotropic support necessary to manage septic shock (see Chapter 5 Understanding the Immune System and the Nature and Pathogenesis of Infection).

Antibiotic therapy should be initiated at the onset of symptoms and the combination prescribed should be recommended by a microbiologist. The bacterial cause of necrotising fasciitis is confirmed by blood culture along with cultures from the wound. In cases caused by severe group A streptococcal disease, 69–97 % of patients will have a positive blood culture, and wound swabs and aspirate taken from the actual site of the infection will be positive in 65 % of cases.[434] Initially it is important that the antibiotic cover provided has a broad spectrum of activity, as the infection may be polymicrobial in origin, so it should cover Gram-positive cocci, facultative anerobic Gram-negative rods and anaerobes. Benzlypenicillin is effective against Gram-positive cocci, as is clindamycin. Flucloxacillin is effective against *S.aureus*. Gentamicin is a potent broad spectrum agent which is not effective if given on its own but has a synergistic effect if given in combination with penicillin. Metronidazole is effective against anaerobic bacteria. The antibiotic regimen can then be modified once the results of blood and wound cultures are known.

STREPTOCOCCAL TOXIC SHOCK SYNDROME

Streptococcal toxic shock syndrome (STSS) is essentially any streptococcal infection associated with the sudden onset of shock and multi-organ failure, with or without necrotising fasciitis, and carries a mortality rate of approximately 45 %.[397,401]

Risk factors

Unlike necrotising fasciitis, in which advanced age is a predisposing risk factor, STSS can affect any age group, with cases documented in children and healthy young adults.[434,435] Many people affected by it do not have a history of any underlying medical conditions. Surgical procedures are a recognised risk factor in both diseases and whereas necrotising fasciitis can be a rare complication following abdominal or perineal surgery, STSS can occur following 'routine' procedures such as hernia repair, bunionectomy, vasectomy and childbirth.[401] It can also occur following infections such as meningitis, septic arthritis, central venous catheter-related bacteraemia, otitis media, urinary tract infection and respiratory tract infection.[433] Blunt trauma resulting in haematoma formation and muscle strain have both been documented as causes of STSS, with clinical signs occurring within 24–72 hours of the injury.

Clinical presentation

Approximately 20 % of patients will complain of a prodromal influenza-like illness, experiencing high fever, chills, muscular aches and pain, vomiting and diarrhoea, along with signs of confusion.[423] These signs may precede the onset of hypotension by 24–48 hours, and by the time the patient is admitted, the signs of shock are either already apparent or follow within 4–8 hours.[401,434] Where there is a defined portal of entry, signs of soft tissue infection may be evident which increases the risk of the patient developing necrotising fasciitis, with the patient complaining of severe pain. A diffuse spreading erythematous rash may also be present over the body. Some patients may just present with overwhelming septic shock and die within 24–48 hours of admission to hospital.[433]

Diagnosis and management

In patients who present with septic shock and early signs of organ dysfunction, STSS should be suspected and a search for the site of infection initiated promptly.[431] Clinically the patient should be treated for septic shock, requiring empirical broad spectrum antibiotic therapy, and respiratory, haemodynamic and renal support in the intensive care unit. Cultures should be taken to determine the source of the infection and the skin examined for signs of a possible portal of entry even if there are no apparent signs of recent skin trauma. If the patient exhibits signs of soft tissue infection, prompt and aggressive surgical exploration and debridement will be necessary.

INFECTION CONTROL PRECAUTIONS FOR INVASIVE GROUP A STREPTOCOCCAL DISEASE

As group A streptococcus is a highly invasive organism, strict adherence to infection control precautions is essential in order to prevent cross-infection not only to other patients but also to healthcare workers. The infection control precautions are summarised in Table 12.3.

INTERIM UK GUIDELINES FOR THE MANAGEMENT OF CLOSE COMMUNITY CONTACTS OF INVASIVE GROUP A STREPTOCOCCAL DISEASE[397]

These guidelines were developed in 2004 by the Group A Streptococcus Working Group of the Health Protection Agency and provide recommendations for the management of individuals who have had close contact with a case of invasive group A streptococcal disease and who are therefore at increased risk of developing the disease themselves. All cases of suspected/confirmed invasive disease should be reported to the relevant consultant in communicable disease control (CCDC), and clinical isolates sent to the relevant national reference laboratory. The appendix to the guidelines contains the necessary information with regard to contact details. A close contact is defined as any person who has had prolonged close contact with the index case in a household-type setting during the seven days before the onset of illness. In the event of an outbreak of invasive disease occurring within a nursing home facility, where the mortality rate may be particularly high given the patient population and increased susceptibility, all residents and staff may be treated as close contacts. In order to prevent transmission, chemoprophylaxis is necessary to eradicate carriage in those contacts at highest risk of invasive disease. This can be achieved by eradicating carriage from established carriers who pose a risk to others, along with the eradication of carriage in those who have newly acquired an invasive strain and are therefore at increased risk of developing invasive disease themselves.

The working party recommend that antibiotic prophylaxis is only prescribed in the following circumstances:

– to mother and baby if either develops invasive group A streptococcal disease within the first 28 days after delivery
– to close contacts if they themselves have symptoms suggestive of localised group A streptococcal infection, such as a throat or skin infection.

Contacts should be made aware that if they develop symptoms suggestive of invasive group A streptococcal disease, such as a high fever accompanied by severe muscular aches or localised muscular pain, they should attend an accident and emergency department for an urgent medical assessment. All other close contacts should be given a group A streptococcal information leaflet which outlines the signs

Table 12.3 Infection control precautions for invasive group A streptococcal disease

Isolation	Patients with invasive group A streptococcal disease should be nursed in a single room with the door kept closed until they have received 48 hours' treatment with antibiotics. In the case of necrotising fasciitis, the patient should continue to remain in isolation until all necrotic tissue has been debrided.
Visitors	Patients with invasive group A streptococcal disease can receive visitors; they should be advised on the importance of keeping any skin breaks covered and to decontaminate their hands with alcohol hand rub on leaving the side room/ward. Visitors who meet the case definition for 'close contacts' will be managed according to the HPA guidelines.
Hand hygiene	All staff should ensure that they decontaminate their hands with alcohol hand rub on entering and leaving the isolation room, after contact with the patient/contaminated equipment and before contact with another patient. If hands are visibly soiled with dirt and/or body fluids, hands should be washed with liquid soap and water.
Personal protective equipment and clothing	Disposable aprons and gloves should be worn if there is any episode of direct contact with the patient or with equipment within the immediate patient environment. They should be removed and disposed of as clinical waste immediately after each activity.
Linen	All linen should be treated as contaminated/infected and disposed of in red linen bags and according to local policy/national guidance.
Waste	Clinical waste should be disposed of according to local policy and national guidance.
Decontamination of equipment	Equipment can harbour bacteria, potentially increasing the risk of the spread of infection. Where possible, the patient should be allocated equipment that is single-patient use and disposable, or equipment that can remain with the patient during their time in hospital and either be disposed of or decontaminated appropriately when the patient has been discharged home. Any equipment which is multi-patient use, such as wheelchairs, commodes, monitors, sphygmomanometers etc must be decontaminated in between each patient use, either using detergent wipes or cleaned according to the manufacturer's instructions.
Decontamination of the environment	Streptococci can survive for long periods in the environment, particularly in dust, and the patient environment should be kept clean and free from dust and dirt, reducing environmental reservoirs and decreasing the risk of the spread of infection to others. When the patient is de-isolated, discharged or if the patient is transferred to another ward, the immediate bed area must be thoroughly cleaned according to local policy, bedside curtains changed and equipment decontaminated. This should include the cleaning of bedside audio-visual equipment.
Care of the deceased patient	A patient who has died of invasive group A streptococcal disease should be placed in a body bag.

and symptoms of invasive disease and be advised to seek urgent medical attention if they develop any of the clinical signs described. Oral penicillin V, 250–500 mgs four times a day for 10 days, is the drug of choice. In the event of penicillin allergy, azithromycin (erythromycin) 12mgs/kg/day for five days is a suitable alternative as long as the index case isolate is sensitive.

Further information on necrotising fasciitis and group A streptococcal infections can be found on the web.[436,437,438]

13 Meningococcal Disease

INTRODUCTION

Invasive meningococcal disease, presenting as meningitis, septicaemia (meningococcemia) or both, with its dramatic clinical presentation and rapid disease progression, is a life-threatening condition which constitutes a medical emergency. Meningococcal disease is endemic across the globe occurring in both developed and undeveloped countries and representing a major public health concern. Globally it is estimated that there are more than one million cases of meningococcal disease every year which result in 135,000 deaths.[439] Children account for the greatest number of cases, and meningitis, with or without septicaemia, is recognised as the leading infectious cause of death in childhood and the third most common cause of death in children outside infancy after cot death, accidents and malignancy.[440,441] It is not surprising that it is the childhood disease that parents fear the most[442], but it can affect any age group and meningococcal meningitis is the second most common cause of community acquired bacterial meningitis in adults, with approximately 900 adult cases reported each year.[443,444]

This chapter provides an overview of invasive meningococcal disease. It begins by looking at the causative organism, *Neisseria meningitidis*, and the epidemiology of meningococcal disease and the scale of the global situation; meningitis and meningococcal septicaemia are then described, along with the pathogenesis of meningococcal infection and the clinical presentation of disease in both children and adults; antibiotic therapy, the infection control precautions, chemoprophylaxis for close contacts and healthcare workers, and vaccination are also discussed.

LEARNING OUTCOMES

After reading this chapter, the reader will be able to:

- Define 'meningitis' and 'septicaemia'
- Discuss the pathogenesis of meningococcal infection
- Describe the clinical presentation in both children and adults
- Identify the infection control precautions that need to be taken, including the administration of chemoprophylaxis to close contacts

THE ORGANISM

Neisseria is the only pathogenic Gram-negative coccus[445,446], and the bacterial cause of invasive meningococcal disease – *Neisseria meningitidis*, also known as the meningococcus – and gonorrhoea – *Neisseria gonorrhoeae*. *Neisseria* grow in pairs (diplococci) and are bean-shaped, with their concave sides facing inwards. They have exacting growth requirements, and are susceptible to inhibitory agents within culture media, growing best in media with heated blood and/or ascitic fluid (CSF) added.[447] This results in growth of grey glistening colonies, 0.5–1.0 mm in diameter, within 18–24 hours although they are relatively slow growers and require a further 24 hours incubation to produce larger colonies.[447] In order to differentiate between the species, which are indistinguishable under the microscope and on culture media, sugar fermentation tests are performed, with *N.meningitidis* fermenting both glucose and maltose, while *N.gonorrhoea* only ferments glucose.[448]

The most important virulence factor of the meningococcus, which accounts for its invasiveness, is the antigenically diverse lipopolysacchaide (LPS) capsule. Meningococci can be segregated into 13 different serogroups – A, B, C, D, X, Y, Z, W135, 29E, H, I, K and L – according to their capsular antigens.[449] Serogroups A, B and C account for approximately 90 % of cases of meningococcal disease, with W135 also causing significant problems in some parts of the world. X and Y account for very few cases, and Z and 29E generally only tend to pose any risk to those who have underlying disease.[447] Serogroup D is no longer recognised as being of any significance.[450] The identification of serogroups is usually only undertaken in a reference laboratory and once the meningococcus has been isolated from a clinical specimen such as blood or CSF, the isolate is sent away to the reference laboratory for typing. This is particularly important in instances where there is an outbreak, or a cluster, of meningococcal disease, and public health measures are required involving chemoprophylaxis for close contacts.

As the meningococcus is a Gram-negative organism, it produces endotoxin in the form of lipid A, which forms part of the lipopolysacchaide capsule (see Chapter 2 Bacterial and Viral Classification, Structure and Function). Blood bacterial loads increase very rapidly and the endotoxin is not only shed in steady amounts from living bacteria, but also released in large quantities when the bacteria is dead.[445,451] Lipid A causes the blood vessels to haemorrhage, visible on the skin or conjunctiva of the eyes as tiny round dots called petechiae[445], and also gives rise to septic shock, a common manifestation seen in meningococcal disease.

EPIDEMIOLOGY

Meningococcal meningitis was first described as epidemic cerebrospinal fever, following an outbreak in Geneva in 1805[449], although *Neisseria meningitidis* wasn't identified as the bacterial cause until 1887 when it was isolated from CSF, and the relationship between the organism and the disease established.[452] The case fatality rate in meningococcal disease varies according to the prevalence of the disease within the community and the serogroup involved and, in some parts of the world, the economic and social infrastructure of the area as many of the worst affected areas are remote and inaccessible.[449,452] The highest burden of meningococcal disease is seen in sub-Saharan Africa, where the African 'meningitis belt' runs from Senegal in the west to Ethiopia in the east, encompassing 15 countries and a population of 300 million people.[452] During 1996, this region saw the largest outbreak of meningococcal disease in history, with more than 250,000 cases and 25,000 deaths. Epidemics within the meningitis belt are caused by serogroups A, C and, in recent years, W135, with attack rates as high as 1,000 per 100,000 population.[452]

In 2000/2001, an international outbreak of meningococcal disease caused by serogroup W135 occurred in Saudi Arabia among 2,000 pilgrims going to the Hajj in Mecca, resulting in 424 cases and 96 deaths spread across 12 countries, and also affecting close family contacts of the pilgrims.[453,454] Prior to this W135 had not been associated with epidemics, so this outbreak was particularly significant. Consequently, public health policy changed and from 2002 it became a visa requirement that all pilgrims entering Saudi Arabia are vaccinated with the quadrivalent (non-conjugated) polysaccharide meningococcal vaccine. This offers short-term protection lasting three–five years in older children and protecting adults[52] against serogroups A, C, W135 and Y, and is recommended for all travellers to countries where possible acquisition of meningococcal disease is considered to be a high risk.[455,456]

In the UK, 50 % of cases of meningococcal disease occur in children under the age of five[457] and the incidence is approximately 5 per 100,000 population.[451] Provisional data from the HPA for 2004-2005 estimates that there were 1,462 confirmed laboratory reports of *N.meningitidis*, of which 1,288 were caused by group B and 43 by group C.[458] Group C used to account for 40 % of all cases of meningococcal infection but following the introduction of the new meningococcal C (MenC) conjugate vaccines and the meningitis C rolling immunisation programme in November 1999, which was the biggest vaccination drive in 40 years, cases fell dramatically, with the overall incidence of group C disease reduced by 90 %.[52] MenC conjugate vaccines are made from capsular polysaccharide (see Chapter 2 Bacterial and Viral Classification, Structure and Function) extracted from cultures of group C *Neisseria meningitides*.[52] They are conjugated, or linked, to a carrier protein such as tetanus toxoid or a non-toxic derivative of diptheria toxin (RM 197)[52,459] which increases the immunogenicity of the vaccine, stimulates a T and B-cell generated immune response and produces immunological memory and long-term protection[459] (see Chapter 5 Understanding the Immune System and the Nature and Pathogenesis of Infection). During the first year of the MenC vaccination programme, approximately 13 million children under the age of 12 months were immunised, followed in 2000/2001 by all other children up to the age of 18. The vaccine was then made available to all young adults up to the age of 25. There is no vaccination against group B disease, which now accounts for 80 % of cases of laboratory confirmed cases of meningococcal disease in the UK, with the greatest burden of disease seen in children under the age of 5.[52]

THE PATHOGENESIS OF INFECTION

The meningococcus is a normal inhabitant of the upper respiratory tract, residing in the nasopharynx, and carried asymptomatically by 10 % of the general population, although only 1 % are estimated to carry an invasive strain.[460] It is transmitted from person to person through prolonged or close contact with a carrier and their respiratory secretions. The average period of meningococcal carriage is estimated to last nine months[461] although there are reports that the carriers fall into three distinct groups – chronic, intermittent and transient, and that the chronic carrier state can persist for up to two years.[449] Carriers rarely go on to develop invasive disease, and although the transition from the carrier state to invasive disease is not clearly understood, it primarily occurs in individuals who become newly infected with meningococcus or in a carrier where the immune defences are weakened through illness.[449] Carriage rates have been found to be high in smokers, in military institutions and among students in their first term at university living in shared accommodation on campus, and may increase in areas where there are epidemics/outbreaks of meningococcal disease. Carriage is associated with the production of natural antibodies[446,447,449] and systemic immunity normally develops within 14 days of acquisition of the organism.[462] In pregnancy, maternal antibodies cross the placenta and provide protection for the first few months of life. However, there is a window period from six months – two years when young children are without protection as their own antibodies are slow to develop, and this explains why infants and young children are so susceptible to meningococcal infection and why the attack rate is so high in this age group.[449]

Risk factors for meningococcal carriage and invasive disease are summarised in Table 13.1

Infection of the central nervous system (CNS) is actually a rare event as the blood-brain barrier inhibits the entry of micro-organisms.[463,464] The barrier is a membrane created by the endothelial cells which line the small blood vessels, or capillaries, of the brain. In other parts of the body, there are gaps between the endothelial cells, allowing soluble chemicals within the tissues to pass into the bloodstream. Within the brain, tight junctions between the epithelial cells prevent the free exchange of substances between the blood and the brain[464,465], but if the CNS is invaded, the

Table 13.1 Risk factors for meningococcal carriage and invasive disease

Smoking.
Residence in overcrowded households and institutions e.g. university campuses and military institutions.
Travel to parts of the world where meningococcal disease is endemic.
Peak incidence in carriage and outbreaks during the winter months.
Lack of immunity to circulating strains.
Age < 1 year.
Recent influenza infection.
Complement deficiency.

attack comes via the bloodstream from organisms which have colonised other body sites and then entered the bloodstream.

MENINGITIS

Meningitis is infection of the meninges and the CSF surrounding the brain and spinal cord. The process of infection begins on the nasopharyngeal surface where the organism uses pili (see Chapter 2 Bacterial and Viral Classification, Structure and Function) to attach to the microvilli of the non-ciliated nasopharyngeal epithelial cells.[446] It then enters the microvilli, passing through the cell and into the submucosa. From there it is transported via the bloodstream to the ventricles of the brain, where it directly infects the choroid plexus and enters the CSF, which contains little in the way of immune defences. The meningococci are lysed into the subarachnoid space and the cell wall toxins induce inflammation of the meninges and stimulate cytokine release (see Chapter 5 Understanding the Immune System and the Nature and Pathogenesis of Infection) which result in the physiological and physical manifestations of headache, fever and raised intracranial pressure, indicating meningitis. Of those patients with meningococcal meningitis, 5 % will die.[456]

MENINGOCOCCAL SEPTICAEMIA

Meningococcal septicaemia carries a fatality rate of 20–50 %.[456] If the meningococci enter the bloodstream, they initiate a massive inflammatory response, which stimulates the release of inflammatory mediators such as tumor necrosis factor (TNF) and interleukin -1 (IL-1), along with neutrophils, monocytes and platelets. The patient displays signs of septicaemia and septic shock (described in Chapter 5 Understanding the Immune System and the Nature and Pathogenesis of Infection). The most important distinguishing sign in meningococcal septicaemia is the appearance of a haemorrhagic rash, caused by haemorrhaging in the capillaries of the small blood vessels as a result of clotting abnormalities.

CLINICAL PRESENTATION

Meningococcal disease presents in two distinct ways – meningococcal meningitis and/or septicaemia – but the presenting signs and symptoms can vary widely. Patients presenting with meningococcal septicaemia alone may have different symptoms to those with meningitis, and those with meningitis may quickly progress to exhibiting signs of septicaemia. Unfortunately it is all too common for the diagnosis of invasive meningococcal disease to be delayed or missed altogether, particularly in cases involving babies and young infants. Deterioration tends to be swift and death can occur within a matter of hours, so rapid diagnosis is absolutely crucial to survival. Healthcare workers should have a high index of suspicion and look for signs of meningococcal disease in any patient who presents with a febrile illness but without any obvious cause of fever.

More often than not it is the non-specific symptoms of meningococcal disease – vomiting, diarrhoea, fever, muscle and joint pain, lethargy and headache, seen in both children and adults – which cloud the picture and hinder the diagnosis. Patients attending the accident and emergency department or the GP surgery may be sent home with a diagnosis of influenza or gastroenteritis or a 'viral infection', only to return in a matter of hours with obvious symptoms of meningitis and/or in profound septic shock. Children in particular may become ill very rapidly.[440,456] As the disease progresses, the clinical features become more specific. If meningitis is present, the patient will complain of a severe headache, associated with neck stiffness and *photophobia* attributable to inflammation and irritation of the meninges covering the brain and the spinal cord. Neck stiffness and *photophobia* may be absent in children, but their absence does *not exclude* meningitis. As the **intracranial pressure** rises, CNS function decreases and patients may exhibit signs of irritability, drowsiness and impaired levels of consciousness.[440,456] They may appear combative and aggressive – signs which could be mistaken for drug abuse. In newborn babies and infants, non-specific signs of meningitis include fever, vomiting, diarrhoea, irritability, distress when handled with babies often giving a high pitched cry, and anorexia, with the baby/infant refusing feeds.[440,456] A specific, although late, sign of meningitis in babies is a bulging fontanelle, which indicates raised intracranial pressure.

Signs of meningococcal sepsis in both children and adults, occurring with or without meningitis, include pallor, tachycardia and tachyapnoea, cyanois, rigors, and cold extremities due to poor capillary refill.[440,456] Changes in conscious level are seen, although in the early stages of shock children are often alert and able to speak. **The presence of a non-blanching peticheal rash in any age group is one of the most important signs to recognise as it indicates septicaemia and patients may have septicaemia with no evidence of meningitis.** The rash may present in a number of ways[440,456]; as red or brown pin-prick marks which may resemble flea bites; purple blotches; bruises (where it can be mistaken for injury, trauma or abuse) or blood blisters. It may be profuse or scanty, and in the very early stages in children, it may be macropapular in appearance and may be mistaken for measles. On dark skin it can be difficult to see but it can be detected on lighter areas such as the palms of the hands, soles of the feet, abdomen, conjunctivae or palate of the mouth. Examination of the entire skin surface is essential, and should be carried out frequently – if there is no evidence of a rash on initial examination, it does not mean that it will not develop. **The most important diagnostic aid in determining whether or not the rash is non-blanching is to press a glass tumbler against it; the rash will not fade and the marks will be visible through the glass.**[440,456]

The presence of shock, an extensive or rapidly progressive skin rash and a reduced level of consciousness, in either adults or children, are strongly associated with a fatal outcome.[460]

ANTIBIOTIC THERAPY

The outcome in meningococcal disease is therefore largely dependent upon swift diagnosis, which may be based on the index of suspicion, and the initiation of the appropriate treatment, although some hold the view that the outcome of meningococcal disease has not improved at all since the 1960s, in spite of the use of antibiotics and the availability of intensive care units for the treatment and management of cases.[443] Early treatment of cases with benzylpenicillin, carried by all GPs, and swift transfer to hospital are the highest priority in order to reduce the case fatality.[466]

LABORATORY DIAGNOSIS

Although a diagnosis of invasive meningococcal disease can be made based on the presenting clinical picture, definitive diagnosis is dependent upon culturing meningococci from CSF (critical in the diagnosis of meningitis) and/or blood. CSF is secreted by the epithelial cells of the choroid plexus within the brain and circulates in the subarachnoid space. A sample is obtained by lumbar puncture, which is performed using a strict aseptic technique to avoid contaminating the specimen and introducing infection from skin flora or other organisms into the site. If antibiotics have been administered prior to either specimen being obtained, the sensitivity of the microbiology results will be reduced[449] but this does not mean that antibiotic administration should be delayed. Lumber punctures are contra-indicated if there are signs of raised intra-cranial pressure, focal neurological deficits or space-occupying lesions, which could induce herniation, or coning, of the brain stem. Although raised intracranial pressure is only seen in the minority of patients, a CT-scan of the head is recommended in the first instance to detect any abnormalities, although these may not necessarily be apparent on the scan.[460,464]

Table 13.2 Signs of raised intracranial pressure

Headache
Hypertension and bradycardia
Fluctuating/decreasing levels of consciousness
Unequal, dilated or poorly reacting pupils
Papillodema (late sign)
Tense/bulging fontanelle in babies

Three specimens of CSF (1–2 mL each) are obtained and sent for microbiology and biochemistry and examined for complete cell count, differential leukocyte count, Gram-stained smear, culture for pathogens, protein and glucose concentrations and PCR[450] (see Chapter 3 The Collection and Transportation of Specimens and Chapter 4 The Microbiology Laboratory). The pressure of the CSF is also measured. Table 13.3 shows the normal values of CSF and the changes seen in bacterial meningitis.

Table 13.3 CSF values

	Normal	Meningitis
Appearance	Crystal clear	Turbid/purulent
Mononuclear cells	<5 mm^3	<50 mm^3
Polymorphonuclear cells	Nil	200–300 mm^3
Protein	0.2–0.4 g/l	0.5–2.0 g/l
Glucose	60–80 % of plasma glucose	<50 % of plasma glucose
CSF pressure	60–80 mm H$_2$O; abnormally low CSF is <50 mm	>200 mm

The appearance of the CSF will give a clue to the likely diagnosis prior to the specimen being processed in the laboratory. Normal CSF is clear and colourless; in cases of meningitis, the specimen will be turbid or purulent due to the presence of white bloodcells. It may also be bloodstained if the lumber puncture has been traumatic. In the microbiology laboratory, the specimen will be Gram-stained in order to identify Gram-negative diplococci on the smear and then cultured, and the number of white bloodcells counted. Generally, the sensitivity of Gram-staining is 65 % depending on the stage of the disease, the number of organisms and whether or not antibiotics have been administered.[466] The biochemistry laboratory will determine the glucose and protein concentrations. The concentration of glucose within CSF is approximately 70 % of the glucose concentration in the blood, and in order to interpret the CSF result, a blood sample should be taken at the time of the lumber puncture so that the results can be compared. The concentration of glucose within the CSF will be lower than the blood glucose concentration if bacteria are present as they metabolise glucose. The concentration of protein in CSF is raised due to an increase in capillary permeability resulting from the meningeal inflammation.

Both blood and CSF should be sent to the meningococcal reference unit for PCR (see Chapter 3 The Collection and Transportation of Specimens). The availability of rapid diagnosis by PCR has revolutionised the diagnosis of meningococcal septicaemia by allowing confirmation of the diagnosis on an *EDTA* blood sample despite any prior antibiotic treatment, which compromises the traditional blood culture method.

If the patient has peticheal skin lesions, a skin scraping or needle aspiration from an affected area can be sent to the microbiology laboratory for Gram-staining and culture. A nasopharyngeal swab should also be taken to detect possible nasopharyngeal carriage/colonisation.[449]

PROGNOSIS AND RECOVERY

While many people recovering from meningitis experience problems in the short term, one in seven are left with a permanent disability which may be neurological or physical. Hearing loss is the most common affliction and anyone who has had bacterial meningitis should have their hearing assessed.[460] Amputation of limbs or digits as a result of gangrene is sometimes required, with patients facing extensive surgery and skin grafting.

INFECTION CONTROL PRECAUTIONS

Meningococci do not survive outside of the nasopharynx, dying quickly once they have left the host[467], and so cross-infection from the environment does not occur.[468] However, as the meningococcus is carried in the nasopharynx and can be acquired via oral and respiratory secretions, secondary transmission to close contacts can occur.

The specific precautions to be taken when caring for a patient with suspected/confirmed meningococcal disease are summarised in Table 13.4.

PUBLIC HEALTH IMPLICATIONS

Meningococcal meningitis and septicaemia are notifiable diseases under the Public Health (Infectious Disease) Regulations 1988, and it is a legal requirement that all cases are reported to the local consultant in communicable disease control (CCDC) at the local health protection unit. The risk of invasive disease in household contacts is increased by 500–1,200 times, with the risk highest in the first seven days after the index case[460] and the CCDC is responsible for organising *chemoprophylaxis* for close contacts of the index case, with the aim of reducing the risk of invasive

Table 13.4 Infection control precautions for cases of suspected/confirmed meningococcal disease[86,467]

Isolation	Patients with suspected/confirmed meningococcal disease should be isolated in a single room with the door kept closed until they have received 24 hours of antibiotic therapy.
Personal protective equipment and clothing	Respiratory droplets/secretions are considered to be infectious from the onset of the acute illness until completion of 24 hours of antibiotic therapy; healthcare workers undertaking exposure-prone procedures such as airway management during resuscitation or intubation prior to mechanical ventilation should wear face/eye protection. Gloves/aprons are required for direct contact with secretions and should be removed on leaving the room and disposed of as clinical waste. HPA guidelines recommend that 'chemoprophylaxis is recommended only for those whose mouth or nose is directly exposed to large particle droplets/secretions from the respiratory tract of a probable or confirmed case of meningococcal disease during acute illness until the index case has completed 24 hours of systemic antibiotics . . . general medical or nursing care of cases is not an indication for prophylaxis'. Staff contacts requiring chemoprophylaxis may be determined by the infection prevention and control team in conjunction with the CCDC.
Visitors	Only family members who have had close contact with the patient prior to admission should be advised to visit the patient. They do not need to wear protective clothing but should be advised to decontaminate their hands prior to leaving the isolation room/ward. A list of close contacts will be forwarded to the CCDC at the health protection unit and the need for chemoprophylaxis determined.

disease through the eradication of nasopharyngeal carriage of *N.meningitidis,* and the prevention of community outbreaks.[460,469] As the index case is likely to have acquired the invasive strain from a close contact who is an asymptomatic carrier, eradicating carriage from unknown established carriers will reduce the risk of infection to other contacts. It will also eradicate carriage in those who may have newly acquired the organism and reduce the risk of invasive disease to themselves. The CCDC will determine who the close contacts are and information will need to be supplied to the local health protection unit with regard to their names and contact details.

The Health Protection Agency[467] defines close contacts as:

a) 'Those who have had prolonged close contact with the case in a household-type setting during the seven days before the onset of illness (i.e. living/sleeping in the same household, including extended household, shared dormitories, university students sharing facilities in a hall of residence, or boy/girlfriends).'

b) 'Those who have had transient close contact with a case only if they have been directly exposed to large particle droplets or secretions from the respiratory tract of a case around the time of admission to hospital.'

The drugs of choice for chemoprophylaxis are rifampicin (taken orally twice a day for two days), ciprofloxacin (one or two tablets given orally as a one-off dose) and ceftriaxone (injection only).[469] Rifampicin is recommended for all age groups, while ciprofloxacin can be used in adults and children over the age of two. Ceftriaxone or rifampicin can be administered to pregnant or breast-feeding women. Drug information leaflets should be given to individuals who require either rifampicin or ciprofloxacin chemoprophylaxis.

The index case will also need to receive chemoprophylaxis as, in spite of receiving treatment with benzylpenicillin, studies have shown that approximately 5 % of cases will carry the invasive strain following treatment.[469,470] If the disease is caused by serogroup C, recommendations are that the index case and close contacts should be offered the conjugate MenC vaccine if they are previously un-immunised, and that the quadrivalent polysaccharide vaccine (ACYW135 vaccine) is given to those exposed to serogroups A, W135 and Y.

Within the community setting, the management of clusters is dependent upon the number of probable or confirmed cases, the serogroup of the invasive strain, the dates of onset of symptomatic illness, links between cases, the population at risk, and the uptake of the MenC vaccine within the community.[469] The CCDC may then take the decision to initiate either a vaccination programme or administer wide-scale oral chemoprophylaxis.[469] Where clusters occur among pre-school groups (i.e. nursery/play groups) chemoprophylaxis is usually offered to staff and children. In other settings such as schools, colleges and universities, wide-scale chemoprophylaxis may be offered if a clear 'at risk' subgroup cannot be identified.

14 Norovirus

INTRODUCTION

Every winter there are reports in the media of ward or hospital closures due to outbreaks of small round structured viruses (SRSVs), 'winter vomiting disease' and norovirus infection, which most commonly occur when community outbreaks are at their height. These outbreaks result in massive disruption to the provision of healthcare services, can potentially result in death amongst elderly, debilitated or immuncompromised individuals, and cost NHS Trusts in the region of £657,000 in terms of lost bed days and staff sickness.[36] Add to that figure other costs arising as a result of extra cleaning requirements, bed blocking from delayed discharges and the impact on waiting list initiatives and government targets and it is easy to see why hospital managers and infection prevention and control teams dread the start of the winter norovirus season; logistically, these outbreaks can be a nightmare to manage for all concerned. However, while it is inevitable that many Trusts will experience problems with norovirus infection, much can be done to limit and control the impact and enable affected hospitals to return to normal working as soon as possible. Early recognition of symptoms and the prompt implementation of stringent infection control measures are key to preventing hospital-wide outbreaks.

This chapter looks at the epidemiology of norovirus infection, its transmission and the management of ward closures, drawing on the recommendations of the Public Health Laboratory Service Viral Gastroenteritis Working Group[470] which were published in 2000. Risk management issues are also discussed.

LEARNING OUTCOMES

After reading this chapter, the reader will:

- Understand the significance of norovirus outbreaks
- Be able to describe the clinical features of norovirus
- Understand the infection control precautions that need to be taken in order to reduce the risk of spread

THE VIRUSES

Noroviruses belong to the virus family *Caliciviridae*; the name is derived from the Latin word *calyx*, meaning goblet or cup, in reference to the 32 cup-shaped depressions on the surface of the capsid.[471,472] They are a group of non-enveloped single stranded RNA viruses and the causative agents of acute viral gastroenteritis in humans.[58] They are also known as small round structured viruses (SRSVs). SRSVs were first identified following an outbreak of non-bacterial gastroenteritis in the town of Norwalk, Ohio, USA, in 1968[58,473] where a range of morphologically identical viruses were later detected in 1972 by electron microscopy from saved stool samples.[471] Additional SRSVs have since been identified and named for the geographical region in which they were first identified[471] but they are often reported as Norwalk-like viruses (NLVs), which is the term adopted by the International Committee on the Taxonomy of Viruses[47], and they are now more commonly known as noroviruses. The media often reports outbreaks of norovirus infection as 'winter vomiting disease', which was first described in 1929[474] and so named because of its seasonal incidence and the dominant symptom of vomiting.

Noroviruses circulate within the community throughout the year, causing small clusters and outbreaks, and peaks in incidence have occurred globally with the emergence of new variant genotypes in 1995, 2002 and 2004.[474,475] There are now at least four different norovirus genogroups, divided into at least 20 different genetic clusters.[473] Large community outbreaks also often affect hotels, cruise ships, schools, colleges and nursing and residential homes.[470,476,477] The Health Protection Agency estimates that between 600,000 and 1 million people are affected in the UK each year[477] but as norovirus is not a notifiable disease, the true figures in relation to the number of outbreaks occurring annually and the number of individuals affected are not known. What cannot be underestimated though is the fact that these viruses are important pathogens, and while outbreaks can be perceived by those who have to deal with them as a nuisance, infection with norovirus is far from trivial.

TRANSMISSION, INCUBATION PERIOD AND CLINICAL FEATURES

Norovirus is highly contagious. It has been estimated that more than 30 million virus particles are released during vomiting[478] and the infecting dose necessary to induce symptoms is astonishingly small, at only 10–100 virus particles.[474,479] The incubation period is relatively short, ranging from 12–48 hours, and the attack rate is often more than 50 %, affecting both patients and staff. Cold foods such as sandwiches and salads, bakery items, liquids (including salad dressing and icing) and food contaminated at source, such as oysters harvested from contaminated waters, have all been implicated in outbreaks.[470,471,480,481] Within the healthcare setting, outbreaks arise as a result of faecal-oral spread and person to person spread following the dissemination of virus particles through the air, which leads to widespread environmental and fomite contamination. Hard surfaces, equipment and soft furnishings readily become contaminated, along with food, particularly if handled by a contaminated or infected food handler, and water jugs.[470] Since contaminated fingers can transfer norovirus on to as many as seven clean surfaces[482], and the virus can remain viable within the environment for up to 12 days[483], controlling transmission presents a major challenge.

There is no prodromal illness before the onset of symptoms, which are typically explosive.[473] Diarrhoea and vomiting are the presenting clinical features, although not all affected individuals experience both symptoms. While vomiting appears to result in greater numbers of individuals becoming infected because of airborne spread, diarrhoea can also be problematic. Norovirus can continue to be excreted in faeces after the symptoms have resolved[404], but it is also thought that virus excretion can occur before the onset of symptoms[485], giving rise to the possibility of norovirus being transmissible prior to the onset of clinical symptoms and after resolution, potentially prolonging outbreaks. Other symptoms, including nausea, abdominal cramps, headache and **myalgia**, are commonly reported following onset of the initial symptoms.[486]

Although the duration of illness is generally short, lasting between 12–60 hours, and symptoms may be mild in some, the elderly often bear the brunt of norovirus infections with prolonged duration of symptoms[485], and may be more severely affected than younger 'healthy' individuals. Immunity to noroviruses is thought to be strain-specific and may only last a few months.[476] It is possible for individuals to be affected several times during their lifetime, and during the course of an outbreak some may be affected on more than one occasion if there is more than one strain of norovirus in circulation. The clinical features of norovirus are summarised in Table 14.1.

Table 14.1 Clinical features of norovirus[470]

Sudden abrupt onset of symptoms
Watery profuse diarrhoea and/or projectile vomiting
Short incubation period of 12–24 hours
High attack rate, affecting > 50 % of patients and staff
Short illness duration of one to three days

PARTICULAR PROBLEMS ASSOCIATED WITH REPORTING 'DIARRHOEA'

It is important that staff understand what is meant by the word 'diarrhoea', as healthcare professionals often rely on their own subjective opinion as to whether or not patients have diarrhoea.[487] To simply report cases of 'loose stools' is particularly unhelpful to the infection prevention and control team, and it is important that the team establishes a case definition (see Table 14.2) and that staff are aware of it. The form of the stool is determined by the faecal transit time and 'true'

Table 14.2 Suggested case definition for norovirus

Sudden onset of profuse watery diarrhoea and/or explosive vomiting in an individual with no other explanation for their symptoms.
OR
A patient with sudden onset of watery diarrhoea only, without any other explanation for their illness, occurring in the context of a cluster of probable cases.

Reproduced by permission of East Kent Hospitals NHS Trust

diarrhoea is the frequent passing of liquid/watery stool with very little, if any, solid contents. The Bristol Stool Chart[488] can be a useful tool in identifying different stool types. In addition, while it can, on occasions, be difficult to completely exclude an infectious cause in a patient with diarrhoea and/or vomiting, to report *all* patients experiencing diarrhoea or vomiting can be misleading, particularly if there is an established or suspected cause for the symptoms seen in that individual; for example, diarrhoea in the post-operative period following bowel surgery; post operative nausea and vomiting; medication; laxative/enema administration; long-standing history of diarrhoea of a chronic nature, as in irritable bowel syndrome or colitis. As the infection prevention and control team have to make decisions with regard to ward closures based on the information that they are given by ward staff, and as ward closure can have implications for patient care, it is absolutely crucial that the information given to them is accurate and reliable.

LABORATORY DIAGNOSIS

Ideally, samples of unformed stool should be obtained within 48 hours of the onset of symptoms and sent to the laboratory immediately. However, in spite of the infectious nature of norovirus, relatively low numbers of virus are actually shed in faeces (10^6 viruses/g faeces[486]) so detection of virus particles in faecal specimens is not always particularly reliable. Electron microscopy has traditionally been the first-line diagnostic tool for identifying SRSVs but although it is rapid, it is not particularly sensitive and less than 50 % of all faecal stool samples tested will be negative. Other diagnostic methods such as PCR and ELISA are more reliable (See Chapter 4 The Microbiology Laboratory) but may still yield a negative result. Infection prevention and control teams generally make a diagnosis of norovirus infection based on the clinical features and the attack rate.

MANAGEMENT OF OUTBREAKS

In 2000, the PHLS Viral Gastroenteritis Working Group[470] issued guidance on the management of SRSV outbreaks, which are generally regarded as the UK standard for management of outbreaks. Many Trusts have since adapted these guidelines for their own use, and used them as the basis for their own norovirus outbreak policy. This section looks at the recommendations of these guidelines in detail, focusing on ward closures and control of spread, staffing issues, and decontamination.

WARD CLOSURES

The closure of hospital wards is always controversial and unpopular given the pressure on beds, particularly during the winter months which generally see an increase in admissions, particularly on medical wards. If any patient suddenly develops vomiting and/or diarrhoea, and there is no other explanation for their symptoms, viral gastroenteritis should be suspected. Similarly, reports of illness among healthcare staff working on a ward should be reported and treated with suspicion. Norovirus should also be suspected in patients admitted to wards with a history of diarrhoea and vomiting, and such patients should be isolated in a single room until an infectious cause is disregarded. The decision to close a ward will be based on the clinical features and the numbers of patients, and possibly staff, affected, and will be made by the infection prevention and control team in conjunction with the hospital managers. Given the low infectious dose and widespread environmental contamination that arises once patients become symptomatic, several cases may be seen on a ward within a matter of hours. Although a patient who is symptomatic on admission can be immediately isolated, there is probably little to be gained from moving a symptomatic patient in an open bay or ward into a side room, unless it takes place immediately after the onset of symptoms and stringent cleaning measures are initiated. A bay of potentially infected patients can be closed to new admissions and watched carefully over the next 12–48 hours; if a case occurs in the open ward, it is more difficult to manage.

If the ward is closed, it is because of the necessity of preventing not only the introduction of susceptible patients into an infected environment, but also to reduce the risk of spread to other areas. If unrestrained patient movement occurs between affected and unaffected wards and departments, it could quite quickly result in a hospital-wide outbreak with potentially enormous repercussions.

Transfers to other wards, departments and even other hospitals should be avoided unless medically urgent and any non-urgent investigations should be cancelled. The decision to cancel patient investigations ultimately rests with the medical team and should never be made by anyone else. The restriction of patient movement applies to all patients on the ward. Those who are not initially affected will have been exposed to infected patients and could potentially be in the incubation phase of the illness and they could become symptomatic at any time and without warning. In the event of clinically important investigations being required, it should be the responsibility of the medical team and the nurse in charge of the ward to ensure that the receiving departments are informed and that the appropriate arrangements are in place. Wards should remain closed until 72 hours after the onset of the last new case, and any remaining symptomatic patients are recovering. Ideally, anyone remaining symptomatic at the time the ward is due to re-open should be moved into a single room. The '72 hour rule' takes into account the typical incubation period of 24 hours, and the maximum period of infectivity, which is usually 48 hours.

MANAGEMENT OF STAFF

The guidelines[470] recommend that staff working on an affected ward should not work on an unaffected ward until 48 hours after the end of their shift, although staff who have had norovirus and returned to work can move between wards if required. Unfortunately, given that outbreaks often decimate the workforce, staff movement between affected and unaffected wards may have to occur following a risk assessment. The use of agency or bank staff is often increased during outbreaks, and if working on an affected ward, they should be block booked where possible, although this may be easier said than done.

Essential healthcare staff will still need to visit the ward, and given the complexities of patient care, medical teams in particular often work across wards. If at all possible, staff such as physiotherapists and occupational therapists should either be allocated to the closed ward, or advised to visit it last, and non-essential personnel discouraged from visiting the ward altogether. However, as well as taking steps to reduce the spread of infection, it is important to remember that patient care overall takes precedence and should not be compromised, and staff movement and ward visits need to be risk assessed by the infection prevention and control team in conjunction with the staff involved.

If *any* member of staff becomes symptomatic while on duty, they should be sent home and not return to work until they have been asymptomatic for 48 hours. Similarly, staff who become ill at home should refrain from working until they have been asymptomatic for 48 hours.

INFECTION CONTROL PRECAUTIONS

These centre on hand decontamination, isolation or cohorting of patients, the use of protective clothing, the cleaning up of vomit and faeces and the restricting of visitors to closed wards.

Hand decontamination

As with all infections, hand decontamination is the single most important preventative measure when controlling cross-infection.[86] Although alcohol hand rubs are effective against a wide range of organisms with the exception of *Clostridium difficile* they are ineffective against organic material such as dirt, blood and body fluids, and if hands are visibly soiled they should be washed with liquid soap and water. Patients should be offered the opportunity to wash or decontaminate their hands[125], particularly before eating, as they may acquire norovirus via the faecal-oral route due to the environmental contamination that arises. Hand wipes offer a suitable alternative to hand washing or alcohol hand rub, the application of which may be beyond some patients. Visitors to the ward should also be asked to decontaminate their hands with alcohol hand rub on entering and leaving the ward.

Isolation or cohort nursing of symptomatic patients

Depending on the size and layout of the affected ward, together with the patient group involved, it may be possible to cohort the patients, dividing them into those who are symptomatic, those who are directly exposed to a symptomatic patient but currently asymptomatic themselves, or those who are asymptomatic and who haven't been directly exposed. This may allow the ward to function in a relatively normal fashion for a period of time. However, unless the ward has bays with doors that can be closed, effectively sealing it off from the rest of the ward, airborne transmission of norovirus particles and spread to the rest of the ward is probably inevitable, followed by complete ward closure.

Symptomatic new admissions via the A&E department or elsewhere can be admitted into closed wards. The admission of patients, symptomatic or otherwise, is discussed later in this chapter under Risk Management.

The use of protective clothing

Disposable aprons and gloves should be worn for, and changed in between, each episode of direct contact with a symptomatic patient or a piece of potentially contaminated equipment.[86] There is no evidence to support the wearing of masks.

Dealing with vomit and faeces

It is important that bedpan washers and macerators are fully functional and any problems should be reported to the estates department immediately. Bedpan washers should be holding their temperature at 80 °C for one minute to ensure that disinfection takes place. Macerators should not be opened until one minute after the cycle has finished, preventing the dissemination of aerosols into the environment and over the healthcare worker who has opened the lid.

Any body-fluid spillages should be dealt with immediately in order to reduce environmental contamination and cross-infection to patients and staff. Removing spillages from hard surfaces such as lino flooring is straightforward as they are easily cleaned. Protective clothing must be worn and paper towels must be used to soak up the excess liquid which, together with any solid waste, must be placed in a yellow clinical waste bag. The contaminated area must then be cleaned using detergent and water and a disposable cloth, and disinfected with a solution of 0.1 % hypochlorite (1,000 ppm). The gloves, aprons and disposable cloths should also be disposed of as clinical waste. A spillage of vomit or diarrhoea in the middle of a bay of patients necessitates cleaning of the entire bay. Contaminated bed linen and curtains should be treated as infected and carefully placed in red soluble alginate linen bags, taking care not to generate aerosols. Pillows with an impermeable cover can be wiped using a solution of 1,000 ppm hypochlorite but if they are impermeable, they should be laundered along with the infected linen.

Patient discharges

From an infection control perspective any patient who is medically fit, including those who are symptomatic, should be discharged from an affected ward as soon as the appropriate arrangements are in place. However, discharges or transfers to other hospitals or nursing and residential homes should be postponed until 72 hours after the onset of the last new case, unless the patient concerned has had norovirus and recovered. If a patient from a closed ward requires transfer to another ward or hospital on medically urgent grounds, the receiving ward must be informed and the infection control and prevention team informed. An asymptomatic patient moving from a closed to an unaffected ward should ideally be isolated for at least 48 hours in case they are incubating the illness.

Visitors

Restricting visiting during norovirus outbreaks can cause considerable upset to patients and their families, but there are a number of very valid reasons for doing so. Firstly, relatives entering a closed ward are at risk of contracting the virus themselves. In addition, as norovirus is essentially a community acquired illness, it is not unknown for symptomatic members of the public to visit friends or relatives, become ill whilst there, and potentially cross-infect patients and healthcare staff. Representing even more of a challenge is the explosive onset of norovirus and the fact that individuals are not aware that they have the infection until the symptoms are upon them; members of the public could unexpectedly be taken ill in the middle of a clinical area and again infect patients and healthcare staff. Where possible then, visiting should be restricted or discouraged altogether, although some discretion may need to be applied in the event of relatives wishing to see a dying patient. Children should certainly be discouraged from visiting the ward. The working group guidelines[470] contain information and guidance for patients which can be adapted to form a patient and visitor information leaflet.

Decontamination of equipment and the environment

There is much written in the literature about the role environmental contamination plays in prolonging outbreaks and increasing cross-infection.[482,483,489] The amount of environmental contamination that occurs on a ward as a result of norovirus infection really cannot be underestimated and the use of cleaning and hotel services will be increased considerably during outbreaks, particularly if several wards are closed at the same time. The working group guidelines recommend that hypochlorite

1,000 ppm is used for the disinfection of hard surfaces, but not for carpets or soft furnishings which are not bleach-resistant and would require prolonged contact. Although these items can be steam cleaned, vacuum cleaning of carpets and buffing of floors is not recommended as these activities can increase the circulation of virus particles. If clinical areas are carpeted, the carpet should be washed with detergent and water then either disinfected with a solution of 0.1 % hypochlorite if bleach resistant, or steam cleaned.

Any items that are handled frequently, such as door handles, taps, toilet chains, and toilet and bath rails should be cleaned frequently; they are likely to be heavily contaminated and norovirus could be transmitted to other patients via the faecal-oral route. Consideration also needs to be given to cleaning items such as telephones and computer keyboards and accessories, since these are often overlooked generally in day-to-day cleaning and yet they are also sources of infections. Patient equipment such as dynamaps, drip stands, infusion pumps and monitors should be cleaned daily with detergent wipes (hypochlorichite may be damaging) or in between each patient depending on how often they are used. Before the ward reopens, it should be thoroughly deep-cleaned and domestic staff should be given the time to do this before new patients are sent to the ward; if this process is not thorough, the environment will serve as a reservoir of norovirus and new cases are likely to be seen on the ward with the potential for ward closure again. There are reports that ozone gas can successfully inactivate norovirus, but because of its potential toxicity its application is restricted to environments that can be closed off or sealed, such as hotel rooms or cabins on cruise liners.[490]

COMMUNICATION

Informing the infection prevention and control team of any patients with diarrhoea and/or vomiting where there is no other explanation for their symptoms is perhaps key in preventing an outbreak. It is important that all healthcare personnel who may have cause to visit the ward are informed of the problem, together with departments where patients on the closed ward may be scheduled for appointments or investigations. This is normally something that the nurse in charge of the ward, or ward clerk/receptionist can do. The infection prevention and control team will be busy liaising with the hospital management team, the consultant in communicable disease control (CCDC) at the Health Protection Agency, dealing with general enquiries from other clinical areas, assessing new patients and maintaining and updating their records. As ward closures attract local media interest, particularly if more than one ward is affected, they may also be involved in dealing with media enquiries. The education of staff, patients and visitors is important and written information should be disseminated to all wards and departments, giving a simple explanation of norovirus, its signs and symptoms, incubation period and routes of spread, and the preventative measures that should be taken. The infection prevention and control team may also convene an outbreak committee and hold an outbreak meeting, as norovirus has the potential to disrupt the provision of healthcare services considerably and there will be operational and strategic issues to discuss. This is where the affected patients and clinical areas are discussed, a containment plan is agreed and roles and responsibilities are decided and allocated. The constitution of an outbreak committee can vary but will generally consist of the infection prevention and control team, a representative from hospital management, a bed manager, matron, a nursing representative from the affected ward(s), hotel services staff, the hospital communications department and the HPA. Depending on the size and duration of the outbreak, the committee may need to meet several times.

RISK MANAGEMENT

Risk management is a recurring theme during outbreaks, with infection prevention and control teams continually having to assess the risk to patients of being admitted and acquiring norovirus, against the risks of not receiving medical treatment because the ward or hospital is closed. A single ward closure will have an impact on the activity of the A&E department and the smooth running of the rest of the hospital; multiple ward closures have an even bigger impact. Closure of the hospital on the other hand (a decision that must be approved by the Strategic Health Authority) has massive resource implications for neighbouring Trusts. As outbreaks inconveniently tend to occur during the winter months when bed occupancy is at its height, the turnover of patients is slower, and there is increasing pressure to admit patients, the threat of a major hospital outbreak can loom large.

Symptomatic patients in A&E can be admitted to closed wards, as can a symptomatic patient from an unaffected ward who is being transferred out of the ward swiftly in the hope that problems there can be averted. Obviously the admission of symptomatic patients into a closed ward will prolong its closure, but that is preferable to infecting the patients and staff on an unaffected ward. Complications arise whereby a symptomatic patient may require the specialist services provided by intensive care and cardiac care units, renal units, and wards providing specialist respiratory or cardiac support. Unlike general wards, these specialist areas cannot be closed if they become affected and they will have to remain open to admissions requiring specialist care. Under no circumstances should a symptomatic patient be admitted into the middle of an unaffected ward, unless it is either into a side room or the patient requires specialist care. Similarly, asymptomatic patients should never be admitted to closed wards unless their medical condition warrants admission and the only bed available is on a closed ward. In these circumstances, the infection prevention and control team should be contacted as soon as possible (most Trusts now provide infection control advice out of hours), and the patient and relatives should be informed by the medical team that they are being admitted to a closed ward where there is a significant risk that they could contract norovirus, and the reason why they are being admitted there. This should be documented in the nursing and medical notes. It should be remembered that if a symptomatic patient is admitted into an unaffected ward, other patients are likely to contract norovirus and the worst case scenario is that a patient could die as a result. The infection control precautions/actions that should be taken during norovirus outbreaks are summarised in Table 14.3.

Table 14.3 Infection control actions/precautions to be taken during norovirus outbreaks

Inform the infection prevention and control team promptly of any patients or staff who meet the norovirus case definition.

Implement precautions requested by the infection prevention and control team in respect of ward closure.

Restrict patient movement to other areas of the hospital.

Do not transfer patients to other wards/hospitals unless their transfer constitutes a medical emergency (on medical advice).

Do not discharge patients to nursing or residential homes until the ward has been re-opened by the infection prevention and control team.

Advise that visiting is restricted.

Keep ward doors closed to prevent airborne dissemination of norovirus to other wards.

Decontaminate hands in between patient contacts and after contact with potentially contaminated equipment/environmental objects.

Obtain stool samples as advised by the infection prevention and control team.

Liaise with domestic services with regard to enhanced frequency of ward cleaning using hypochlorite solution.

Keep fruit bowls/water jugs covered to prevent contamination.

Staff working on a norovirus affected/closed ward should not work on an unaffected ward until 48 hours after their shift on the affected/closed ward has ended.

Symptomatic healthcare workers should refrain from working until they have been asymptomatic for 48 hours.

15 Campylobacter and Salmonella

INTRODUCTION

Food poisoning, defined as any disease of an infectious agent or toxic nature caused by the consumption of food or drink, is often regarded as an unpleasant but trivial illness and one that often goes unreported, although it is a notifiable disease. The reality is that it is a big public health concern, and the true incidence is difficult to determine as so many cases go unreported. In 2000, the World Health Organization estimated that 2.1 million people died each year from diarrhoeal disease, largely attributable to the consumption of contaminated food and water.[491] In 2005, 34,642 cases of food poisoning in England and Wales were formally notified to the Health Protection Agency, with another 35,000 cases reported via other channels.[492] Undercooked food, poor standards of hygiene in the kitchen, and lack of knowledge around food safety are the main causes of food poisoning, although person to person spread as a result of poor personal hygiene can occur.[493] This chapter examines the two most common causes of bacterial food poisoning in the UK – *Campylobacter* and *Salmonella*. The pathogenesis of infection and clinical features of each organism are discussed, along with the measures necessary for the prevention and control of food-related illness. Within the section on *Salmonella,* one of the most spectacularly mismanaged outbreaks of communicable disease within the NHS is discussed – the Stanley Royd Hospital *Salmonella* outbreak in 1984[494], in which 19 patients died. Salmonella also causes enteric fever, commonly known as typhoid/paratyphoid fever, or traveller's diarrhoea, and these two illnesses are examined within this chapter. The infection control precautions required to prevent the transmission of infection via the faecal-oral route are summarised at the end of the chapter.

LEARNING OUTCOMES

After reading this chapter the reader will:

- Be able to describe the clinical features of *Campylobacter* and *Salmonella* food poisoning
- Understand the measures to prevent/reduce the risk of food poisoning

- Be able to describe the clinical features of typhoid/paratyphoid fever, risk factors for acquisition and prevention of infection
- Understand the infection control precautions necessary to prevent the risk of cross-infection via the faecal-oral route

CAMPYLOBACTER

Campylobacter is a common bacterial cause of diarrhoea in humans and is considered to be the most common bacterial cause of gastroenteritis in the world, causing more cases of diarrhoea in developed countries than other food-borne organisms such as *Salmonelleae*, and is the commonest identifiable cause of gastroenteritis in the UK.[495,496,497] The word *Campylobacter* is derived from the Greek word *campylos*, meaning curved, and *baktron*, meaning rod[498], and they are microaerophilic, motile, non-spore forming, comma-shaped Gram-negative rods, possessing a single flagellum at either one or both ends of the organism[499] (see Chapter 2 Bacterial and Viral Classification, Structure and Function). They were originally isolated from aborted sheep fetuses in 1909, and it was not until the 1970s that the organism was associated with diarrhoea in humans and isolated in faecal specimens.[498,500,501,502] Compared to other enteric bacteria, they multiply slowly under laboratory conditions. They are thermophilic, growing at temperatures of 37 °C and 42–43 °C.[503] Although visible colonies can be seen within 24–48 hours[498], they require selective techniques in the laboratory in order to isolate them from other bacterial species, and they are grown on a selective culture medium which contains antibiotics to inhibit the growth of other pathogens.[503] There are 16 species of *Campylobacter,* of which *Campylobacter jejuni* is the most prevalent human pathogen causing enteric disease, accounting for approximately 90 % of *Campylobacter* associated infections.[504,505]

Campylobacters are commensals of the gastrointestinal tract in wild/domestic cattle, sheep, swine, goats, cats, dogs and rodents, along with commercially raised poultry, and the primary source of transmission in humans is via ingestion of contaminated food and water, or direct contact with pets.[499] It has been suggested that 20–40 % of sporadic *Campylobacter* disease might be due to the consumption of chicken, with 50 % of chicken on retail sale in the UK affected.[3] Animal meat can become contaminated during the slaughtering process, and soil and water can be contaminated with excreta from infected animals. As *Campylobacter* does not multiply in food, food-borne outbreaks are rare, although large outbreaks have been reported arising from raw and inadequately pasteurised milk and contaminated water supplies.[493]

Raw clams, raw/undercooked beef and under-pasteurised cheeses and goats' milk have also been implicated, and cases have arisen whereby bottled milk has become contaminated from birds pecking at the silver foil.[498,502]

PATHOGENESIS OF INFECTION AND CLINICAL FEATURES

Campylobacteriosis is the name given to the disease caused by *Campylobacters*. The number, or inoculating dose, of organisms reaching the intestine, the virulence of the infecting strain and the immunity of the host to the pathogen appear to be related to the development of onset of illness.[498] Once the organism has been ingested, either through eating contaminated meat or via the faecal-oral route on contaminated hands from contact with infected animals, it colonises the jejunum, ileum and colon, with the flagella assisting its motility through the gastrointestinal tract. Fimbriae on the surface of the organism facilitate its adherence to the mucosa enabling it to invade the epithelium.

The incubation period is between one to eleven days, with the onset of symptoms generally occurring within two to five days of ingestion, and the illness is generally self limiting, lasting from three to five days, although symptoms may persist for up to two weeks. The cardinal clinical features are fever, diarrhoea and abdominal fever. Nausea is common, and vomiting can also occur. In some individuals, a non-specific prodromal illness lasting 12–24 hours, consisting of high fever, headache and myalgia, may occur before the onset of the intestinal symptoms.[498] The severity of the diarrhoea experienced may vary, and blood is frequently present in the stools, which may manifest as a frank gastrointestinal haemorrhage, although this is rare.[498] In the majority of cases, it is clinically difficult to distinguish *Campylobacter* from *Salmonelleae* on clinical grounds, but the abdominal pain experienced with *Campylobacter* infection is generally more severe.[503] If diarrhoea is absent, and abdominal pain and fever are the main presenting symptoms, the illness may be mis-diagnosed as appendicitis, as the pain is often localised in the right lower quadrant.[498,503] Nausea is a common feature, but vomiting is rare.

Table 15.1 summarises the clinical features of *Campylobacter* food poisoning.

Table 15.1 Clinical features of *Campylobacter* food poisoning

Incubation period 1–11 days.
Illness duration 3–5 days (may persist for two weeks in some cases).
May experience flu-like prodromal symptoms 12–24 hours before onset of main symptoms.
Fever, diarrhoea and abdominal pain cardinal signs; often nausea but vomiting is uncommon.
Diarrhoea – severity varies but may be massively watery and contain blood.
Diarrhoea may be absent in some cases; abdominal pain and fever are predominant symptoms – possibility of mis-diagnosis.
Abdominal pain – generally severe.

DIAGNOSIS AND TREATMENT

Stool culture and the isolation of *C.jejuni* is the definitive diagnostic tool, although negative results can sometimes be obtained because selective media is required for culture of the organism. A diagnosis of *Campylobacter* food poisoning may therefore be made on the basis of the clinical symptoms and food history or contact with infected animals. Most cases resolve spontaneously but patients with severe infection may lose large volumes of fluid, requiring intravenous hydration to correct fluid and electrolyte imbalances. Antibiotic treatment is not usually indicated unless the illness is severe and erythromycin or ciprofloxacin are the most widely used antimicrobial agents. Available evidence suggests that early treatment may shorten the duration of illness by one–two days at most. However, recent reports of increasing quinolone resistance suggest that antibiotic resistance is a significant problem.[498,506]

COMPLICATIONS

Although most cases resolve spontaneously, complications can occur. The two most common sequalae are reactive arthritis (also known as Reiters Syndrome), a self-limiting inflammatory response involving the ankles, knees and wrists, and Guillain-Barre Syndrome, where demyelination of the nerve sheaths occurs, possibly as a result of an auto-immune reaction, resulting in a severe paralysis which may last for several months.[503] Deaths have been reported in both developed and undeveloped countries among young adults, children, the immunocompromised and the elderly as a result of fluid depletion.[498]

PREVENTION

It is difficult to reduce the reservoir of bacteria as *Campylobacters* are so widely distributed in nature, so measures to control the transmission of *Campylobacter* infection have to centre around preventing contamination in water, milk and food. As wild and domestic animals shed *Campylobacter* into lakes, rivers, streams and reservoirs, water for consumption has to be properly treated and chlorinated. Food should be cooked thoroughly, and hands washed before handling/preparing food and after contact with pets or other animals, particularly before eating. *C.jejuni* infection has a tendency to be seasonal[507], and increases during the summer months may be linked to the barbecue season and the consumption of undercooked poultry.

SALMONELLAE

Salmonellae belong to the family of bacteria known as *Enterobacteriaceae*, and they are facultative anaerobic Gram-negative bacilli, causing food-borne illnesses and enteric fevers.

The organism, of which there are 2,501 species, was first isolated in 1885 from porcine intestine by a veterinary surgeon/pathologist named Daniel Salmon.[508,509] The genus *Salmonelleae* has since been divided into two species, *S.bongori* and

S.enterica, with multiple subspecies and serotypes, which have been further divided into 2,501 serotypes according to their antigenic differences (bacterial cell wall and flagella) and habitats. *Salmonella enterica* contains the serotypes that are classified as human pathogens.[509]

They are commensals and pathogens of the gastrointestinal tract in humans and animals such as wild and domestic birds (poultry), reptiles, and amphibians (especially terrapins), and their widespread distribution in the environment and the food chain has enormous public health implications.[509,510] *Salmonellosis* is the term used to describe the spectrum of disease caused by *Salmonella* species, such as *Salmonella gastroenteritis* or food poisoning, enteric fever, *Salmonella bacteraemia*, and the asymptomatic carrier state. It is important to understand and appreciate the difference between the food poisoning organisms, and those causing enteric fevers. The common food poisoning organisms (such as *Salmonella enteritidis*, *Salmonella typhimurium* and *Salmonella virchow*) affect both humans and animals, and the enteric strains are human pathogens mainly associated with travel (*Salmonella typhi* and *Salmonella paratyphi* A and B).

As the presence of *Salmonelleae* in the gastrointestinal tract is often outnumbered by the normal bowel flora, they need to be cultured in the microbiology laboratory on selective media and enrichment culture, which will select for salmonella species and inhibit the growth of other bowel pathogens.

SALMONELLA FOOD POISONING

Salmonelleae account for the second most common cause of bacterial gastroenteritis after *Campylobacter*[511], with illness arising through the consumption of contaminated food of animal origin (meat, poultry, eggs and milk), the contamination of cooked food by raw food, inadequate cooking temperatures, and poor standards of hygiene in relation to food preparation. Asymptomatic chronic human carriers of the disease may also transmit *Salmonellae* if they are involved in food handling and preparation.[512] Outbreaks are often associated with a 'point-source' such as a wedding, a party, or a meal at a restaurant, where large numbers of people can become infected at the same time having eaten contaminated food from the same source. An outbreak at a residential home in 1995, in which two elderly residents died, was associated with the consumption of prawns in mayonnaise, vol-au-vents, sausage rolls, sausages and corned beef sandwiches which were contaminated with *S.enteritidis* phage type 5a, and was caused by poor and inadequate food hygiene.[513]

Salmonellosis has also been associated with exotic pets, such as reptiles, and exposure to pet birds, rodents, cats and dogs.[509]

The strong association between *Salmonella enteritidis* and hens' eggs has been widely publicised over the last 20 years. The principle site of contamination with *Salmonella* in eggs is the outside of the yolk membrane or the albumen surrounding it, although the shell can also be contaminated, and *Salmonella enteritidis* associated with raw eggs in cooking has been a common problem. In 1988, the junior health minister Edwina Currie, was forced to resign after she stated that 'Most of our (UK) egg production is infected with *Salmonella*', and the resulting furore blighted UK egg production, with many egg producers going out of business as sales of eggs fell by 60 %.[514] The government ordered the slaughter of between two and four million hens to control the spread of *Salmonella* and introduced new legislation in 1989 with regard to improved standards of hygiene within hen houses and the tighter controls around the sale of eggs. In 1993, the Government Advisory Committee on the Microbiological Safety of Food made a series of recommendations and changes in practice regarding egg production, distribution, storage and handling, and advised that eggs should be stored at temperatures below 20 °C and consumed within three weeks of purchase.[515]

In the UK, hens are now vaccinated against *Salmonella* and the Lion Brand, which accounts for 80 % of the egg sales in the UK, has its lion quality mark stamped on the shell and the egg box, indicating that the eggs have been produced to the highest standards of food safety in the world, under the Lion Code of Practice. In 2002–2004, an investigation was initiated by the Health Protection Agency in England and Wales in response to outbreaks of *S.enteritidis* associated with raw egg shell[516]; historically, Spain has been one of the biggest exporters of eggs to the UK, and *Salmonella* species were isolated from 5.6 % of Spanish eggs used in UK catering premises.[516] Although the vast majority of eggs produced in the UK are *Salmonella* free, the HPA investigation highlighted the need for greater control and regulation with regard to imported eggs.

Eggs aside, the consumption of chicken is often implicated in *Salmonella* food poisoning. It is believed that battery chickens are often fed food that is contaminated with mouse droppings (*S.enteritidis* has been cultured from the spleens of mice on farms)[517], which then colonises the chicken's gut, forming part of their normal gut flora. When the birds are slaughtered and eviscerated, the gut contents spill onto the carcass. They are then dipped into a 'scald bath' at a temperature of 60 °C to facilitate plucking and de-feathering, which results in a 'bath water' of faeces, blood and body fluids, and results in the possible contamination of the carcass with *Salmonella* or other pathogens such as *Campylobacte*r. The chickens are sealed and frozen, but in 80 % *Salmonella* can be found on the surface and in deep muscle. Provided that the chicken is well-cooked and cooked right through to the centre of the bird, food poisoning is unlikely, but if the cooking temperature is inadequate, problems may arise.

THE PATHOGENESIS OF *SALMONELLA* FOOD POISONING AND CLINICAL FEATURES

Following ingestion, the organism has to evade host immune defences in order to colonise the caecum and the ileum, and the presence of fimbriae on the surface of the organism enables it to adhere to the intestinal epithelium. It binds to receptors on the epithelial cell surface, degenerating the microvilli so that it can invade the mucosa and intestinal epithelium and replicate within it. Once in situ, cytokine release and enterotoxin production (see Chapter 2 Bacterial and Viral Classification,

Structure and Function and Chapter 5 Understanding the Immune System and the Nature and Pathogenesis of Infection) result in acute inflammation, which leads to excess fluid secretion and fluid production in the small and large bowel, and the onset of diarrhoea.[509]

The resulting illness is usually a self-limiting acute gastroenteritis, of varying severity. Following an incubation period ranging from 6–48 hours, the onset is abrupt with a high fever(lasting 48–72 hours), abdominal pain, nausea (rarely vomiting), headache and myalgia, along with diarrhoea which becomes the main feature within 24 hours.[518] This may be described as 'loose'and of moderate volume, or watery and of large volume and typically persists for three to seven days, although the acute stage of the illness is over within two to three days. Unlike *Campylobacter* infection, blood in the stools is not a clinical feature. In very severe cases, fluid loss can result in hypotension and renal failure which can be life-threatening, and the very young, the elderly, and immunocompromised individuals are most at risk of severe infection.[510] Table 15.2 summarises the main features of *Salmonella* food poisoning.

Table 15.2 Clinical features of *Salmonella* food poisoning

Incubation period 6–48 hours; illness self-limiting.
Abrupt onset; varying severity of symptoms.
High fever, abdominal pain, nausea (rarely vomiting), headache and myalgia.
Diarrhoea the main feature within 24 hours – can persist for 3–7 days; severity/volume of diarrhoea can vary. No blood in stools.
If illness is severe, fluid loss can be potentially life-threatening in high risk patients.

DIAGNOSIS AND TREATMENT

Diagnosis is by stool culture, and also blood culture if the fever is very high or persists for longer than 48 hours. Rehydration and the correction of electrolyte imbalances may be required for 12–24 hours. Treatment with antibiotics is sometimes clinically indicated, but should be avoided where possible because of development of antibiotic-resistant strains, particularly to sulphonamides, tetracyclines, aminoglycosides and broad spectrum penicillins and cephalosporins.[519] This has partly arisen because *Salmonelleae* can colonise animal and human gastrointestinal tracts and have been exposed to antibiotics before through previous antibiotic administration and the inclusion of antibiotics as additives in animal feed (see Chapter 8 The Problem of Antimicrobial Resistance). Where antibiotics are indicated on clinical grounds, ciprofloxacin 500mg twice daily for three to five days is generally considered to be the drug of choice.

CARRIAGE

Excretion of *Salmonelleae* in the stool usually ceases after one to four weeks. Prolonged excretion is rare but can sometimes be seen in individuals with gastrointestinal tract disease, such as diverticulitis, and irritable bowel syndrome, and diseases affecting the immune system such as AIDS. Although it is generally not a problem, it can pose a significant risk if the 'excretor' works in the food industry and is involved in food preparation and food handling, where outbreaks of food-borne illness can occur.

THE STANLEY ROYD HOSPITAL *SALMONELLA* OUTBREAK 1984[494]

In 1984, an outbreak of *Salmonella typhimurium* at the Stanley Royd Psychiatric Hospital in Wakefield, Yorkshire, affected 355 patients and 106 members of staff. 19 patients died and the outbreak resulted in the first ever public enquiry into the running of a hospital, and the removal of **crown immunity** from NHS premises. Stanley Royd originally opened in 1818 as the West Yorkshire Pauper Lunatic Asylum, designed to accommodate 150 patients; by 1971 the addition of further buildings had expanded its capacity to 1,865 beds. At the time of the outbreak in 1984 it was a psychogeriatric hospital with 850 inpatients, who were largely elderly and severely mentally infirm, on 35 wards. There had been two outbreaks of food poisoning at the hospital prior to 1984. The first, in 1974, affected nine patients and resulted in the death of one. The second outbreak occurred in 1979, affected 33 patients and highlighted numerous food safety issues.

The 1984 outbreak began at 7am on Sunday the 26th August with one patient; within two hours, there were 36 affected patients reported on eight wards, and by 9.15pm, the number of patients affected had increased to 94. Fourteen hours after the outbreak began, the first patient died. New cases were seen over subsequent days and the scale of the outbreak, which was not recognised at first by those involved, and the speed with which it occurred, were frightening.

There were serious allegations of mismanagement of the outbreak, which became the focal point of both local and national media interest and led to a public enquiry. The Committee of Inquiry, which was announced by the Secretary of State for Health on the 14th September 1984, revealed several serious failings. *Salmonella typhimurium* phage type 49, cultured from the stool of symptomatic and asymptomatic patients and members of staff, was isolated from the roast beef which had been served to patients the evening before the outbreak began. It was thought that the beef had become contaminated with *Salmonella* from a chicken source after it had been cooked, possibly transmitted to the beef on the hands of catering staff or via kitchen equipment and utensils, and poor kitchen hygiene was subsequently highlighted. Kitchen staff regularly 'sampled' the food and prepared their own meals which they ate in the hospital kitchen; the machinery used for slicing and mincing meat was rarely cleaned properly in between use; cleaning cloths were often re-used; food was stored for long periods before consumption; and there was a shortage of refrigerator capacity, particularly for separating cooked and uncooked meats. The kitchen had originally been built in 1865, and along with other buildings at the hospital was described as Dickensian. Its structure had never been altered, and it was ill-equipped to cope with catering for the patient population. The kitchen floor was cracked and worn, with deep open drainage channels under the metal grills which were impossible to clean properly. When high pressure disinfection jets used for cleaning were directed over the metal grills, an aerosol effect was generated which possibly increased the risk of environmental contamination. In addition, the kitchen was understaffed and the management of the kitchen was largely left to those who worked in it as there was no real supervision by managers, and kitchen practices were therefore unsupervised and went unchallenged.

Several general recommendations were made for the management and control of outbreaks of food poisoning in a hospital setting as a result of the Stanley Royd outbreak. These included the appointment of an infection control nurse in every health authority who should be a full time member of the infection control committee; a major outbreak plan for dealing with a major outbreak of food poisoning or other communicable disease, and the immediate involvement of the Public Health Laboratory and the Communicable Disease Surveillance Centre; the preparation of food history questionnaires so that detailed food histories could be obtained from affected individuals; and the appointment of a medical consultant as the control of infection officer, responsible for co-ordinating and investigating outbreaks of infection. In respect of the Stanley Royd itself, the inquiry recommended, among other things, a review of the staffing ratios on the wards and in the kitchen and catering departments, and a withdrawal of funds from the hospital as the patient population decreased, leading to its eventual closure.

PREVENTION OF FOOD POISONING AND INFECTION CONTROL PRECAUTIONS

Table 15.3 lists the food handling precautions that should be taken to reduce the risk of food poisoning.

Table 15.4 summarises the infection control precautions that should be taken when caring for patients with *Campylobacter/Salmonella* food poisoning.

Table 15.3 Food handling precautions

Wash hands before preparing/handling food.

Food handlers should have good standards of personal hygiene, and not work if they have signs of gastrointestinal infection.

Kitchen surfaces must be maintained, seals and fixtures/features must be intact, and standards of cleanliness must be high.

Separate kitchen utensils should be used when preparing/handling raw and cooked foods and they should be cleaned thoroughly.

Raw food must not come into contact with cooked food.

Ensure that food is cooked thoroughly – hot through to the centre.

Eat cooked food immediately or keep at 70 °C and eat within a maximum of two hours.

Chill food below 5 °C, and cook food above 63 °C; reheated food should reach a temperature of 70 °C.

Table 15.4 Infection control precautions to prevent cross-infection via the faecal-oral route

Isolation	Patients should be isolated in a single room, preferably with en suite facilities, if they have signs of gastrointestinal infection (diarrhoea and/or vomiting of unknown cause; presumptive diagnosis of bacterial/viral gastroenteritis). If en suite facilities are not available, either a separate toilet or commode should be allocated for the patient's use. Patients can generally be de-isolated once they have been asymptomatic for 48 hours and have had a 'normal' stool, but in cases of *Salmonella* food poisoning, negative stool cultures may be required and should not be obtained if/while the patient is taking antibiotics.
Hand hygiene	Hands should be decontaminated with alcohol hand rub in between each episode of patient contact; if hands are visibly dirty or contaminated with blood/body fluids, they should be washed with liquid soap and water. Educate the patient on the need for hand washing after using the toilet and before eating.
Personal protective equipment and clothing	Gloves and aprons should be worn for contact with stool/body fluids, changed immediately after patient contact and before leaving the patient's room, and disposed of as clinical waste according to local policy/national guidance.
Visitors	Visitors do not need to wear protective clothing but should be advised to decontaminate their hands on leaving the isolation room.
Linen	Linen should be treated as infected and disposed of according to local policy/national guidance.
Clinical waste	Clinical waste should be disposed of according to local policy and national guidance.
Bed pan washer/macerator	Ensure bedpan washer reaches temperature of 80 °C and holds for one minute.
	If using a macerator keep the lid closed for one minute after the cycle has finished to minimise aerosol dispersal.
Decontamination of equipment	Equipment should be single-patient use or disposable, or allocated to the patient for the duration of their stay or until they are no longer infectious, when it can be disposed of/decontaminated appropriately. Any equipment that is multi-patient use must be decontaminated in between each patient use, either with detergent wipes or cleaned according to manufacturer's instructions.
Environmental cleanliness	The patient's isolation room and en suite toilet facilities should be cleaned daily according to local policy and a thorough clean of the room should take place on de-isolation/discharge. If the patient is using a toilet/bathroom on the main ward, special attention must be paid to cleaning, particularly fixtures and fittings. If the patient is using a commode that cannot be dedicated for use solely by that patient, it should be thoroughly cleaned with detergent wipes, and wiped with a solution of 1000ppm available chlorine after use.

THE ENTERIC FEVERS

Salmonella typhi and *Salmonella paratyphi* are known as the human typhoid and paratyphoid enteric fevers, and are severe systemic illnesses characterised by abdominal pain and fever. As these serotypes only colonise humans, disease can only be acquired through close contact with an individual with typhoid fever, or with someone who is an asymptomatic carrier, with ingestion of faecally contaminated food or water implicated in the acquisition.[509] Typhoid fever is a bacterial infection of the gastrointestinal tract and bloodstream and is recognised as a global health problem, with 17 million reported cases each year, and a case fatality of 10 % unless treated promptly.[520]

Paratyphoid fever, caused by serotypes of *Salmonella paratyphi enteritidis* A, B and C tends to result in a milder disease, although the clinical features are very similar. In the UK, cases of enteric fever are largely associated with foreign travel and are endemic in high risk countries such as the Indian sub-continent (India, Pakistan and Bangladesh), South East Asia and parts of Latin America and Africa. Where it is endemic, risk factors for acquisition include eating and drinking contaminated food and water, inadequate sanitation, poor/inadequate living conditions, poor personal hygiene and close contact with an infected individual or carrier.[521] Attack rates among travellers to endemic areas are estimated at 10 per 100,000 population.[522]

PATHOGENESIS OF INFECTION AND CLINICAL FEATURES

The incubation period is variable and depends on the inoculating or infectious dose (the bigger the dose, the shorter the time until the onset of symptoms) and various host factors.[523] After ingestion, the organism replicates in the gastrointestinal tract, penetrating the ilieal mucosa before passing into the mesenteric lymph nodes via the lymphatic system. It then multiplies, invading the bloodstream via the thoracic duct, resulting in a primary bacteraemia which tends to go unnoticed as it is often asymptomatic. During this phase, which lasts seven to ten days, the liver, gall bladder, kidneys, spleen and bone marrow become infected.[523] Thereafter the onset of symptoms is insidious, with affected individuals experiencing a non-specific flu-like illness. An increasing fever, peaking at 38–39 °C heralds the onset of a secondary bacteraemia as more bacilli pass into the bloodstream, and systemic signs of illness begin to become apparent. Headache, abdominal pain, constipation and a dry cough develop, along with confusion which can range from mild to full-blown delirium. As the fever peaks, rose coloured spots appear on the costal margins, flanks or buttocks, and diarrhoea begins. Further intestinal invasion from the gall bladder results in an inflammatory reaction in the peyers patches and other intestinal lymphoid tissue and can lead to necrosis and sloughing of the intestinal mucosal and the development of ulcers.[509,510] Complications can arise from week two onwards and occur in 10–15 % of patients, with intestinal bleeding which may be catastrophic, and perforation the most common, in some cases with a fatal outcome.[522] Paratyphoid fever results in a less severe disease. With paratyphoid A, rose coloured spots are absent. Infection with paratyphoid B, which has an incubation period of four to five days, results in watery diarrhoea from the outset, which becomes increasingly bloody as the illness progresses, along with a widespread rose rash.

Table 15.5 summarises the clinical features of typhoid and paratyphoid fever.

Table 15.5 Clinical features of typhoid and paratyphoid fever

---

Typhoid fever
Non-specific flu-like illness.
Headache (may be severe), fever, dry cough, abdominal pain, constipation.
Confusion – may range from mild to full-blown delirium.
Fever increases and peaks – rose coloured spots on costal margins, flanks or buttocks.
Diarrhoea begins.
Fever pattern changes – sustained high temperature and then gradually rising and falling for a period of weeks.
Intestinal perforation as a result of intestinal ulceration/necrosis can occur as a complication.

Paratyphoid fever
Incubation period 4–5 days.
Watery diarrhoea the main feature, becoming increasingly bloody.
Rose coloured spots absent.

DIAGNOSIS AND TREATMENT

Diagnosis of enteric fever is made by isolation of *Salmonella typhi* or *Salmonella paratyphi* from blood (first week of illness) stool specimens (second and third weeks of illness), rose coloured spots or bone marrow. A positive blood culture is found in 80 % of patients, and is most likely in those who have a 7–10 day history of fever. Failure to isolate the organism may be due to using inappropriate laboratory media, the commencement of antibiotic therapy, the volume of the sample obtained, and the time at which the sample is obtained.[523] Enteric fever is one of the few bacterial infections which may require examination of the bone marrow, and is considered to be the gold standard for the diagnosis of typhoid fever; this is because there are higher colony counts of the bacteria in bone marrow than there are in blood.[518,523] The isolation of *S.typhi* from stools is also indicative of typhoid fever, and the quantity of stool specimens obtained increases the likelihood of obtaining a positive result.

TREATMENT

Although 90 % of patients can be successfully managed at home with appropriate antibiotic therapy and medical follow-up, enteric fevers in endemic countries carry a mortality rate of 30–50 %, where multi-antibiotic resistant strains and delayed treatment increase the risk of death.[509,523] In very severe cases, where intestinal haemorrhage is a complication, intensive care support may be required and possibly surgical intervention in the event of intestinal perforation. Oral ciprofloxacin 500mg twice daily for ten days is the first-line treatment for typhoid fever, although chloramphenicol, co-trimoxazole and high dose amoxicillin can also be used. For paratyphoid fever, ciprofloxacin or chloramphenicol can be prescribed. Relapse is experienced by 5–20 % of patients after apparently successful treatment, with fever returning soon after the completion of antibiotic therapy. Patients generally experience a milder illness the second time round, and antibiotic treatment remains the same.[523]

CARRIER STATES

A carrier can be defined as a person without symptoms who has excreted pathogenic organisms in faeces or urine, either continuously or intermittently, for more than 12 months.[493] Most individuals infected with *Salmonelleae* excrete the bacilli in their stools for days or weeks after they have recovered from the illness and symptoms have resolved, but some can become chronic carriers of *Salmonella typhi*, harbouring the enteric bacilli in the gall bladder and excreting it in faeces and urine. In cases of gall bladder disease, cholecystectomy may be required.[510] The risk of carriage increases with age and biliary tract abnormalities, with women affected more than men. Ciprofloxacin 750 mg twice daily for 28 days can successfully treat 80 % of chronic carriers.[523] Typhoid fever is a notifiable disease, and suspected/confirmed cases should be notified to the local health protection unit by the doctor responsible for the patient. Symptomatic individuals and asymptomatic carriers should be excluded from any activities involving food preparation and handling, and should refrain from work until they have had three negative stool specimens obtained at least one month apart.[523] Staff working in healthcare facilities should be excluded from work until they have had negative stool culture, as should children under the age of five who attend nurseries or other similar environments, and older children/adults who are unable to maintain an adequate standard of personal hygiene.[52]

PREVENTION OF TYPHOID FEVER

Measures to prevent typhoid fever are summarised in Table 15.6.

Table 15.6 Measures to prevent typhoid/paratyphoid fever[52]

Vaccination if travelling to areas where enteric fever is endemic.
Drink only 'safe' water – boil water if in a rural area where there is no piped/chlorinated or bottled water.
Wash hands before preparing/eating food.
Avoid raw foods/shellfish/ice.
Eat only cooked/still-hot food.
Appropriate facilities for disposable of human waste must be available.
Maintain good personal hygiene.

Vaccination against typhoid fever is available and is recommended for those travelling to countries where it is endemic and where they will have prolonged exposure to potentially contaminated food and water, especially if they are staying with or visiting the local population, and in situations where exposure to sanitation and food handling hygiene are likely to be poor.[52,509,524] Among the target groups for vaccination are those residing in high risk countries, displaced populations living in refugee camps, children, sewage workers, and laboratory staff who may handle *S.typhi*.[52,523] There is no vaccination available for paratyphoid fever.

16 Blood-borne Viruses

INTRODUCTION

Blood-borne viruses (BBVs) are carried in the bloodstream and unlike most other infections which can be transmitted by normal, everyday social contact, they are spread via direct contact with contaminated blood or high risk body fluids. The Human Immunodeficiency Virus (HIV), hepatitis B (HBV) and hepatitis C (HCV) pose a significant threat to public health as many people with BBVs are undiagnosed, and people can become infected through high risk behaviours such as unprotected sex, and intravenous drug abuse. Viruses can pass through breaks/lacerations in the skin and mucous membranes and in the transmission of HIV infection, heterosexual transfer of HIV now accounts for 90 % of the global HIV total.[525] Injecting drug abusers often share needles and other injecting equipment that is contaminated with blood, and this has accelerated the transmission of HIV and HVC considerably. Acupuncture, tattoos and body piercing have been implicated in the transmission of HCV through the use of contaminated equipment.[526] In order to prevent the transmission of BBVs via donated blood and blood products for transfusion, screening was introduced in the UK in 1985 for HIV and in 1991 for HCV so the incidence of BBVs transmitted by this route remains low.

Healthcare workers are exposed to BBVs every day through the handling of clinical waste, contact with blood and high risk body fluids (see Table 16.1), procedures such as cannulation and venepuncture, and surgery. A significant exposure is classed as a percutaaneous exposure to blood and body fluids from a source that is known to be, or as a result of the incident found to be, HIV, HBV or HCV positive.[527] Within the healthcare setting percutaneous and mucotaneous exposes commonly occur as a result of a skin puncture or scratch with a used needle or other sharp instrument, glassware or item which may be contaminated with blood or body fluids; a splash of blood or body fluids onto non-intact skin or the mucous membranes of the eyes and mouth; contamination of a cut, graze or break in the skin with blood or body fluids; or a human bite which breaks the skin.[528] The risk of transmission of BBVs is greater from patient to healthcare worker than from healthcare worker to patient, and non-compliance with local protocols and procedures is one of the most common contributing factors leading to accidental exposure.[527]

This chapter looks at the risks posed by blood-borne viruses and the importance of safe working to minimise the risks of occupational exposure and potential

Table 16.1 High and low risk body fluids

High risk	Low risk
Blood	Urine
Semen	Faeces
Vaginal secretions	Saliva (unless bloodstained
Saliva (only if	or if exposure occurs during
bloodstained or if	dental work)
exposure occurs	Vomit
during dental work)	
CSF	
Synovial fluid	
Amniotic fluid	
Breast milk	
Pleural fluid	
Pericardial fluid	

transmission to both patients and staff in the workplace. The pathogenesis of infection with HIV, HBV and HCV is discussed, along with diagnosis and treatment, followed by the management of BBV infected healthcare workers, including post-exposure prophylaxis, infection control precautions to prevent the transmission of BBVs, and the safe handling and disposal of sharps. Reference is made to key documents and Department of Health guidance.

LEARNING OUTCOMES

After reading this chapter the reader will:

- Understand the risk factors for the acquisition and transmission of blood-borne viruses
- Understand the pathogenesis of HIV and HBV infection
- Understand how HIV and HBV are diagnosed, and the diagnosis principles of antiretroviral therapy for the treatment of HIV and HBV

HIV

The greatest threat to public health seen so far, which heralded the onset of a world-wide pandemic, came out of nowhere and silently began to emerge between 1979 and 1981, when the Centre for Disease Control (CDC), Atlanta, USA, was alerted to an unusual number of opportunistic infections and rare skin cancers occurring among homosexuals in Los Angeles and New York.[529,530] These infections were notable in that they were normally seen in individuals who were immunocompromised. It was clear that these men, who had previously been fit and healthy, were all suffering from a common syndrome and on investigation they were found to be profoundly immunodeficient with no underlying cause. Cases were subsequently identified at an alarming rate across America, Africa and other parts of the world, including the UK, throughout 1981 to 1983, and it was becoming evident that this was both a blood-borne and a sexually transmitted disease, not only affecting the homosexual population, but also injecting drug users, and those who had received blood transfusions. The term AIDS, or acquired immune deficiency syndrome, was first used by the CDC in 1982 to describe the collection of opportunistic infections that had been seen in these cases. AIDS was defined as 'a disease at least moderately predictive of a defect in cell-mediated immunity, occurring with no known cause for diminished resistance to that disease'.[531]

In 1983 at the Pasteur Institute in France a new virus was discovered which was associated with AIDS, and research at the National Cancer Institute in Washington DC the following year further established that it was indeed the causative agent.[532] It wasn't until 1986 that the AIDS-associated virus was named the human immunodeficiency virus (HIV). HIV is a retrovirus, and retroviruses have been associated with cancers in animals; the HIV retrovirus is believed to be linked to the simian immunodeficiency virus (SIV-1) which causes disease in chimpanzees, and human retroviral infections are believed to have originated as a result of the virus jumping the species barrier.[533] They differ from other viruses in that they are not transmissible by ordinary routes, instead requiring contact with blood and body fluids in order to infect the host. Another distinguishing feature is that they are encoded for an enzyme called reverse transcriptase, which converts viral RNA into a DNA copy which becomes integrated into the DNA of the host cell.[534] HIV, of which there are two subtypes, belongs to the group of retroviruses known as lentiviruses (*lenti* – slow), so named because they cause slow, progressive disease and can persist for long periods of time in a latent state before there are any clinical manifestations.[534] HIV-1 is largely responsible for the AIDS pandemic. HIV-2, although also associated with opportunistic infections and progression to AIDS, is less pathogenic; immunodeficiency tends to develop more slowly and infected individuals may not develop a high viral load for as long as 15–20 years after infection.[535] It is prevalent in Western Africa, with Senegal, the Ivory Coast, Nigeria, Mozambique, Sierra-Leone, Benin, Burkino Faso, Cape Verde, Liberia and the Gambia all reporting cases.[536]

The HIV virus consists of a viral envelope made out of host cell membrane, which is studded with 72 spikes consisting of transmembrane and surface proteins. These proteins aid the binding of the virus to CD4+ T-lymphocytes. Within the icosahedral capsid there are three viral proteins which are essential for the process of viral replication; reverse transcriptase, integrase (which splices the DNA into the host cell gene) and protease (which aids the processing of virus particles). Also contained within the capsid are genes, which assist in the formation of new virus particles and produce 'copies' of the virus, and are believed to play regulatory or accessory roles during infection.[534] HIV-1 is inactivated by heat, gluteraldehyde 2 %, hypochlorite 10,000 ppm and alcohol, and can survive in the environment for up to 15 days at room temperature.[525]

THE PATHOGENESIS OF HIV INFECTION

Within 24–48 hours of the virus entering the body, a period of intense viral replication takes place within the regional lymph nodes and the blood. HIV specifically targets the CD4+ T-helper cells[534] which carry surface receptors for antigens or foreign material, and the transmembrane and surface proteins on the HIV cell membrane enable the virus to adhere to the cell membrane of the CD4 cells. There, the viral envelope fuses with the CD4 cell, releasing its contents, and reverse transcriptase begins the process of converting viral RNA into DNA.[534] CD4+ T-helper cells belong to a group of specialised cells essential to the functioning of the immune system called lymphocytes. The 'normal' healthy adult has two billion lymphocytes, which are found throughout the body.[79] They are produced in bone marrow, thymus gland and fetal liver and they migrate to secondary organs such as the spleen and lymph nodes, as well as other areas of lymphoid tissue around the body, via the peripheral circulation. T-lymphocytes are lymphocytes which have passed through the thymus gland and then re-entered the peripheral circulation before settling in the lymph nodes and the spleen.[79] CD4+ T-helper cells assist the lymphocytes with antibody responses, and assist in the overall immune response. The complex workings of the immune system are explained in Chapter 5 Understanding the Immune System and the Nature and Pathogenesis of Infection.

During this phase of primary infection and intense viral replication, which occurs two to twelve weeks after infection and is known as seroconversion, 50–70 % of infected individuals may experience what is known as an acute seroconversion illness lasting two–four weeks.[537] This can manifest as a non-specific flu-like illness with symptoms which may include a generalised rash and lymphadenopathy, fatigue, sore throat, nausea, weight loss, diarrhoea and mouth ulcers and is generally self-limiting. If symptoms are severe and significant illness is experienced during this time, it is associated with a more rapid progression to end-stage AIDS.[536,537,538]

THE SIGNIFICANCE OF CD4+ T-LYMPHOCYTE COUNT AND VIRAL LOAD

After diagnosis of HIV, the CD4+ count (the number of CD4+ T-lymphocytes in a cubic mm of blood) is initially checked at 3–6 monthly intervals to monitor the immune response and determine when to start anti-retroviral therapy. A typical CD4+ count in a healthy adult ranges from 400–1,600 cells mm³, and can fluctuate for a variety of reasons[536], none of which affect the competence of the immune system. A count of 200–500 indicates that damage has occurred to the immune system. In someone infected with HIV, it is estimated that the CD4 count can decrease by 45 cells per month, and although thousands more are produced every day as the immune system is very resilient, there comes a point where the immune system is unable to keep up with the rate of destruction. Viral load measures the number of copies of HIV RNA per ml of blood, and viral replication can exceed 10,000 new viral copies a day.[534] In terms of measuring the viral load, more than 100,000 viral copies per ml/blood is considered to be a high viral load, and below 10, 000 copies is considered to be low. Ideally the viral load should be undetectable (less than 50 copies), as the higher the viral load, the faster CD4+ cells are likely to be destroyed and the faster the progression to the onset of AIDS. Once anti-retroviral therapy has begun, the aim of treatment is to get the viral load down to an undetectable level within six months.[536]

In the majority of people though, the CD4+ count increases after this episode of primary infection, although the damage has been done and it does not return to baseline values.[537] The individual then enters a long asymptomatic period often referred to as clinical latency which can last 9–10 years, and during this time the immune system very slowly deteriorates. When an individual is first infected, the viral load increases and the CD4+ T-lymphocyte count falls as the immune system tries to fight the infection by producing antibodies. However, as the infection progresses, the proportion of infected CD4+ cells increases, as does the circulating viral load, immune function decreases, and the individual eventually develops signs of early symptomatic disease. These include malaise, weight loss, fever, night sweats and chronic diarrhoea[538] and may also include minor opportunistic infections such as oral thrush (candida), shingles (VZV), herpes simplex virus (HSV 1 or 2) and listeria.[537]

PROGRESSION TO AIDS

As the immune system starts to fail, and the viral load increases and the CD4 count decreases, the end-stage of the disease begins, with the development of opportunistic infections known as AIDS-defining illnesses, as defined by the Centre for Disease Control, Atlanta[539] (see Table 16.2).

THE TREATMENT OF HIV

The aim of antiretroviral therapy is to reduce the viral load to non-detectable levels as quickly as possible and for as long as possible, and the British HIV Association recommends that antiretroviral therapy should be commenced before the CD4 count has fallen below 200 cells/mm^3 because of the increased risk of death or rapid progression to AIDS.[540] The recommendation is that the decision to start treatment should be based on an assessment of the risk of disease progression over the medium term if it is not started, versus the potential risk of toxicity and drug resistance if the treatment is commenced too soon; the risk of disease progression is largely determined by the CD4 count, viral load and the age of the person infected.

The first drug used in the treatment of HIV was zidovudine (AZT or ZDV), but by the mid 1990s other drugs had been developed and highly active antiretroviral

Table 16.2 Some AIDS-defining illnesses[531,537]

Lymphocytopenia – CD4 count $< 200/mm^3$
Recurrent pneumonia
Toxoplasmosis
Cryptosporidiosis
Pnemocystis carinii pneumonia
Kaposi's sarcoma
HIV encephalopathy
HIV wasting syndrome
Histoplasmosis
Invasive cervical cancer
Lymphoma of the brain
Salmonella septicaemia
Disseminated or extra-pulmonary *Mycobacterium avium* complex or
   Mycobacterium kansasii disease
Pulmonary tuberculosis
Other mycobacterial infections, either pulmonary or extra-pulmonary

---

therapy, or HAART, was introduced.[541] Antiretroviral therapy works by targeting the viral enzymes which are responsible for HIV replication and drugs are classed as reverse transcriptase inhibitors, which includes AZT, lamivudine (3TC), didanosine (ddl) and stavudine (d4T) or protease inhibitors such as indinavir, ritonavir and nelfinavir. There are numerous drug combinations, and also clinical trials, and it is not clear which combination is the most effective. Treatment may need to be changed because of treatment side effects or treatment failure, which may be attributable to drug resistance. HIV drug resistance has numerous serious consequences which aside from treatment failure include direct and indirect healthcare costs associated with the need to start more costly second-line treatment, the spread of drug-resistant strains of HIV, and the need for new drugs to be developed.[542] If compliance and adherence to antiretroviral therapy is monitored carefully, poor compliance will be detected early on and could be addressed.

HEPATITIS B

Hepatitis is a general term meaning inflammation of the liver which can be caused by a variety of different hepatitis viruses. Hepatitis B is of huge global significance and like HIV it is a sexually transmitted and blood-borne disease and represents a risk to public health.[543] It has infected two billion people worldwide, with more than 350 million experiencing chronic, or lifelong, infection and at high risk of death from cirrhosis and primary liver cancer.[544] The highly infectious virus particles in the blood of symptomatic and asymptomatic infected individuals poses a serious health risk, with healthy asymptomatic carriers the main reservoir of infection. In an infected individual it will be present in the blood and also body fluids such as semen and vaginal secretions, although the concentration in body fluids is only about 1:1000 of that in blood.[545]

THE VIRUS AND THE PATHOGENESIS OF INFECTION

Hepatitis B belongs to a group of viruses known as *Hepadnaviruses*, which although unrelated to other human hepatitis viruses, also include the woodchuck, ground squirrel and Pekin drug viruses.[545,546] It is a small enveloped double-stranded DNA virus, and it is the smallest known DNA virus.[546] The intact virus is known as the Dane particle; the nucleocapsid core (hepatitis B core antigen, or HBcAg) and the viral envelope which contains hepatitis B surface antigen (HBsAg) are of great clinical significance, as is the soluble component of the core, HBeAg. A diagnosis of hepatitis B is based on the detection of the various viral antigens and antibodies in the blood:

- hepatitis B surface antigen (HBsAg) and antibody (anti HBs)
- hepatitis B core antigen (HBcAg) and antibody (anti HBc IgM and anti HBc IgG)
- hepatitis B e antigen (HBeAg) and antibody (anti HBe).[543]

HBsAg is produced in excessive quantities and is seen in the blood of infected individuals in the form of filamentous and spherical particles.[543] It can be detected before and after the onset of symptoms, and is at maximum titre in the blood at the height of liver damage.[545] Detection of HBsAg is a sign of early infection but if it is detected for longer than six months, it indicates chronic infection. The specific antibody, anti-HBs, does not appear until one–four months after the onset of symptoms; it replaces HBsAg, and indicates clinical recovery and immunity.[543] HBeAg, which is indicative of high infectivity, is produced when the virus is replicating and appears after HBsAg. The first antibody to be detected in the blood is anti-HBc, which indicates either current or past hepatitis B infection; anti HBc IgM usually disappears after six months, but anti HBc IgG can be detected for life.[554] The specific antibody to HBeAg, anti-HBe, appears after anti-HBc and indicates recovery and immunity.[543,545]

CLINICAL FEATURES OF HEPATITIS B INFECTION

Hepatitis B has a long incubation period of between 45–120 days (the duration of which is affected by the size of the inoculum and the route of infection), and it is during this time that HBsAg and HBeAg may be detected in the blood.[547] Following this a pre-jaundice or pre-icteric phase occurs, which can last from days to weeks and is characterised by malaise, anorexia, nausea, mild fever and right-sided upper abdominal discomfort. The jaundice or icteric phase follows on from this, and clinical features include bilirubinuria (dark urine caused by the jaundice) and an enlarged tender liver, as well as jaundice of the skin, mucous membranes and conjunctivae. Recovery usually takes several months.

Transmission of hepatitis B can occur through[543]:

- percuataneous exposure – transfusion of unscreened blood or blood products; sharing drug injecting equipment; haemodialysis, acupuncture, tattooing and inoculation from needlestick injuries
- mucous membrane exposure – sexual and perinatal transmission as a result of exposure to high-risk body fluids
- indirect exposure – via inanimate objects such as toothbrushes, razors and eating utensils that are contaminated with blood, and hospital equipment.

Table 16.3 highlights Hepatitis B high risk groups.

IMMUNISATION AGAINST HEPATITIS B

Protection against hepatitis B infection can be given by the administration of a vaccine, which confers active immunity. It can be administered as pre-exposure prophylaxis in high risk groups, or as post-exposure prophylaxis, and is given as an accelerated course at zero, one and two months followed by a fourth dose at twelve months for those who remain at continued risk. The Department of Health 'Green Book'[52] recommends that vaccination against HBV is given to the following categories of people who are high risk of exposure (Table 16.4)

Where exposure to HBV has occurred following an inoculation or contamination incident, specific immunoglobulin (HBIG) is given at the same time as the vaccine to provide immediate but temporary protection against HBV while the vaccine takes effect. It is also used to give protection to those who have a failed response to the vaccine but who have been exposed to HBV.

Antibody responses to the vaccine are variable and should be checked one to four months after the primary course has been given in order to confirm that the recipient is adequately protected against HBV. Ideally, anti-HBs levels should be above 100 IU/ml, and if the anti-HBs level is between 1 –100 IU/ml, an additional dose should be administered. Non-responders have antibody levels of below 10 IU/ml and a further course of vaccine should be given, followed by further checking of the antibody titre at one to four months.[52]

Table 16.3 Hepatitis B high risk groups

Babies born to infected mothers.
Sexual/household contacts of infected individuals.
Healthcare workers.
Patients and staff in haemodialysis centres.
Injecting IV drug mis-users.
Acupuncture/tattooing using unsterile devices.
Sexual activity – heterosexual/homosexual.
Unsterile medical/dental instruments or equipment.

Table 16.4 Department of Health recommendations for vaccination against Hepatitis B in individuals at high risk of exposure[52]

Injecting drug users:
    all current IDUs
    those who inject intermittently
    those likely to progress to injecting
    non-injectors living with injecting partners
    sexual partners of injectors
    children of injectors.
Those with frequent sexual partners.
Close family contacts of a case/individual with chronic HBV infection.
Families adopting children from countries where there is a high prevalence of HBV.
Foster carers.
Those receiving regular blood transfusions/blood products.
Patients with chronic renal failure.
Patients with chronic liver disease.
Travel to/residence in areas of high/intermediate prevalence.
Prisoners in the UK.
Those at risk of occupational exposure to BBV.
All healthcare workers who may have contact with blood, blood-stained body fluids and
    tissue.
Laboratory staff.
Staff of residential accommodation for people with learning difficulties.
Other occupational at risk groups, such as the police, fire and rescue services.
Post exposure.
Accidental inoculation/contamination.
Sexual partners of infected individuals.
Pre term babies.
Babies born to mothers who are chronically infected with HBV or who had acute HBV
    infection during pregnancy.

HEPATITIS C (HCV)

The hepatitis C virus was first identified in 1989 as the cause of post-transfusion non-A-non-B hepatitis[548], and the World Health Organization has compared it to a 'viral time bomb' that has infected 3 % of the world's population, and induced the chronic carrier state in 130 million people, putting them at high risk of developing cirrhosis and liver cancer.[549] It is estimated that there are 3.4 million new cases each year, and that 200,000–250,000 people in England and Wales have been infected.[550] In 2002, the Department of Health published the *Hepatitis C Strategy for England*[551], in response to the action areas identified in the Chief Medical Officer's report published by the Department of Health in 2002.[3] The strategy highlighted the need for robust prevention, diagnosis and treatment services in order to prevent new cases from occurring and to identify and treat new carriers. As injecting drug users represent the biggest high risk group in the UK, the strategy made several recommendations for this target group, including the setting up of needle exchanges, increased treatment for drug dependent persons to prevent them from progressing to injecting drugs, national campaigns to raise public awareness of hepatitis C and the avoidance of high risk behaviours, and education and health promotion in prisons and schools.

THE VIRUS: CLINICAL FEATURES, TRANSMISSION, DIAGNOSIS AND TREATMENT

HCV belongs to the genus *Hepacivirus*, and is a member of the virus family *Flaviviridae,* of which there are six genotypes and multiple subtypes.[546]

It is a small-enveloped single-stranded RNA virus, 50 nm in diameter. It has an incubation period of 6–12 weeks, and while fatigue and jaundice have been reported, most infected individuals are completely asymptomatic. Although disease progression can be variable, infected individuals may be asymptomatic for anything from 20–50 years, and it is not until the liver has been extensively damaged that symptoms become apparent. Of those infected 80 % will develop chronic hepatitis C, of whom 30 % will develop cirrhosis within 30 years of infection, and chronic infection and hepatocellular cancer are the leading indicators for liver transplantation.[552]

During this long period of undiagnosed and asymptomatic infection, countless other people may become infected through certain high risk behaviours and practices. In both developed and undeveloped countries, high risk groups for the acquisition and transmission of HCV include injecting drug users who share contaminated needles and other drug-related equipment, and who constitute the greatest high risk group in the UK at the present time[551]; recipients of unscreened blood donations prior to 1991, and anyone who may have received blood products such as factor VIII, anti-D and immunoglobulin which were manufactured before virus inactivation procedures were implemented in 1986[548]; dialysis patients; and men and women with multiple sexual partners who have unprotected sex. Transmission can also occur from infected mother to child during delivery although this is rare[553], and potentially high risk practices such as sharing toothbrushes and razors that are contaminated with blood, tattooing and skin piercing.[551] Healthcare workers are now at increasing risk of contracting HCV through occupational exposure, and data collated by the HPA between 2002 and 2005 has shown that out of 755 percutaneous exposures to BBVs that occurred to healthcare workers, 369(49 %) involved HCV source patients.[527]

Clinically, infection with HCV is indistinguishable from other hepatitis viruses, and diagnosis is dependent upon the detection of antibodies through serological assays, and molecular techniques such as PCR for the detection of viral RNA (see Chapter 4 The Microbiology Laboratory). The aim of treatment is to eradicate HCV RNA in order to prevent progressive viral fibrosis occurring, and the duration of treatment varies according to the serotype and the viral load.[552] For mild chronic hepatitis C in adults over the age of 18, combination therapy with weekly subcutaneous injections of peginterferon alpha and daily oral ribavirin is the recommended regimen; in moderate to severe chronic disease, peginterflora alfa-2a or pegininterflora alfa-2b in conjunction with ribavirin is prescribed.[550]

THE MANAGEMENT OF BBV INFECTED HEALTHCARE WORKERS

The first documented seroconversion of a healthcare worker to HIV arising from an occupational exposure occurred in the UK in 1984, and in 2005 two patient-to-healthcare worker cases of hepatitis C occurred in the UK, bringing the total number of occupationally acquired HCV transmissions to 11.[527,554] The risk of acquiring HIV through occupational exposure is considered to be very low. It has been estimated that the average risk for HIV transmission after percutaneous exposure to infected blood is 1 in 300 injuries, although percuataneous exposures involving large volumes of fluid can exceed that risk if the index patient has a high viral load; the risks are higher with HBV (1 in 3) and HCV (1 in 30).[528,555] However, although as previously mentioned the risk of transmission of BBVs from patient to healthcare worker is greater than that of healthcare worker to patient, transmission of both HBV and HCV to patients has occurred.[556] Healthcare worker-to-patient transmission is generally limited to exposure-prone procedures whereby injury to the healthcare worker could result in contamination of the patient's open tissues with blood ('bleed-back'). Exposure-prone procedures (EPPs) are defined as invasive procedures where the gloved hands of the healthcare worker are in contact with sharp instruments, needles or sharp tissue such as spicules of bone or teeth, or inside an open body cavity or wound, or confined anatomical space where hands or fingertips may not be visible all the time.[556]

Revised guidance on the management of HIV infected healthcare workers was re-issued by the Department of Health in 2005[556], and on the management of HBV infected healthcare workers in 2007[557], in order to protect patients and also to ensure that infected healthcare workers receive the appropriate support and treatment.

Healthcare workers with HIV should be restricted from performing EPPs and may need re-training or redeployment.[556] With regard to hepatitis B, the most recent recommendation from the Department of Health is that infected healthcare workers with HBV should be allowed to perform EPPs if their baseline viral load does not exceed 10^5 geq/ml, and if their viral load is adequately suppressed.[557] Healthcare workers who have antibodies to HCV and who carry out EPPs should be tested for viral RNA and, if positive, restricted from carrying out EPPs until they have successfully responded to therapy (HCV RNA negative after six months).[558]

POST-EXPOSURE PROPHYLAXIS (PEP) FOR HEALTHCARE WORKERS

In the event of an accidental occupational exposure to BBVs, the healthcare worker is likely to require post-exposure prophylaxis, and it is essential that all staff are aware of local arrangements for access to urgent advice so that the incident can be risk assessed and the appropriate treatment can be given. Where exposure to HIV is deemed to be significant, a 28-day course with a triple combination of antiretroviral drugs is recommended by the Expert Advisory Group on AIDS[555] which consists of zidovudine 250 mg or 350 mg (twice daily), plus lamivudine 150 mg twice daily and nelfinavir 1250mg twice daily (or 750mgs three times a day), and this should ideally begin within one hour of the injury occurring.

If the healthcare worker has potentially been exposed to HBV and has not been vaccinated, they will need to commence an accelerated course of HBV vaccine and HBIG which should be given within 48 hours of exposure[52]; if they have received a full vaccination course and are a known responder, no further treatment is required. As there is no vaccination against HCV, antiviral treatment is commenced if symptoms of liver disease develop.

Table 16.5 summarises the immediate precautions to be take following an occupational exposure to a BBV.

Table 16.5 Action to be taken in the event of an inoculation injury or mucous membrane exposure to blood/body fluids

For **WOUNDS**
- **Wash** the site of injury thoroughly with soap and water; **encourage** bleeding by **gently** squeezing the site of the injury but **do not** rub. Cover with a waterproof dressing.

For **MUCOUS MEMBRANES**
- **Irrigate** contaminated areas thoroughly with normal saline or water.

THEN AS SOON AS POSSIBLE
- **Inform** the person in charge, who should make a **risk assessment** of the incident, and ensure that the appropriate advice is sought and action taken immediately. Staff should be aware of the local arrangements for reporting. An incident report should also be completed and sent to the appropriate person as per local policy.

HIGHEST RISK BLOOD EXPOSURE
- Deep injury with a hollow needle, especially if previously in source patient's vein or artery **or**
- large volume of blood **and**
- high titre of virus (acute retroviral illness or end stage AIDS).

INCREASED RISK BLOOD EXPOSURE
- Suture needle **and**
- large volume of blood **or**
- high titre of virus.

Post-Exposure Prophylaxis (PEP) should be considered urgently if:
- the source is known or highly suspected to be HIV positive
- the healthcare worker has not been immunised against hepatitis B, or is a non-responder to the vaccine.

PROTECTION AGAINST BBVS IN THE HEALTHCARE SETTING

In order to protect both patients and staff from BBVs, it is essential that avoidable exposure is prevented. Guidance for healthcare workers on the prevention of infection with blood-borne viruses was published jointly by the Expert Advisory Group on AIDS and the Advisory Group on Hepatitis in 1998.[528] Together with the revised EPIC guidelines[86] which contain recommendations for best clinical practice in the prevention and control of infection, these documents provide a robust evidence-based framework for ensuring that best practice is implemented for the protection of the healthcare workers and patients. The EPIC guidelines are discussed in Chapter 6 The Principles of Infection Prevention and Control, but the basic precautions that should be taken are summarised in Table 16.6. The safe handling and disposal of sharps is summarised in Chapter 6, Figure 6.1.

Table 16.6 Precautions to prevent transmission of BBVs in the healthcare setting[86,528]

Hand hygiene
Decontaminate hands in between each and every episode of direct patient contact or after contact with contaminated equipment. If hands are visibly contaminated with dirt, blood or body fluids, wash hands using liquid soap and water.

Gloves
Wear disposable gloves where contact with blood/body fluids is anticipated. They should be worn as single-use disposable items, changed in between each patient contact and discarded as clinical waste as soon as the patient activity has been completed. Hands must be decontaminated/washed following removal of gloves.

Aprons
Disposable plastic aprons should be worn when contact with blood/body fluids is anticipated, and changed in between each patient contact and discarded as clinical waste. Where there is a risk of heavy contamination or splashing with blood/body fluids, full length fluid repellent gowns should be worn.

Face protection
Where there is a risk of blood/body fluids splashing into the face and eyes, face protection such as visors and goggles must be worn to protect the mucous membranes.

Protect broken areas of skin
Broken areas of skin on the hands of healthcare workers, including skin lesions and wounds, should be covered at all times with a waterproof dressing.

Sharps safety
All staff should ensure that they handle and dispose of sharps safely (see Figure 6.1).

Spillages of blood and blood-stained body fluids
All blood and blood stained body fluids present a potential hazard and should be dealt with immediately:

- cordon off the area where the spill has occurred
- gather together disposable non-sterile gloves and a disposable plastic apron, plus eye/face wear if required, paper towels, a yellow clinical waste sack, sodium dichlorisocyanurate solution 10,000 ppm, and sodium dichlorisocyanurate granules

---

Table 16.6 (continued)

- wearing protective clothing, cover the surface of the spill either with dichlorisocyanurate granules, or cover the spill with paper towels and gently pour a solution of 10,000 ppm sodium dichlorisocyanurate over the towels
- wait until the granules solidify, or leave the solution for two minutes to take effect, and then gather up the towels and dispose of them into the clinical waste sack
- wipe over the area with detergent and warm water
- dispose of gloves and apron as clinical waste and decontaminate/wash hands.

Decontamination of equipment
Decontaminate equipment according to manufacturer's instructions/local policy.
Organic material such as dirt and blood should be removed with detergent and warm water prior to disinfection or sterilisation.

17 Severe Acute Respiratory Syndrome (SARS)

INTRODUCTION

In 2002 a report by the Chief Medical Officer[3] acknowledged that it was inevitable that new infectious diseases would emerge, and that it was 'essential to expect the unexpected'. In November of that year, one such new disease began to emerge in South East Asia, leading to a global outbreak between March and July 2003. It affected more than 4,300 people in 32 countries, with an additional 8,400 probable cases, and resulted in more than 800 deaths.[559] It caused widespread fear and panic, badly affected trade and the travel industry, overwhelmed the provision of healthcare services where the highest burden of cases was seen among healthcare workers, and took advantage of the fact that the world is now a highly mobile society by efficiently spreading across the globe. That new disease was severe acute respiratory syndrome, otherwise known as SARS, and it was the first new viral disease threat of the 21st century. In July 2003, the World Health Organization issued a global statement declaring that the last human chain of transmission had been broken and the first global outbreak of SARS had been contained[560] and in May 2005 it declared that SARS had been eradicated, although whether it has gone forever remains to be seen. This chapter looks at the emergence of SARS, the development of the global outbreak and how it was successfully halted before it became endemic throughout the world. The new SARS virus, pathogenesis of infection and clinical features and infection control precautions are discussed, along with accounts of some of the nosocomial outbreaks that occurred within healthcare settings.

At the time of writing, there are no confirmed cases of SARS anywhere in the world. In October 2004, WHO published updated guidelines and recommendations[561] following four incidents in which cases occurred following breaches in laboratory biosafety or from exposure to an animal or environmental reservoir, demonstrating the potential for SARS to re-emerge again. This document, which supersedes all other recommendations, provides a revised definition of the WHO SARS Global Alert, clinical case definition, case exclusion and laboratory diagnosis, and preparedness planning in the event of the re-emergence of SARS, and describes the ongoing need for global surveillance. The World Health Organization[562], the Health Protection Agency[563] and the Centres for Disease

Control[564] websites also provide a wealth of information on SARS and the reader is encouraged to explore the fascinating SARS story further.

LEARNING OUTCOMES

After reading this chapter the reader will:

- Understand the extent of the global threat posed by SARS and how the 2003 global outbreak evolved and was contained
- Be aware of the revised case definition for SARS in the event of a re-emergence of the disease
- Understand the stringent infection control precautions required to prevent the spread of disease, particularly among healthcare workers who are most at risk

BACKGROUND

'We do not mark the end of SARS today but we observe a milestone: the global SARS outbreak has been contained. At this point we should all pause and give thanks to the scientists, public health and hospital workers who took risks in the face of a new and unknown disease. And we must remember those frontline workers who died of SARS. Their daily dedication, courage and vigilance averted a global catastrophe.' Dr Gro Harlem-Bruntland, Director General of WHO. 5th July 2003.[565]

In November 2002 the first cases of a new acute infectious respiratory disease, characterised by fever, dry cough, shortness of breath and pneumonia, were seen in Foshan, Guangdong province, China. Cases were subsequently seen in neighbouring Heyan, affecting healthcare workers and family contacts of the index case, who was a chef in an exotic game restaurant. It was later discovered that many of those initial cases had links to the live animal trade, an epidemiological link that would become increasingly significant in the weeks and months to come.[566] By January 2003, the disease had spread to Guangzhou, the capital of Guangdong province, presenting as a rapidly progressive atypical pneumonia associated again with outbreaks among families and healthcare workers. On the 11th of February, WHO was informed by the Chinese authorities of 305 cases from Guangdong province, and more than 30 % of those cases were among healthcare workers working in hospitals in urban areas.[566] In total, there were 1,512 clinically confirmed cases of atypical pneumonia in Guangdong province, with healthcare workers alarmingly accounting for 27 % of those. WHO officials, in collaboration with other experts, worked around the clock to identify this mysterious illness and by the 14th February they had excluded pneumonic plague, anthrax, influenza, leptospirosis and hemorrhagic fever.[567]

One single event on the 21st February 2003 resulted in the spread of this new disease outside China, spreading it via international air routes to Hong Kong,

Vietnam, Singapore and Toronto[567], where the full horror of SARS was unleashed. A doctor who had treated patients in Guangdong province developed respiratory symptoms and spent one night at a hotel in Hong Kong, where it is believed that he infected at least 16 other guests staying on the same floor. From that one index case however the disease spread to local hospitals and communities in other countries. Again, healthcare workers were primarily affected – they were in the front line and at enormous risk from this as yet unidentified and potentially fatal disease, working without respiratory barrier protection. The doctor died of respiratory failure. Also staying at the same hotel, and on the same floor as the doctor, was a Chinese-American businessman. He died in March in the Vietnam French Hospital in Hanoi, and was the index case for the cases subsequently seen in Hong Kong, and cohorts in Canada, Vietnam, Singapore, the USA, Thailand and Germany. The doctor looking after the businessman was Carlo Urbani, a WHO official based in Hanoi. He had been contacted by hospital officials and was asked to examine the businessman as there were concerns that the atypical pneumonia that he had presented with was actually avian influenza. Dr Urbani was subsequently instrumental in alerting the Vietnamese authorities to a new disease, which resulted in heightened global awareness and surveillance. His work at the Vietnam French Hospital in Hanoi, when he initiated stringent infection control precautions, led to the early identification and isolation of new cases and contained an outbreak that threatened Vietnam as well as other countries. Dr Urbani died of SARS on the 29th March 2003. Information about Dr Urbani and his work in Hanoi is available on the WHO website.

On the 12th March 2003, WHO issued a global health alert warning the world of a severe respiratory illness presenting as an atypical pneumonia, which had been causing outbreaks in Vietnam, Hong Kong and Guangdong province, China, and was spreading among healthcare workers.[568] The decision to issue a global alert was made for a number of reasons; the causative agent and its potential spread had yet to be identified, but the disease had already spread from Asia; it posed the greatest risk to healthcare workers and the close contacts of those infected; antibiotics and antivirals had been used to treat those affected but with very poor response and little indication that they would be effective in treating this new disease, and there appeared to be rapid progression to adult respiratory distress syndrome (ARDS) among some patients, and particularly among affected healthcare workers.[567]

As yet, the disease had not been named but it was referred to as a severe respiratory illness. Data collected from the cases so far revealed that early symptoms in patients progressing to SARS were fever, malaise, chills, rigor, headache, myalgia, malaise, dizziness, and a cough, sore throat and runny nose [569] – all fairly non-specific respiratory symptoms. Chest x-ray tended to reveal small unilateral patchy shadowing, which over the course of 24–48 hours progressed to bilateral infiltrates. Abnormal changes could sometimes be seen in the absence of chest symptoms, and in the end stages of the illness some patients progressed to ARDS. In the early stages, the patient's blood picture was normal but by days three and four of the illness, lymphopenia was seen, along with raised liver function tests

(LFTs) and C-reactive protein (CRP). The alert confirmed that there was no link between this new respiratory disease and avian influenza (A/H$_5$N$_1$ – see Chapter 18 Pandemic Influenza) which had caused an outbreak of bird flu in Hong Kong in February 2003.[567]

On the 15th March, just three days after the global alert was issued, the Singapore authorities contacted WHO with an urgent request for assistance; a doctor who had treated the first cases seen in Singapore was himself reporting respiratory symptoms and was on board an aeroplane from New York, where he had been attending a medical conference, returning to Singapore via Germany. The doctor and his wife were removed from the plane in Frankfurt.[570] WHO then announced that this new disease, which was named severe acute respiratory syndrome, or SARS, was indeed a 'worldwide health threat'[567], and they issued global response plans, case definitions for probable and suspected cases and infection control guidance for hospitals. They also mobilised GOARN, the Global Outbreak And Response Network which had been launched by WHO in 2000 to closely monitor evidence of evolving infectious disease and monitor response to outbreaks. On the 16th March, 150 new suspected and probable cases of SARS were reported globally, and on the 24th March, Hanoi in Vietnam reported that 63 % of cases there were in healthcare workers.

A report from one of the first WHO investigative teams brought in to investigate the outbreak in Guangdong province, China, made the following statement.

'If SARS is not brought under control in China there will no chance of controlling the global threat of SARS. Control of a new and rapidly disseminating disease like SARS is challenging, especially in a country as large and diverse as China. Effective disease surveillance and reporting are key strategies in any attempt to control the spread of a serious new communicable disease such as SARS.'[567]

CONTROLLING THE 2003 GLOBAL OUTBREAK

The aim of the World Health Organization was to halt further international spread of SARS and prevent it from becoming endemic.[567] It was an unprecedented global response that brought SARS under control, breaking the last chain of human transmission in June 2003.

During the outbreak hospitals, schools and borders were closed; police in Hong Kong adapted and modified the electronic tracking systems that they used to track criminal activity and used them for contact tracing and monitoring compliance with quarantine. In Singapore, the army assisted with contact tracing and enforcing quarantine. As every country with an international airport was considered by WHO to be at potential risk of an outbreak, health screening was introduced for passengers travelling on international flights and in Taiwan, infra-red body temperature screening devices were introduced that accurately measure body temperature, and any traveller with a fever was prevented from boarding aircraft.[571] Guidance for travellers was issued in the form of advisory notices detailing the typical clinical features of

SARS, along with guidance for airlines on the action to be taken if passengers were taken ill on board flights. Although air travel was not suspended initially, when evidence emerged that SARS was spreading WHO then recommended postponing all but essential travel to those areas.[567]

The issuing of global alerts, which were amplified by the media, resulted in global vigilance, promoting the reporting and detection of cases in new areas; specialist teams went into the worst affected areas with supplies of respiratory equipment for the healthcare workers battling to save lives, and specialist WHO teams also investigated and monitored potential environmental sources. Eleven WHO affiliated laboratories worked 24 hours a day to identify the virus and develop rapid and reliable diagnostic methods and within a month the causative agent was identified.[567] Case definitions, guidance on the clinical management and infection control precautions were communicated worldwide and were refined as more became known, facilitating the implementation of precautions and assisting the global response.

CORONAVIRUSES

The SARS virus was found to be a novel coronavirus (later named SARS-coV), and was initially independently isolated by three laboratories working within the WHO network from clinical specimens obtained from patients with SARS.[572,573] Coronaviruses are single stranded RNA viruses, 60–220 nm in diameter, with an outer envelope. They have a 'crown-like' appearance (corona), which creates a halo effect around the virus.[574] They are primarily responsible for causing upper respiratory tract infections, along with viral gastroenteritis, in humans but they are also pathogens in animals and have been known to mutate and infect new species.[574] Early in November 2002, when the first cases of SARS emerged in Guangdong province, there were reports that some of those affected had been exposed to live wild game animals in markets. Some of these animals were subsequently tested and were found to carry a virus that was very similar to the human SARS coronavirus, most notably the Himalayan palm civet cat (*Paguma larvata*) (73 % of the market traders primarily trading in palm civet cats were found to be seropositive[575]), the racoon dog (*Nyclereutes procyonoides*), and the Chinese ferret badger (*Melogale moschata*) – all regarded as delicacies in southern China. The virus was therefore presumed to be zoonotic in origin, arising from the animal kingdom with the palm civet cat as the most important animal reservoir.[576] The live market setting, offering a diversity of animal species, is believed to have given the virus ample opportunity to amplify and over a period of time jump hosts, eventually infecting humans and resulting in human-to-human transmission.[576] In September 2005, a study from China confirmed that 40 % of horseshoe bats near Hong Kong were infected with a coronavirus similar to SARS-coV, raising the question: did the horseshoe bats infect the palm civet cats?

TRANSMISSION AND CLINICAL FEATURES OF SARS

Coronaviruses replicate in the ciliated epithelial cells of the nasopharynx, and the route of infection is therefore via the respiratory tract, giving rise to systemic flu-like symptoms and fever. Transmission occurs via exposure to respiratory droplets, close contact with an infected individual, or contact with contaminated environmental surfaces and fomites.[570,577] The outbreak at the hotel in Hong Kong, in which 16 guests were infected from one index case, also suggests that airborne spread is implicated.[578] An outbreak at the Amoy Gardens, a private housing estate in Hong Kong, in March 2004 affected more than 300 residents, and is believed to have originated from one index case who had diarrhoea, which was a prominent clinical feature amongst local cases. An investigative team from WHO concluded that virus-laden aerosols arising from a bathroom were driven by an exhaust fan within the room and carried on air currents, entering other apartments within the complex.[575] Local problems with sewerage systems were also identified but faecal-oral spread was not considered to be as significant as airborne spread.[579] Although SARS is considered to be less infectious than influenza, there is documented evidence of spread from one index case to 100 others, and there are reports that one infected person could go on to infect three other people, who in turn could go onto infect hundreds more.[580]

The incubation period ranges from 2 to 10 days, although 13 days has been reported.[581,582,583] The earliest clinical features are a non-specific influenza-like prodromal illness but generally without coryzal symptoms or a sore throat (although the preliminary description of SARS issued by WHO in 2003 included these symptoms), with those affected reporting a high fever ($>38\,°C$) lasting at least 24 hours, along with rigors, a headache, malaise and myalgia. This is followed within a week by the onset of a non-productive cough and dyspnoea, together with difficulty in breathing. Diarrhoea also occurs in 25–70 % of cases.[561,574] The symptoms are generally severe enough to justify admission to hospital, and x-rays reveal patchy consolidation indicative of pneumonia or acute respiratory distress syndrome (ARDS).[584] Approximately 25 % of patients develop rapidly progressive respiratory distress and oxygen desaturation, which may resolve or result in death from respiratory failure[574], with 1 in 10 patients requiring ventilatory support.[585] The risk of developing ARDS increases with age and co-morbidities such as cardiac disease and diabetes[574], and carries a fatality rate of 50 % in those over the age of 65.

DIAGNOSIS

A diagnosis of SARS infection is based upon a combination of the clinical features and epidemiological links to other people or areas affected by SARS, and the identification and isolation of SARS-coV from clinical specimens using investigative laboratory methods such as PCR, ELISA and cell culture[579] (see Chapter 4 The Microbiology Laboratory). Tables 17.1 and 17.2 give the UK case definitions for a

Table 17.1 Case definition for a probable case of SARS

An individual with a respiratory illness requiring hospitalisation on clinical grounds and characterised by:
Fever of >38 °C
AND
Cough or difficulty breathing
AND
Radiographic evidence consistent with SARS i.e. radiographic evidence of infiltrates consistent with pneumonia or respiratory distress syndrome (RDS)
OR
Autopsy findings consistent with the pathology of pneumonia or RDS without an identifiable cause
AND a potential epidemiological link – i.e. in the 10 days before the onset of illness a history of travel to an area classified by WHO as having recent local transmission (http://www.who.int/csr/sars/areas/en/).
OR
A history of exposure to laboratories or institutes which have retained SARS virus isolates and/or diagnostic specimens from SARS patients
OR
Close contact* with a probable or confirmed SARS case
AND no alternate diagnosis to fully explain their illness.

---

* Close contact means healthcare worker or persons having cared for, lived with or had face-to-face (within one metre) contact with, or having had direct contact with, respiratory secretions and/or body fluids of a person with SARS.
Case definition for a probable case of SARS. www.brit-thoracic.org.uk/c2/iploads/SARS0304.pdf (30th May 2007), with permission from The British Thoracic Society

Table 17.2 Case definition for a confirmed case of SARS

An individual with symptoms and signs that are clinically suggestive of SARS
AND
With laboratory evidence of SARS-coV infection based on one or more of the following:

a) PCR positive for SARS-coV using a validated method from:
   at least two different clinical specimens (e.g. respiratory and stool) **OR**
   the same clinical specimen collected on two or more occasions during the course of the illness **OR**
   two different assays or repeat PCR using new RNA extract from the original clinical sample on each occasion of testing.
b) Seroconversion by ELISA or IFA
c) Virus isolation
   Isolation in cell culture of SARS-coV from any specimen, plus PCR confirmation using a validated method.

Case definition for a confirmed case of SARS, www.brit-thoracic.org.uk/c2/uploads/SARS0304.pdf (30th May 2007), reproduced with permission from The British Thoracic Society

Table 17.3 Other investigations for SARS

Chest x-ray
Pulse oximetry
Blood gasses if oxygen saturation $< 95\,\%$ on room air
Blood tests – full blood count (FBC), and urea, creatinine and electrolytes liver function
   tests, creatinine, C-reactive protein (CRP), and lactate dehydrogenase

---

probable and confirmed case of SARS based on the 2004 updated British Infection Society, British Thoracic Society, and the Health Protection Agency guidance.[586] In the UK, specimens should only be sent to the HPA reference laboratory once the Communicable Disease Surveillance Centre (CDSC) has been notified and a standard reporting form completed. All specimens sent for microbiology should be double bagged and labelled with a biohazard sticker. Samples include expectorated sputum, 20–30 mL of urine, stool, EDTA blood (20 mL for PCR) and 20 mL of clotted blood for acute serology.[586] Table 17.3 details other investigations that need to be undertaken.

MANAGEMENT OF SARS

The re-emergence of SARS would potentially result in high demand for critical care beds. Studies from Canada and Singapore highlighted that approximately 20 % of patients with suspected or probable SARS required critical care support and that 66–76 % required mechanical ventilation.[587] In terms of drug therapy, the recommendations are that patients should be treated with an antibiotic regimen consisting of intravenous (IV) co-amoxiclav 1.2g tds or cefuroxime. 1.5g tds, together with either erythromycin 500mg qds or clarithromycin 500mg bd.[584] Moderate doses of prednisiolone (30–40 mg/day or IV equivalent) can be given in severely ill patients with deranged blood gases/oxygen saturation. There is insufficient evidence to support the administration of antiviral therapy such as ribavirin.

INFECTION CONTROL PRECAUTIONS

The HPA[588] provides detailed information in relation to the infection control precautions required, and the overall management of patients with SARS, and these are summarised in Table 17.4.

The wearing of protective clothing and equipment – long-sleeved fluid repellent disposable gowns, tight-fitting latex/latex-free gloves with high cuffs, visors and goggles and FFP3 respirators – is discussed in detail in Chapter 18 Pandemic Influenza.

The majority of the outbreaks during the 2003 global outbreak centred around hospitals which amplified the transmission of the virus, predominantly to healthcare workers, and also provided a portal of entry for SARS into the wider community, enabling it to spread from patients to visitors and their close contacts, including close contacts of infected healthcare workers. It is now known that SARS-coV can survive in the environment for up to 24 hours, and result in wide spread

Table 17.4 Infection control precautions to prevent the transmission of SARS[588]

Isolation	Patients with suspected/confirmed SARS must be admitted to a single room with the door kept closed; preferably, the room should be negative pressure (see Chapter 10). If there is more than one patient affected and insufficient isolation facilities, patients may be cohort nursed following a risk assessment by the infection prevention and control team. Side rooms or bays that have air conditioning should have the air conditioning system switched *off* until the patient has been discharged and the room decontaminated.
Personal protective equipment and clothing	*All* staff entering the room must wear protective clothing consisting of a long-sleeved fluid-repellent disposable gown, latex or latex-free gloves with tight long-fitting cuffs, goggles and/or visors, and an FFP3 respirator conforming to EN 149:2001. Protective clothing should be removed before leaving the room and disposed of within the room as clinical waste, along with the FFP3 respirator. Visors/goggles should be decontaminated either according to the manufacturer's instructions or with a solution of hypochlorite 1,000 ppm and rinsed thoroughly.
Equipment	Dedicated equipment should be used and reusable equipment avoided where at all possible. If reusable equipment has to be used it should be decontaminated after use with a solution of hypochlorite 1,000 ppm. Closed circuits should be used and ventilators protected with filters. Equipment such as fans should not be used as they re-circulate air and can re-aerosolise settled particles. Disposable crockery is not required: crockery should be washed in a dishwasher.
Hand hygiene	Hands can be decontaminated using alcohol hand rub but if visibly contaminated with dirt, blood or body fluids they must be washed with liquid soap and water. Hand decontamination must take place on leaving isolation rooms/cohort bays, in between each episode of patient care, after removing personal protective equipment/clothing and after contact with and following decontamination of contaminated equipment.
Linen	All linen should be treated as infected and bagged inside the isolation room/cohort bay.
Waste	All waste should be disposed of as clinical waste according to local policy/national guidelines.
Visitors	The number of visitors should be limited to include only next of kin; visitors should wear protective clothing as described above; close contacts of a probable or confirmed case of SARS should be screened for symptoms before being permitted to enter the hospital; a record of all visitors to the ward should be kept.

Table 17.4 (continued)

Staff	Staff should be restricted to essential staff only and a record of all staff having patient contact kept and sent to the occupational health department every day; bank and agency staff usage should be avoided; staff working with SARS patients should avoid working with non-SARS patients until 10 days after they last had contact with a suspected or probable case; staff should be vigilant for symptoms of SARS in the 10 day period following their last exposure and report any symptoms immediately to the infection prevention and control team and the occupational health department.
Specimen collection	Specimens must be double bagged and labelled as a bio-hazard risk
Last Offices	Mortuary and funeral directors should be informed of the bio-hazard risk; staff should carry out last offices wearing full protective clothing and the body should be placed in a body bag.

environmental contamination, and as well as encompassing respiratory and contact precautions, infection control precautions need to incorporate high levels of environmental hygiene and decontamination.[586]

There is documented evidence that staff undertaking high risk exposure-prone procedures that generate aerosols are at enormous risk themselves from acquiring SARS, or even pandemic influenza[589,590]; nebulised therapy, humidification, bronchoscopy induced sputum, non-invasive (NIV) pressure ventilation via a face mask, suctioning, cardio-pulmonary resuscitation, intubation and extubation should be undertaken in a single room, preferably one with negative pressure, and with the door kept closed; the procedure should ideally be planned in advance and controlled, the number of staff present should be kept to the absolute minimum, and all staff present should wear full protective clothing.[586]

NOSOCOMIAL OUTBREAKS OF SARS

There were several hospital outbreaks of SARS during 2003, which demonstrated how easily the virus was transmitted within healthcare settings. Hospitals in China and Taiwan experienced outbreaks as a result of patients being admitted with unrecognised SARS. In Toronto, Canada, a cluster of cases of SARS was seen among healthcare workers who were undertaking high-risk exposure-prone procedures with SARS patients but being inconsistent in their compliance with infection control precautions. These three nosocomial outbreaks are discussed here.

TIANJIN, CHINA

An outbreak occurred in a general hospital in Tianjin, China, where a single patient directly infected 33 other people.[591] The index case for the Tianjin outbreak was a patient who left a hospital in Beijing where he was being treated for cardiovascular problems on the 15th April 2003 after sharing a hospital room with a patient who was diagnosed with SARS. Although SARS contacts were advised not to leave Beijing this patient did leave out of fear, and he sought treatment that very same day for his medical conditions in the cardiovascular department at a hospital in Tianjin. He was admitted for further examination and investigations. His initial clinical examination revealed nothing untoward, but on the 16th April he developed a pyrexia, sore throat, myalgia and a productive cough. His temperature peaked that afternoon and a chest x-ray showed some abnormal changes, but his blood count was within normal parameters. However, one doctor did suspect SARS and the patient's exposure to SARS at the hospital in Beijing became apparent on questioning and investigation. He was immediately diagnosed with probable SARS and transferred to a specialist chest hospital in Tianjin, where he was treated for two days before being transferred to the infectious diseases hospital where he died on the day of admission. Cases were seen at the hospitals where the patient was treated and out of the total of 175 cases of SARS in Tianjin, 164 were directly linked to this index case. The outbreak lasted for approximately four weeks and during that time the hospital in Tianjin where the patient first sought treatment was more or less quarantined and the hospital sealed and guarded by armed police.

KAOHSIUNG, TAIWAN

An outbreak of SARS involving a medical centre in Kaohsiung, Taiwan, resulted in 55 cases of SARS arising from the index case, two deaths and led to 227 health-care staff being quarantined between the 26th April and the 26th May 2006.[592] The index case was admitted to hospital with respiratory symptoms but denied any SARS contact and was diagnosed with pneumonia. When her condition dramatically worsened, staff learnt that she had in fact been exposed to SARS at a hospital in Teipi, which had been closed due to a nosocomial outbreak. She was immediately diagnosed with SARS and isolated in a negative pressure isolation room; two other patient contacts were also isolated and 48 members of staff who had been exposed to the index case before the diagnosis of SARS was made were quarantined. The ward was closed and all remaining patients on the ward were screened for SARS. Wards above and below the affected ward were also closed; one was converted into 15 negative pressure rooms, while the other underwent modification with the installation of window-mounted exhaust fans. 16 members of staff developed SARS, and out of those initially looking after the index case, one nurse and two doctors were diagnosed with probable SARS. There were two fatalities – a doctor and a mortuary worker. Staff had been involved in high risk procedures with the index case before the diagnosis of SARS was made, but were not wearing full personal protective equipment and clothing.

TORONTO

Out of 442 probable and suspected cases of SARS seen in Canada during the global outbreak, the majority were seen in Ontario, and 44 % of the probable cases in Canada were in healthcare workers. A study was undertaken[593] to identify the factors that led to an increase in the incidence of SARS among healthcare workers who developed the disease *after* the implementation of SARS-specific infection control precautions, and highlighted multiple contributing factors which facilitated the spread of SARS among healthcare staff.

In March 2003, staff at all hospitals in Ontario had been instructed to implement SARS-specific infection control precautions, which included the wearing of personal protective equipment and clothing, using dedicated or disposable equipment, and hand washing in between patient contacts, to halt the progression of SARS among healthcare workers. However, between the 28th March when these precautions were implemented and the 24th April, 17 cases of probable SARS were seen among healthcare workers at six different hospitals in Toronto. The affected staff were interviewed and it became apparent that there had been breaches in infection control practice and that compliance was inconsistent. Examples included failure to wear personal protective clothing and equipment, including respiratory protection, some of which was not fit-tested, and failure to dispose of contaminated respiratory equipment and protective clothing appropriately or change it in between patients; failure to decontaminate hands in between patient contacts, after removing gloves and aprons or handling contaminated equipment; reusing items of equipment that should either have been disposed of after use or decontaminated; and having direct contact with respiratory secretions from SARS patients while failing to wear protection against respiratory droplets. There were other contributing factors. Staff were exhausted from caring for so many patients with SARS and they took shortcuts. They were confused about the use and removal of personal protective clothing and equipment which some staff found time-consuming. Staff working in dedicated SARS units, emergency departments and intensive care units were expected to wear protective clothing and respirators throughout their shift, and many reported experiencing nausea, dizziness and shortness of breath when wearing respirators for long hours. Infection control training was felt to have been inadequate.

THE FUTURE

SARS has already demonstrated that it has the potential to re-emerge so a further outbreak at some point in the future cannot be discounted. The containment of the 2003 outbreak demonstrated that human-to-human chains of transmission could be interrupted. However, a commitment to ongoing global surveillance and international collaboration and partnership between governments, agencies and health authorities is absolutely crucial to ensuring that robust systems remain in place and that the capacity is there to launch another successful global response against a threat to the world's health.

18 Pandemic Influenza

INTRODUCTION

Every year there are reports of seasonal epidemics of influenza, which are estimated to kill between 500,000 and 1 million people globally[594], and in the UK alone 10–15 % of the population are affected, with 12,000 deaths occurring predominately among the elderly and those with pre-existing respiratory disease. Influenza viruses have an amazing ability to change their genetic make-up and essentially recreate themselves, and they are described as 'the chameleons of the microbial world'.[594] Pandemics of influenza have been reported since the sixteenth century, and are associated with high morbidity, excess mortality and social and economic disruption. Pandemic influenza is now regarded by many experts as the most significant global public health emergency caused by a naturally occurring pathogen[595], and the problems seen in Asia and other parts of the world since 2003 with the highly pathogenic H_5N_1 avian influenza virus, now capable of causing severe disease in humans, suggests '. . . that the world is closer now to a pandemic than at any time since the 1960s'.[596] Pandemic influenza has the potential to circle the globe within three months, kill between 2–50 million worldwide, cause massive social and economic disruption by adversely affecting trade and industry, and completely overwhelm healthcare services everywhere.[594,595,596,597] However, two 'modelling' studies undertaken in 2005 (to assess the potential impact of a pandemic and examine the extensive containment measures required) suggest that containment of a pandemic, which would possibly prevent global spread, may be possible if antiviral drugs are rushed to the region where the pandemic strain first emerges, and if stringent public health measures are implemented.[598]

This chapter looks at the influenza virus, and its clinical features; the three great influenza pandemics of 1918, 1957 and 1968 and the problem of pandemic influenza are discussed, along with the link with avian influenza, or 'bird flu'; pandemic outbreak management, based on the latest WHO/DoH guidance, and treatment, are also discussed. It should be emphasised here that as pandemic influenza has yet to become a reality, all national and international guidance is very much a work in progress and the reader should bear in mind that guidance will be revised and updated as the situation and the threat changes. Documents relating to the UK can be found on the Department of Health[599], the Health Protection Agency[600] and the World Health Organization websites.[601]

LEARNING OUTCOMES

After reading this chapter the reader will:

- Understand the differences between pandemic and seasonal influenza
- Understand the terms 'antigenic drift' and 'antigenic shift' in relation to the evolution of new strains of influenza
- Understand the significance of avian influenza and its link to the pandemic threat
- Know the clinical features and route of transmission/mode of spread of influenza
- Understand the principles of both the Department of Health UK Influenza Plan and the World Health Organizsation Global Influenza Preparedness Plan

THE VIRUS

The influenza virus belongs to the virus family *Orthomyxoviridae*[602,603], and was first identified in 1933. There are three serotypes which are based on antigenic differences and differences in genetic make-up, structure, host susceptibility, epidemiology and clinical features.[604] Influenza A viruses, while mostly prevalent among humans, also circulate among many mammalian and avian species, and it is this ability to jump the species barrier that makes this serotype the biggest threat in terms of the evolution of new influenza viruses and a potential influenza pandemic. While influenza B can cause severe disease in the 'at risk' groups, and influenza C causes mild disease throughout the year, neither of these serotypes have been linked to previous pandemics, although that does not rule out the possibility of a new B or C strain evolving that has pandemic potential.

The virus is covered with surface projections or spikes, which consist of two types of antigen – HA antigen and NA antigen. HA antigen – hemoglutinin – plays an important role in initiating infection by enabling the virus to attach to receptor sites on the respiratory cell surface in the host. NA antigens – neuraminidase – assist fusion of the viral cell envelope with the surface of the host respiratory cell and aid the release of newly formed virus particles from infected cells, which go on to enter and replicate within other cells.[605]

INFLUENZA A

Influenza A consists of eight segments of viral RNA and is the only influenza virus broken down into subtypes dependent upon its HA and NA antigens. There are at least 15 different and antigenically distinct HAs (H_1 to H_{15}) and 9 NAs (N_1 to N_9), of which H_1, H_2 and H_3 and N_1 and N_2 are the most medically significant.[602] Currently there are three subtypes of influenza A in circulation – A/H_1N_1, A/H_1N_2 and A/H_3N_2.[606]

Influenza viruses are able to mutate and swap genes, undergoing frequent changes in their surface HA and/or NA antigens which may be minor (antigenic drift) or major (antigenic shift). Antigenic drift, caused by a single mutation in the viral RNA, occurs constantly among flu A viruses and is responsible for annual flu epidemics, with new strains emerging every year. Generally with antigenic drift there is some kind of serological relationship between new and the old HA and NA antigens, so although the virus is 'drifting' and changing subtly, it does not differ too drastically from previous strains. Some of the population will have immunity to the virus and vaccination is an effective preventative measure in those with no immunity or who are in one of the at risk categories.

Antigenic shift poses much more of a problem, whereby major changes to actual gene segments on the surface antigens lead to the creation of a 'new' virus and ultimately give rise to a pandemic. As the population will not have previously been exposed to this virus in any shape or form, no preventative vaccine will have been developed and immunity will be virtually non-existent. Antigenic shift can occur either as a sudden 'adaptive' change during replication of a normal virus, or from genetic exchange between a human and an animal strain of influenza A. With genetic exchange, an animal is co-infected with both a human and an animal strain and serves as a 'mixing vessel' for the virus, allowing it to genetically 're-assort' itself and create a new virus capable of causing disease in humans.

THE PATHOGENESIS OF INFECTION, CLINICAL FEATURES AND TREATMENT OF SEASONAL/'ORDINARY' INFLUENZA

Influenza is transmitted from person to person by respiratory aerosols and droplets. Depending upon the size of the inhaled virus particles, they are either deposited on the mucous membrane lining the respiratory tract, or they directly enter the alveoli.[603] Once the influenza virus has successfully penetrated the respiratory epithelial cells, viral replication occurs within hours, causing functional and structural damage to the cells, and releasing virus particles into the airways which go on to infect neighbouring cells.[602,607] The damage to the respiratory epithelium initiates an acute inflammatory response, impairing both mechanical and cellular host responses and giving rise to the classic flu-like symptoms (see Chapter 5 Understanding the Immune System and the Nature and Pathogenesis of Infection).

Influenza typically begins with the abrupt onset of systemic symptoms after a short incubation period of one to two days. Although respiratory symptoms, particularly a dry cough and severe pharyngeal pain, are present at the outset, they are dwarfed by the systemic symptoms, with the illness reaching its maximum severity within six to twelve hours. The systemic symptoms include fever and rigors, with fever lasting intermittently for four to eight days, myalgia, malaise and headache; myalgia and headache are often the most troublesome features, and their severity is related to the height of the fever.[607] Myalgia typically affects the long muscles of the back or calves, and may also involve the muscles of the eyes. Many patients with influenza exhibit signs of both lower and upper respiratory tract infection, and by the fourth day of the illness, the respiratory symptoms tend to be predominant, although the acute systemic symptoms persist for three to five days.

Recovery tends to begin after a week but it may actually take several weeks. Complications following influenza are not uncommon and can result in death. Patients with underlying respiratory and cardiac conditions are particularly susceptible to secondary respiratory infection, as they do not have the necessary respiratory or cardiac reserves to be able to combat it. In some instances, the viral infection rapidly progresses and leads to an overwhelming viral pneumonia. More commonly, bacterial superinfection caused by *Staphylococcus aureus, Streptococcus pneumoniae* and *Haemophilus influenzae* results in pneumonia and disseminated bacterial infection. Other respiratory complications include croup and exacerbation of chronic pulmonary diseases. Non-respiratory complications include cardiac complications, toxic shock syndrome, Guilliain-Barre syndrome, and **Reyes Syndrome**, which predominantly affects children.[604]

The UK annual influenza immunisation programme has become one of the major public health programmes[52,608], with approximately 12 million doses of influenza vaccine administered each year, primarily to those over the age of 65 and those in the at risk groups.[594] Each year the World Health Organization Global Influenza Surveillance Network advises on the most suitable vaccination against flu depending on the strains which are likely to be in circulation, and annual immunisation is recommended against currently prevalent strains to provide ongoing protection.[52] The strains in the vaccine match the strains in circulation as closely as possible, and the vaccine is a trivalent preparation, made up of an influenza A (H_1N_1) virus, influenza A (H_3N_2) virus, and an influenza B virus.[594,604] There are numerous vaccine manufacturers who supply the UK market. Patients in the at risk groups and who are a priority for vaccination include those with chronic respiratory disease, including asthma, chronic heart disease, chronic liver disease, diabetes which requires control with insulin or oral hypoglycaemic drugs, and patients who are immunosupressed.[608]

THE PROBLEM OF AVIAN INFLUENZA

Of the 100 subtypes of avian influenza, only four strains of avian flu are known to cause disease in humans – H_5N_1, H_7N_3, H_7N_7 and H_9N_2. The highly pathogenic avian H_5N_1 strain, which has a 100 % mortality rate among infected birds, has infected 307 people and killed 186 worldwide since 2003[609], when the most serious outbreak of avian influenza ever reported originated in southeast Asia and subsequently spread to the European Union. Prior to 1997, when the first cases of avian influenza affecting humans were seen in Hong Kong, avian H_5N_1 had only caused mild disease in birds, with symptoms such as ruffled feathers and reduced egg production which often escaped detection. Months later it mutated into a highly pathogenic strain which was fatal within 48 hours of acquisition and which then jumped the species barrier causing severe disease in humans, infecting 18 people and killing six.[607] The deaths were linked to an outbreak of the disease among birds in a live bird market, where the risk of exposure is significantly high during activities such as slaughter, defeathering, butchering and preparation of the carcass for cooking.[610] Currently, the main route of transmission to humans is by direct contact with infected poultry, or surfaces and objects contaminated by their faeces. As infected birds shed large quantities of virus particles in their faeces – 1gram of faeces contains sufficient virus particles to kill one million birds[594] – there is plenty of opportunity for exposure to infected bird droppings or to environments which have become contaminated.[611] Hong Kong's entire poultry population – in the region of 1.5 million birds – was culled within three days of the human cases being diagnosed, an action which reduced further opportunities for the disease to infect humans and which may have averted a pandemic.[598]

H_5N_1 is a huge public health concern and poses the biggest risk to humans in terms of pandemic threat, for although it does not spread from person to person, it fulfils two out of the three conditions necessary to cause a human pandemic; it can jump the species barrier and infect humans and it can cause severe disease.[594,611] If an individual infected with avian flu were to be co-infected with a human strain of flu A, genetic exchange or re-assortment with the human as the mixing vessel could occur, leading to the creation of a new pandemic strain. Pigs could also be the mixing vessel for a pandemic strain as they are susceptible to flu A and they possess receptors for avian flu, and in October 2004 evidence emerged that H_5N_1 had jumped the species barrier again and expanded its host range within mammals, infecting captive tigers in Thailand.[595] Alternatively, avian flu could simply adapt itself to the human body and evolve into a transmissible human strain. The more avian influenza outbreaks there are amongst poultry, and the greater the geographical areas covered, the greater the risk that H_5N_1 will infect humans.

All birds are susceptible to avian flu, and there is a significant risk of migratory birds carrying H_5N_1 over long distances and affecting domestic flocks along flight paths. Therefore it is subjected to global surveillance and stringent legislation and control measures. In England, the *UK Avian Influenza and Influenza of Avian Origin in Mammals (England) Order 2006* came into force following the discovery of avian influenza in poultry in Norfolk on the 26th April 2006.[611] In February 2007, an outbreak of H_5N_1 on a turkey farm in Suffolk was linked to the importation of turkey meat from a sub-clinically infected turkey flock on an associated turkey farm in Hungary.[612] In the event of suspected cases, control and surveillance zones are erected around the index case in order to prevent lateral spread, with the quarantining of infected poultry farms, the rapid culling of all infected and exposed birds, and the disposal of carcasses. In southeast Asia, where there is strong evidence to suggest that H_5N_1 is now endemic, there are plans (at the time of writing) for the mass vaccination of domestic poultry.

PREVIOUS INFLUENZA PANDEMICS

Recent evidence suggests that the worst ever influenza pandemic, which occurred in 1918 and which is discussed next in this chapter, was caused by direct mutation of a highly pathogenic avian strain without any recombination with a human influenza strain.[594,595,607,613,614] This information heightens the global concern that the current H_5N_1 strain may do the same and cause the next pandemic.

Influenza A has undergone antigenic shift three times in the last century, resulting in three pandemics of varying pathogenicity.

THE 1918–1919 'SPANISH FLU' PANDEMIC

The 1918–1919 influenza pandemic was a global disaster of epic proportions and has been cited as the most devastating outbreak in recorded history. It is estimated that the pandemic killed at least 50 million people worldwide[615] (although that figure is now believed to be considerably more), was responsible for more deaths than World War 1, and that more people died from influenza in a single year than in four years of the bubonic plague, which killed 25 million people between 1347–1351.[616] The 1918–1919 pandemic was known as the 'Spanish flu' – not because it had originated in Spain but because it received more media coverage in Spain than it did anywhere else, since Spain was not involved in the war and was not subject to wartime censorship. It circled the globe, spreading along trade routes and shipping lines, decimating populations and wreaking havoc on the economy. It had an unusual pattern of morbidity, predominantly affecting those in the 20–40-year-old age group, who represented the greater part of the workforce. Of those who died 99 % were under the age of 65.[595] Life expectancy in many parts of the world was decreased by 10 years.

The first outbreaks began simultaneously in Europe and states within the USA during March 1918, and spread to Asia and Africa with the movement of wartime troops. Although the influenza was highly contagious, the mortality rate was not significantly high, but when the second wave struck in August 1918, the world was unprepared. Explosive outbreaks with massive attack rates saw a ten-fold increase in the death rate, and happened simultaneously in France, Sierra Leone and the USA. Although secondary bacterial infections accounted for many of the deaths, 'Spanish flu' also caused a form of primary viral pneumonia, with extensive haemorrhaging of the lungs which killed previously fit and healthy people in less than 48 hours and caused 'healthy' individuals to drop down dead in the street.[595] It is now believed that the excessive mortality rate was caused by a cytokine storm[617] – an exaggerated, inappropriate and overwhelming immune response generated by the host with potentially fatal results (see Chapter 5 Understanding the Immune System and the Nature and Pathogenesis of Infection). As the course of the disease was so severe, its presentation so marked, and the mortality rate so excessively high, influenza was not at first suspected, and there were fears that this was a return to the days of the black death.[595] No countries escaped the pandemic unscathed, although by the time Australia was affected in 1919, the virulence and pathogenicity of the virus had somewhat decreased, and the country experienced a milder, although more prolonged, period of influenza activity. Control measures focused on quarantine and isolation, which would have delayed the spread of the disease for a time but ultimately had very little impact on the number of people who were infected, given that everyone was susceptible. Many countries introduced the wearing of gauze masks in public, and in some countries people who coughed and sneezed in public, without taking steps to protect against aerosols, were fined or jailed. Curfews and restrictions were imposed on public gatherings and travel, and theatres, churches, dance halls and other public places were closed.[595,616]

THE 1957 H_2N_2 ASIAN INFLUENZA PANDEMIC

By the time of the 1957 pandemic, the world was better prepared; influenza viruses had been discovered, effective vaccinations had been developed, antibiotics for the treatment of secondary bacterial infections were available, and the World Health Organization had been established since 1948. Reports of extensive influenza outbreaks in Hong Kong and Singapore, which had originated in China in February 1957 were received by WHO in May, and by the end of that month WHO had identified a new virus subtype, sent samples of the virus to vaccine manufacturers, and alerted the world to the onset of an influenza pandemic.[595] Every country in the world experienced cases within six months of the virus being identified in Hong Kong. The pattern of spread varied between countries, with some experiencing peaks and troughs of disease. Similar to the 1918 pandemic, the first wave was explosive but fatality rates were low, and predominantly affected young school-aged children. The second wave, which occurred one to three months after the first wave, caused very high rates of illness and fatalities, and affected the elderly.

Vaccines were available in the USA, UK and Japan by the end of November 1957, but the quantities were inadequate for widespread use, and no country had sufficient production capacity to cover its entire population, or to consider exporting vaccines elsewhere.[595] Quarantine measures were imposed in some countries, and international travel and trade were subject to severe restrictions but were largely ineffective. The total global mortality was estimated at 1–2 million.[607]

THE 1968 H_3N_2 HONG KONG INFLUENZA PANDEMIC

The world was alerted to yet another pandemic caused by a novel influenza virus in August 1968, a month after the onset of a widespread outbreak of acute respiratory disease which originated in China.[595] Although the pattern of spread was similar to previous pandemics, clinical symptoms were milder and the mortality rates were lower, with the exception of the USA which experienced the highest burden of cases and deaths. The 1968 H_3N_2 pandemic occurred only 11 years after the 1957 H_2N_2 pandemic, and the N_2 subtypes were the same. It is now believed that this conferred protection by previous exposure, as many of those populations affected by the 1957 pandemic would still have been alive in 1968.[595]

THE PROBLEM WITH PANDEMICS

These three influenza pandemics have all been caused by influenza A, which makes this subtype the most likely to cause problems in the future. Historically, most pandemics have originated in Asia, where dense populations of humans live in close proximity to pigs and birds, all susceptible to influenza A viruses. If the world is faced with another influenza pandemic, it is likely to arise from Asia and be caused by a new influenza A subtype, possibly the highly pathogenic H_5N_1 [607], although it is not improbable that another influenza virus will be the culprit. The viruses responsible for the 1957 and 1968 pandemics were reassortments of avian and human influenza viruses. The 1957 subtype obtained three of its eight genes from an avian virus, and five from the strain which was responsible for the 1918 pandemic. The 1968 virus had taken three genes from an avian virus and the rest from the 1957 H_2N_2 strain which was in circulation.[595]

The behaviour of influenza viruses cannot be predicted and their real pathogenic potential can only be estimated as the mortality rate, severity of illness and pattern of spread can vary greatly; until it starts circulating, its full effects won't be known. As pandemics tend to occur in waves, it is likely that the age groups and geographical areas that are unaffected initially will be particularly vulnerable during the second wave, and the attack rate and mortality rates will be much higher; it is also possible that during the interval in between waves, the virus will mutate into a far more virulent form.[595] Global spread is likely to occur quickly, within a matter of months, given the expansion of international air travel, so once cases have been detected in one country, pandemic influenza will have started to arrive in many more.

People of all ages will be susceptible to pandemic flu, not just those in the at risk groups, and although it is likely to cause the same symptoms as 'ordinary flu', these are likely to be more severe. As so few of the population will have any immunity to this novel strain, the spread of disease and the severity of symptoms are going to be far in excess of what would normally be expected during the worst seasonal epidemic. It is possible that at the peak of the pandemic, there could be in excess of one million new cases of influenza per day in the UK, and pandemic-related occupancy of intensive care beds could be over 200 % of total current capacity.[595] The excess mortality in the UK, based on the clinical attack rates and fatality rates of the last three pandemics, is estimated to be in the region of 50,000, and it is also estimated the greatest mortality rates will be seen in people less than 65 years old, again based on statistics from previous pandemics.[618] Vaccination against seasonal influenza will offer no protection against a pandemic strain. There will be no vaccine available until the subtype of influenza virus is identified, and the DoH and WHO estimate that it will take at least six to eight months to produce a vaccine. Even then, there will only be sufficient quantities initially available to vaccinate the high priority groups, such as healthcare workers, essential services workers and high risk patient groups, rather than the general population.[595]

PREPARING FOR A PANDEMIC

In 2005, the World Health Organization published its *Global Influenza Preparedness Plan*[619], which summarises the role of WHO and its recommendations with regard to the measures to be undertaken globally before, during and after a pandemic. Each country has been urged to either update an existing national plan or develop a new one in concordance with WHO's recommendations. The document describes three phases, each with a series of sub-phases, which cover the interpandemic phase, the pandemic phase, and a return to the pandemic phase when the global outbreak is over. Within these phases, the overarching goals, objectives and actions for both WHO and national authorities are discussed in detail, with each phase focusing on different aspects in relation to planning and co-ordination, situation monitoring and assessment, prevention and containment, health system responses, and communications.

In England, the DoH is the lead government agency for co-ordinating a pandemic response, and takes overarching responsibility for the UK response. *The UK Influenza Pandemic Contingency Plan*[618] has been devised by the Health Protection Agency in order to provide a framework through which individual divisions of the HPA can develop more detailed operational plans, and describes in considerable detail the responses that will be undertaken at a national, regional and local level within the UK. The Department of Health's *UK Influenza Contingency Plan*[597] describes four levels of pandemic influenza alert for the UK:

- Alert level 1 – cases due to pandemic virus only outside the UK
- Alert level 2 – new pandemic virus isolated in the UK (pandemic imminent in the UK)
- Alert level 3 – outbreak(s) due to new pandemic subtype in the UK
- Alert level 4 – widespread pandemic activity across the UK.

In the event of a new influenza virus with pandemic potential being isolated by WHO, the Secretary of State, advised by the Chief Medical Officer, will convene the National Influenza Pandemic Committee, which will in turn cascade the information to all other relevant departments, agencies and organisations, including the HPA and the National Health Service. In order to facilitate planning by NHS Trusts in advance of a pandemic, the DoH, in conjunction with the HPA, issued *Guidance for Pandemic Influenza in Hospitals and Primary Care Settings* in 2005[620], and in March 2007 further guidance was published by the Department of Health.[621] The way in which the health service functions will alter drastically during a pandemic and exceptional and extraordinary infection control precautions will have a major impact on operational issues. All NHS Trusts have been required to develop their own pandemic influenza contingency plan, based on guidance issued by WHO, the DoH and the HPA.

INFECTION CONTROL PRECAUTIONS FOR HEALTHCARE SETTINGS

NHS and Primary Care Trusts are going to be under unprecedented pressure if, or when, the UK is affected by pandemic influenza. The workload will be increased due to the huge numbers of patients admitted suffering from pandemic influenza and its associated complications; there will be excess demand on critical care and infection control facilities and equipment; the workforce is likely to become depleted through illness; supplies, utilities and transport are likely to be affected; other essential aspects of healthcare provision are likely to be affected and there will be pressure on mortuary facilities.[620]

Since 2005, Trusts have been holding pandemic influenza planning committees, developing guidelines, plans and escalation policies, determining the infection control precautions that will need to be stringently implemented and rigorously adhered to, calculating the huge reserves of personal protective equipment that will be needed, both in terms of numbers and financial cost, stockpiling supplies of antiviral therapy, and participating in local and regional pandemic outbreak exercises to assess how ready the health service is to deal with pandemic flu. These plans are based on possible attack rates, the clinical impact and assumed mortality rates and additional business contingency planning guidance which is issued by the Cabinet Office.[621] The last time that the health service in the UK was faced with a threat of this nature was with the advent of severe acute respiratory syndrome (SARS) (see Chapter 17 Severe Acute Respiratory Syndrome (SARS)), which threatened the world in 2003.

The 2005 DoH/HPA guidance[620] details the infection control precautions that will need to be in place in acute care and primary care settings and they are discussed briefly here. These precautions include the segregation and cohorting of influenza patients; the environmental infection control considerations around decontamination of equipment and the environment; the management of laundry and the management of waste; specific infection control precautions focusing on hand hygiene; PPE and droplet precautions; and the deployment of staff. Any pandemic influenza management plan or outbreak policy will include these precautions.

The segregation/cohorting of symptomatic influenza patients

The routine day-to-day running and operational issues that govern the provision of healthcare services will have to change significantly in order to accommodate the exceptional infection control arrangements that will be in place. All healthcare providers, whether hospitals or community settings, which includes GP surgeries, health centres and nursing/residential homes, will have to be able to segregate influenza patients from non-influenza patients, and this will place an immense strain on resources, including staff and equipment, and the facilities available. Staff will have to be very innovative, as the layout and facilities, particularly in the community, may not easily support patient segregation.

A designated self-contained area of the hospital, or GP surgery/health centre, will need to be identified and allocated for the care of patients with pandemic influenza, with its own reception area, entrance and exit separate to the rest of the building. It should not be in an area of the building that is used as a thoroughfare by patients, staff or members of the public, and appropriate signage will need to be in place that clearly identifies this area as a pandemic influenza zone. In the hospital setting, the hospital engineers should be consulted as the pandemic management plans are devised so that any design considerations can be taken into consideration, including ensuring that mechanical ventilation systems will not dilute from segregated to non-segregated areas of the building. Influenza patients will need to be cohorted in segregated areas of the hospital to avoid the risk of cross-infection to other patients, and side rooms will need to be allocated for those patients who have to undergo aerosol generating procedures. Consideration will also have to be given to the separate cohorting of patients with pandemic influenza and other pathogens such as MRSA and *C.difficile*, and this will be dependent on the number of isolation rooms available, the numbers of patients who are co-infected, and staffing levels. Patients will be required to remain in the segregated area until they are discharged. If the pressure on beds is extreme, convalescing patients can be transferred to another area of the hospital but they will have to be segregated with other convalescent patients.

Areas such as accident and emergency departments, and community care settings, will need to establish triage areas for the rapid assessment of patients presenting with pandemic influenza, and designate segregated areas within the department for the treatment of influenza and non-influenza patients.

On entering the designated pandemic influenza area, staff will be required to sign in so that contact details are available in the event of contact tracing being required. The number of staff entering the area should be limited to only essential personnel, and a sign displaying the infection control precautions to be taken should be displayed at the entrance. Equipment stations containing supplies, personal protection equipment (PPE) and alcohol hand rub should be available at the entrance to segregated areas and cohort bays.

Patients with pandemic influenza should not be transferred to other hospitals unless they require specialist care as a result of complications or other health-associated events. The staff will have to liaise closely with the receiving hospital, including the infection prevention and control team, to ensure that all of the necessary infection control precautions are in place and understood by everyone concerned. If a patient requires an intra-hospital transfer to another ward or department, communication with the receiving area and the infection prevention and control team is essential. Patients who are moving between areas should wear a surgical facemask while they are in transit in order to prevent cross-infection to others via droplet transmission.

Environmental infection control considerations

Soft furnishings in healthcare settings should be easily cleanable and not retain any moisture, and non-essential furniture should be removed from the area in order to prevent heavy contamination. Surplus equipment and supplies should also be removed and dedicated patient equipment should be available where possible. If there are inadequate supplies of patient equipment and equipment has to be shared, it must be thoroughly decontaminated with neutral detergent and hot water in between patients. The distance between bed spaces should be in excess of one metre, with beds separated by a curtain, and the environment cleaned thoroughly at least once a day as a minimum standard. Frequently touched surfaces (i.e. door handles, telephones, bathroom taps) will require cleaning twice a day. Damp dusting as opposed to dry dusting should be carried out, to avoid generating dust particles and disseminating them throughout the environment, and vacuuming of floors should be avoided. Environmental cleaning issues require close liaison with domestic services as there will be resource implications, and domestic staff will need to be allocated to the segregated areas for the duration of the pandemic.

At the time of writing, no special precautions are required for the segregation of clinical and non-clinical waste, and the disposal of used and infected linen beyond local policy, and they should be managed as per standard infection control principles (see Chapter 6 The Principles of Infection Prevention and Control). However, new legislation governing the segregation and disposal of clinical waste generated from healthcare settings has been the subject of debate and may be subject to reforms and new guidance. Waste and linen bags should be handled safely to avoid exposure to and contamination from respiratory secretions and gloves and aprons worn for handling contaminated linen and waste, following which hands should be decontaminated following the removal of PPE.

Hand hygiene

With hand hygiene the single most important component of infection control practice to prevent the spread of infection, strict adherence to hand hygiene guidelines is another crucial element in preventing the spread of pandemic influenza. Studies have suggested that influenza A can be transmitted from contaminated surfaces to hands and although the virus will only be viable for approximately five minutes, that is sufficient time in which self-inoculation of the conjunctiva and/or mucous membranes can take place.[622] Hands must be decontaminated on entering patient areas, in between each episode of patient contact, following contact with contaminated equipment, following the decontamination of equipment, immediately following the removal of any item of PPE, and immediately after handling linen and waste. Providing hands are not visibly soiled with dirt or organic material, alcohol hand rubs can be used in place of hand washing. Patients and visitors will need to be advised to decontaminate their hands.

Personal protective equipment (PPE)

The wearing of PPE (gloves, aprons, masks and eye protection) is essential in order to protect the healthcare worker, as far as possible, from unnecessary exposure to body fluids, secretions and excretions, and to prevent the transmission of infection to other patients or members of staff (see Chapter 6 The Principles of Infection Prevention and Control). With regard to pandemic influenza, the aim of PPE is to prevent its transmission, and in order for this to be effective it is absolutely essential that all PPE is worn appropriately, fitted correctly and disposed of properly. Staff will require training in the use of some PPE.

Masks

In day-to-day infection control practice masks are generally only routinely worn when looking after patients with bacterial meningitis, drug-resistant pulmonary tuberculosis and SARS, where there is significant risk of the transmission of infection via droplet spread, particularly where aerosol generating procedures are being undertaken with these patients. As pandemic influenza is highly contagious and spread by respiratory droplets, masks will be an essential component of PPE, protecting the facial mucosa from contamination by respiratory droplets.

For close patient contact, defined as within three feet, surgical facemasks should be worn by healthcare workers, and care should be taken to ensure that the mask covers both the nose and the mouth. It should be put on immediately prior to entering the bay, removed after exiting and disposed of immediately after removal as clinical waste.

Surgical facemasks should be changed in between patients, or when the mask becomes moist, but if the healthcare worker is caring for pandemic influenza patients in a cohort bay, or an 'influenza clinic' in a community setting, one mask can be worn for the duration of the activity within that bay.

While the wearing of a mask will help to prevent droplets being expelled into the environment by the person wearing them, and also protect the wearer against splashes of blood or body fluids, they are not generally designed to effectively filter airborne particles. When aerosol generating procedures are performed, including intubation, suctioning and nebulised therapy, a higher level of respiratory protection is required, and in these situations staff should wear disposable respirators that conform to the European Standard EN149 2001, such as the FFP3 disposable respirator. EN149 is the European Respiratory Protection Standard for disposable filtering respirators, worn as facemasks and covering the nose, mouth and chin, which filter particulates including bacteria and viruses. The FFP3 respirator provides 99 % particle filtration efficiency, and affords the highest level of protection under the EN Standard for disposable respirators.[623]

So that the FFP3 respirator can provide the optimum filtration efficiency and protection against airborne particles, it is absolutely essential that the respirator fits the face snugly, and healthcare workers will have to be fit-tested to ensure that there is a tight seal and that no air can enter from the sides. Facial hair such as beards and moustaches, and also stubble, can prevent a tight seal against the skin and so the skin should be clean-shaven. Each time a new respirator is worn, the fit will need to be checked. Although the respirators can be worn for eight hours at a time, they must not be re-used and must be disposed of as clinical waste.

Gloves, aprons and eye protection

Gloves and disposable plastic aprons should be worn for all patient care activities where there is a risk of contamination with blood, body fluids, excretions or respiratory secretions, and must be changed in between each patient use and disposed of as clinical waste. Eye protection, either in the form of goggles or visors, should be worn for aerosol generating procedures; otherwise its requirement should be based on individual risk assessment. It will need to be appropriately decontaminated or disposed of after use.

The allocation and movement of healthcare staff

As staff will be at risk of acquiring pandemic influenza through work-related and community exposure, they will need to be aware of the clinical signs and the action that they need to take, and staff education will need to be undertaken in conjunction with the occupational health department. Symptomatic members of staff should be excluded from work but in exceptional circumstances where there are extreme staffing shortages they may be allowed to work if they are well enough, but only in areas designated for pandemic influenza patients. Staff who have had pandemic influenza and are completely recovered, or who have been vaccinated, should be prioritised to work in pandemic areas, and any member of staff working in a designated pandemic area should not work in non-influenza areas; however, staff from non-influenza areas can move to affected areas but they will be required to remain working there until the end of the pandemic. Bank and agency staff should be managed the same way as permanent staff. The same principles for the allocation/deployment of staff apply to both acute and community settings.

VACCINATION AND ANTIVIRAL DRUG THERAPY

In 2005, the Department of Health announced its proposal to buy two million doses of the existing H_5N_1 vaccine to be used as a first line of defence (prophylaxis) for the immunisation of priority workers, such as those in healthcare, if the threat of a pandemic increased.[624] However, this will only be effective if the pandemic strain is the same as, or similar to, H_5N_1 and is not caused by another avian influenza subtype.[598]

Once a vaccine against the pandemic strain has been manufactured, and this will not be until after the end of the first pandemic wave, groups for vaccination will be ranked from 1–7 according to their priority.[625] The vaccination of healthcare workers will be the first priority, followed by the emergency/essential services (which includes the army, fire brigades and police forces), those with high risk medical conditions, all those over the age of 65, those working in selected industries (to minimise disruption to the economy), selected age groups as advised by WHO and finally the rest of the population.[598] The treatment of pandemic influenza for those with symptomatic illness will be reliant upon the use of antiviral drugs.

Antiviral therapy, which is currently used to treat patients with seasonal influenza, consists of four drugs divided into two classes; M2 inhibitors (amantadine and rimantadine) and nuraminidase inhibitors (zanamivir, also known as relenza, and oseltamivir, known as tamiflu). Unlike a vaccine, which stimulates the production of antibodies to mount an immune response against the virus, these drugs act directly on the virus itself. Amantadine and rimantadine are thought to prevent the virus from entering the host cell, while zanamivir and oseltamivir block the release of the virus from an infected cell.[595,607] Although these drugs are effective in treating influenza if taken within 48 hours of the onset of symptoms, they are more effective if they are used as prophylaxis, to treat those who have been exposed to the virus. Unfortunately, the rapid emergence of resistance to amantadine and rimantadine by H_5N_1 in Asia means that the world is now reliant upon only zanamivir and oseltamivir for the treatment of pandemic influenza, and their effectiveness against a pandemic strain is unknown.[626] However, data from clinical trials based on seasonal influenza suggests that they could reduce the duration of illness by 24 hours, allowing rapid mobilisation of individuals such as affected healthcare workers, possibly reducing the need for admission to hospital in affected individuals along with reduced antibiotic usage.[626]

There are three ways in which zanamivir and oseltamivir could be utilised, and countries all over the world that have the resources to do so have been stockpiling and identifying the priority groups to be targeted. Antiviral therapy could be used only for the treatment of affected individuals, given as 'blanket' prophylaxis, or used as targeted prophylaxis, which could be given to essential workers such as healthcare workers and the emergency services. In terms of who should be treated with these drugs, the recommendation is that they should only be given to affected individuals who have an acute influenza-like illness with a fever of >38 °C and who have been symptomatic for two days or less.[626,627]

In 2005, the government ordered the stockpiling of 14.6 million courses of oseltamivir, based on the assumption that one quarter of the UK's population will be affected, each requiring one course of treatment. This supports the favoured 'treatment only' option but currently does not allow any leeway for usage as blanket or targeted prophylaxis, as the stockpile is too small.[596] If demand outstrips supply, provisional first priority groups to receive antiviral drugs are healthcare workers[598] and those who fall into the at risk groups.[628] One of the major pharmaceutical companies, Roche, has offered to provide WHO with an international stockpile of oseltamivir, equating to three million courses, for use in the country of origin of the pandemic strain in a bid to contain it and stop it at the point of source.

The administration of antiviral therapy to the general population though is not recommended because of the threat of drug-resistance.[598]

THE FUTURE – LESSONS TO BE LEARNED FROM THE SARS OUTBREAK

The spectre of an influenza pandemic looms ever closer. The SARS outbreak caught everyone by surprise and gave the world a wake-up call; pandemic influenza cannot do the same, and there are lessons to be learnt from SARS in relation to infection control.[629] Compliance with infection control precautions and clinical practice will be crucial in limiting spread. Failure among healthcare workers to consistently wear full protective clothing during the SARS outbreak was instrumental in staff exposure to the virus, and aerosol generating procedures are thought to have exacerbated the spread of SARS to other patients. In patients presenting with an atypical pneumonia, there needs to be a high index of suspicion and infection control precautions need to be implemented immediately.

19 Creutzfeldt-Jakob Disease (CJD)

INTRODUCTION

During the 1990s an outbreak of disease among cattle which had begun in the UK in 1986 reached epidemic proportions. Bovine Spongiform Encephalopathy (BSE) or 'mad cow disease' as it was commonly called, has affected more than 170,000 cattle and lead to the slaughter of 4.7 million. It devastated the cattle and meat export industry, and ruined the livelihood of thousands of farmers in the process. The government denied that the outbreak posed any significant threat to public health, assuring the worried public that it was safe to eat beef, but that changed in 1996 when the then Secretary of State for Health, Stephen Dorrell, announced that 10 young people in the UK had developed a variant form of Creutzfeldt-Jakob Disease (vCJD). Both BSE and vCJD are caused by transmissible spongiform encephalopathies (TSEs), otherwise known as prion diseases, which fatally affect the central nervous system in animals and humans. In the 11 years to 2007 there have been 112 confirmed deaths from vCJD, plus another 46 deaths where the diagnosis was suspected but unconfirmed.[630]

Although vCJD is not transmissible from person to person, it is known that transmission of TSEs can occur in specific situations. Between December 1970 and December 2005, there were 58 cases of CJD via iatrogenic (nosocomial) transmission; seven from dura mater implants, 50 from injections of human derived growth hormones, and one recipient of human gonadotrophin.[632] There have also been four cases of vCJD associated with blood transfusion up to the year 2007.[632]

The history of BSE and vCJD is a complicated story to tell. This chapter aims to give a brief overview of the BSE/vCJD 'problem'. Prion diseases are explained, and the clinical features of both animal and human TSEs are described; this is followed by a potted history of the evolution of the BSE epidemic and the emergence of variant CJD, and the precautions necessary to prevent the transmission of CJD in the healthcare setting. The recommendations in the section headed *Infection Control Precautions* are based on the guidance issued from the Advisory Committee on Dangerous Pathogens and the Spongiform Encephalopathy Committee (*Transmissible Spongiform Encephalopathy Agents: Safe Working and the Prevention of Infection*)[631] in 1998. This was updated in 2003 and various appendices have been revised since, and will continue to be updated, giving important information and guidance on the management of TSEs from a health and safety, laboratory containment and infection control perspective. They should form the cornerstone of any infection control policy on the management of TSEs but the reader is reminded that they should consult their own infection prevention and control team for advice and refer to their infection control manual.

LEARNING OUTCOMES

After reading this chapter the reader will:

- Understand the difference between sporadic, familial, iatrogenic and variant CJD
- Understand the link between BSE and vCJD.
- Understand the necessary precautions to be taken in order to reduce the risk of transmitting vCJD in the healthcare setting

PRION DISEASES

Prions, or proteinacious infectious particles, were first identified by Stanley Prusiner[633], an American neurologist and biochemist, as the causative agents of a group of fatal degenerative neurological diseases which affect animals – the transmissible spongiform encephalopathies – causing scrapie in sheep and goats and BSE in cattle. They are thought to be naturally occurring proteins derived from normal body proteins which undergo a rare spontaneous process, affecting normal protein synthesis in the individual. They are unconventional infectious agents which replicate by converting natural prion protein into the abnormal form and can be distinguished from viruses and viroids as they have no detectable nucleic acid.[634] They are also difficult to inactivate as they are resistant to the normal disinfection and sterilisation techniques used to kill bacteria and viruses and can therefore present an infection control risk. Prusiner later made the link between prion disease in animals and prion disease in humans and was awarded the Nobel Prize in 1997 in recognition of his work. The characteristics of prion disease and their clinical features are displayed in Table 19.1.

Table 19.1 Characteristics of Prion Diseases

Long incubation period – months to years (decades).
Unlike bacterial and viral infections, they do not generate either an immune response or an inflammatory process in the affected individual.
They cause degenerative changes in the central nervous system, with microscopic holes or vacuoles in the cortex and cerebellum of the brain giving it a sponge-like appearance.
Death occurs within months of onset of symptoms.

SCRAPIE

Scrapie is an endemic, fatal, progressive neurological disease affecting sheep and goats first identified in 1732, and it is estimated that up to one third of UK flocks are affected.[635] The exact mode of transmission is unclear but research is ongoing and there are suggestions that the prion protein can be transmitted in urine, which can survive within the environment for decades. The disease is named after one of the clinical symptoms, where the affected animals compulsively scrape their fleece off against wood or rocks. Scrapie tends to affect sheep between the ages of two–five and has an incubation period of four years. Clinical features include irritability and excitability, scratching, biting and rubbing of the fleece and skin, tremor, impaired vision, weight loss and weakness of the hind quarters. There is no cure and as scrapie spreads amongst flocks, the only method of control is the slaughter of the affected flock.

BSE

BSE is a new disease of cattle which was first recognised in the UK in 1986 and peaked in 1992, when there were 36,680 cases in Great Britain. Between 1986 and September 2006 there has been a total of 183,139 confirmed cases, and the rate of incidence is now in decline.[636] The cardinal signs of BSE are apprehension, hypersensitivity to touch and sound, and weakness of the legs together with an abnormal gait. Other symptoms include changes in behaviour, tremors and loss of body condition, body weight and milk yield.

The disease is discussed later in this chapter under the section on the BSE outbreak of 1986.

HUMAN TRANSMISSIBLE SPONGIFORM ENCEPHALOPATHIES (TSES)

Most cases of human TSE show disturbances of mood (depression, anxiety or apathy), dementia (impairment of reasoning ability and memory) and motor signs. The motor signs can include involuntary jerky movements (myoclonus), unsteadiness and unco-ordination, involuntary movements of various types, and rigidity. The key features are progressive deterioration with the appearance of all three components: emotional and cognitive deterioration, together with motor signs. The duration of illness and deterioration in the individual varies according to the type of TSE. Decline may be so rapid that the presentation is suggestive of viral encephalitis, but it usually occurs over months or years. Disturbances of behaviour and mental abilities usually precede motor disturbance, and patients are often initially referred to psychiatrists. A wide variety of other neurological features may appear during the course of the disease.[637]

KURU

Kuru affected the Fore people of New Guinea and reached epidemic proportions during the 1950s but is now almost extinct. It is a disease that is linked to cannibalism, where family members were cooked and eaten after death, with the closest female relatives and children eating the brain.[638] The onset of symptoms occurred anything from 4–20 years following exposure, with those affected exhibiting clumsiness, headache, emotional instability, and progressive wasting.

CREUTZFELDT-JAKOB DISEASE (CJD)

CJD is a rare, degenerative and fatal disorder and the most commonly occurring human TSE. It was first identified in the 1920s and takes one of three forms. 85–90 % of all cases of CJD are classed as sporadic, or classic, occurring in a random distribution with no known genetic or environmental cause, but are believed to arise as the result of a spontaneous conversion of a normal cerebrellar prion protein into an abnormal shape or configuration, resulting in degeneration of the brain tissue.[639] It is a worldwide illness, affecting one in one million people, and 50 cases are reported in the UK each year. It tends to affect adults between the ages of 50–75 but it can affect any age group, and presents as a rapidly progressive neurological illness that typically lasts 3–4 months. Iatrogenic, or acquired, CJD was first reported in 1973 following the case of a patient who had received a corneal graft 18 months previously from a donor who died of CJD but who wasn't known to have had the disease at the time of the donation.[640] Inherited CJD is extremely rare and occurs as the result of an abnormal inherited gene.

NEW VARIANT CJD (vCJD)

New variant, or vCJD, is a human disease acquired through the consumption of contaminated beef from cattle with BSE. The first cases were detected in 1995, 10 years after the onset of the BSE epidemic.[641] It typically tends to affect those between the ages of 14–50, although the youngest 'victim' was 12 at the age of onset and the oldest was 74.[631] Clinical illness lasts on average 14 months, although illness duration can be less or more. It initially presents as a psychiatric illness, with the infected individual exhibiting behavioural changes and depression, which may cloud the diagnosis. These symptoms are then followed by progressive neurological signs, including gait disturbances, ataxia and tremors and resulting in dementia. At the time of death, sufferers are often mute and immobile.

Table 19.2 summarises the characteristics and common clinical features of human TSEs.

It can be difficult to accurately diagnose vCJD. Definitive diagnosis depends on pathological examination of brain tissue (biopsy or post mortem), although clinical features and other investigations such as MRI, may allow a 'probable' diagnosis to be reached.[637]

Table 19.2 Characteristics and clinical features of human TSEs

Sporadic CJD	Familial CJD	vCJD
Onset – late middle age	Onset – average age 52	Onset – young adults
Illness duration – 4–6 months	Illness duration – years	Illness duration – 14 months
Presents as a rapidly progressive dementia with focal neurological signs	Presents as memory lapses, depression and fatigue, or initial symptoms may be unsteadiness/lack of co – ordination. Progresses to dementia (may be rapid progression)	Presents as a psychiatric illness, often with behavioural changes and depression, then followed by neurological signs

THE BSE OUTBREAK AND THE ORIGINS OF VCJD

In December 1997, it was announced in Parliament that an inquiry was to take place in order to establish and review the history of the emergence and identification of BSE in cattle and new variant CJD in humans, and the overall management of the crisis. What follows in this chapter is a very brief history of the BSE outbreak. A copy of the official report is available on the web[642] and makes fascinating, if somewhat disturbing, reading.

The first cow to die from BSE in September 1985 came from a herd in Sussex, where a number of other cows were exhibiting similar symptoms. A spongiform encephalopathy of the brain was identified at post mortem but the cow had underlying pathologies, and death was attributed to kidney disease. Then, throughout 1986, pathologists at the pathology department of the Central Veterinary Laboratory began receiving brain samples from herds in Kent and Bristol, all showing degenerative changes to the brain. At the end of 1987, it was decided that the cause of the transmissible spongiform encephalopathy in cattle, named Bovine Spongiform Encephalopathy, was the consumption of meat and bone meal in cattle feed which consisted of animal carcasses derived from sheep infected with conventional scrapie.

Once contaminated cattle feed had been identified as the probable vector of BSE, the government introduced a ban on the inclusion of ruminant protein in bovine feed in 1988, but they allowed a five week period for farmers and food suppliers to clear existing stocks, unaware that the rate of infection in cattle was silently and swiftly progressing. Some farmers continued to use up their existing supplies after the ban had been introduced, unaware of the gravity of the situation, and feed mills and feed mill merchants continued to sell cattle feed containing animal protein after the ban had been imposed. Subsequently, nearly 12,000 cattle born after the ban in 1988, and more than 12,000 born in 1989, developed BSE. However, ruminant protein in cattle feed wasn't the crucial issue; it was later discovered that ruminant feed was contaminated with feed for pigs and poultry which contained meat and bonemeal from cattle incubating BSE at the time of slaughter. Specialised bovine offal, consisting of high risk tissues such as the spinal cord and dorsal root ganglia, were not always cleanly removed from the parts of the carcass that went to be rendered for animal feed, and this was subsequently banned from inclusion in animal feed. This ban was followed in 1989 by a human specialised bovine offal ban, banning the use of those tissues most likely to be highly infectious in food for human consumption. However, infected cattle had been entering the animal and human foodchain long before either of these bans came into effect.

Throughout the late 1980s and early 1990s, questions were being asked about the safety of mechanically removed meat (MRM) entering the human food chain. These questions focused on the practicalities of removing all of the spinal cord from the carcass during the abattoir process, and the practices of the mechanical recovery of scraps of spinal cord and peripheral nerve tissue, which included dorsal route ganglia, for inclusion in human food. A paper on slaughterhouse practices had been sent to the Spongiform Encephalopathy Advisory Committee (SEAC) for information, and the paper identified that small pieces of spinal cord could remain attached to the vertebral column, not all nerves were removed from between the vertebrae, and the carcass would be contaminated from high risk materials during splitting. Unfortunately, a breakdown in communication between various committees and officials led to the belief that the 'odd' piece of spinal cord slipping through the net was not a problem and there was an assumption that all spinal cord could be removed from the carcass if slaughterhouses conformed to good practice.

Bovine material was extensively used in pharmaceutical, medical and veterinary products such as heparin, insulin, vaccine cultures and suture material. Joint guidelines were issued in the late 1980s by the Committee on the Safety of Medicines and the Veterinary Products Committee on the exclusion from these products of brain or neural tissue, spleen, thymus and other lymphoid tissue, placental tissue or cell cultures of bovine origin.

The risk of infection to humans, however, was considered to be low and as there was no evidence that BSE could be transmitted to humans, it was considered unlikely that BSE posed any risk to public health, and that beef was safe to eat. There were, however, concerns from scientists, neurologists and other members of the medical profession who were of the opinion that BSE *could* be transmitted to humans, that infection could take years to become clinically apparent, and infected individuals would be likely to exhibit symptoms similar to that of CJD. In 1990, a 'scrapie-like' spongiform encephalopathy was diagnosed in a domestic cat – the first case of FSE (feline spongiform encephalopathy), raising concerns that BSE had jumped the species barrier. This case was played down although there were huge concerns behind the scenes. Meanwhile, newspaper headlines were proclaiming that BSE posed the biggest threat to public health that had ever been seen, but still the risk was played down, and the general message continued to reiterate that British beef was safe to eat.

The first reported case of human CJD associated with a farm was made in 1989. Then, in 1992 and 1993, two cases were reported of farmers whose herds had been infected with BSE. Although both cases were publicly reported as classical or sporadic CJD, behind the scenes they were viewed as 'disquieting'. These cases were followed in 1994 by that of CJD in another herd and a reported case of 'undiagnosed brain disease' in a 16-year-old girl. The chief medical officer continued to state that there was no evidence to demonstrate a causal link between BSE and CJD. But then, in 1995, three suspected cases of CJD in people under the age of 50 were referred to the CJD surveillance unit (CJDSU) in Edinburgh. The CJDSU had been set up in 1990 as a research project, initially to run for four years, with the dual aims of identifying any changes in the epidemiology of CJD and assessing to what extent, if any, the changes were linked to BSE. It was becoming increasingly difficult to explain these cases as 'chance phenomena', especially as more cases were reported during 1995. In 1996, a paper was published in *The Lancet*, reporting on the emergence of a new variant form of CJD in the UK, causally linked to BSE.[641] It was considered that these cases were likely to have occurred as a result of exposure to bovine offal before the bovine offal ban came into effect in 1989.

The Report of Inquiry surmised that in all likelihood the BSE epidemic originated in the 1970s when the first cow became infected. The head and offal were sent to the renderers and the parts containing BSE contaminated a batch of meat and bonemeal (MBM) produced from the rendering. The MBM was sold to a compounder and mixed into cattle feed. It was ultimately this widespread practice of using bovine offal to produce meat and bonemeal for use in animal feed which resulted in the recycling and widespread distribution of BSE among cattle where it was to take root, infecting thousands of cattle over the next decade, and ultimately humans too.

PREVENTING THE NOSOCOMIAL TRANSMISSION OF CJD

The Department of Health estimates that up to several thousand people within the UK could be infected with vCJD at a subclinical level[643], and one of the greatest risks in the transmission of vCJD continues to be associated with the use of high risk surgical instruments contaminated with prion protein. After the 1998 guidance was issued by the TSE Advisory Committee, a 'snapshot' survey of the decontamination of surgical instruments was commissioned by the Department of Health in 1999. The survey reviewed numerous examples of poor practice, highlighting that not only was there a failure to decontaminate equipment appropriately, but that traceability of used instruments was poor[644], and this further highlighted the urgent need for a comprehensive review of decontamination services across the whole of the NHS. Prion protein still resists standard decontamination methods, and inappropriate decontamination processes still need to be addressed, along with the design of surgical instruments.[645]

The probable transmission of vCJD via contaminated blood has been a worrying development. The first case was identified in 2003, when the recipient developed signs of CJD six-and-a-half years after a transfusion of red cells from a donor who developed symptoms three-and-a-half years after donating blood. A second case was reported in a patient who also received red cells from a donor who died 18 months after donation; the patient died from unrelated causes but abnormal prion protein was found in the spleen and one cervical lymph node at post mortem. In March 2004 the then Health Secretary John Reid announced that people who had received a blood transfusion would no longer be able to donate blood, and later that year this exclusion was extended to include those who were unsure if they had received a previous blood transfusion, along with donors who donated certain blood components on a regular basis. The current practice of leucodepletion (removing white bloodcells from donated blood) was introduced in 1998 to reduce the risk of transfusion associated vCJD.[646]

INFECTION CONTROL PRECAUTIONS[640]

General management of patients in the 'risk' groups

In most routine clinical contact, no additional precautions are needed for the care of patients in the risk groups (see Table 19.3). However, when certain invasive interventions are performed, there is the potential for exposure to the agents of TSEs, and it is essential that control measures are in place to prevent the iatrogenic transmission of CJD or vCJD.

* Isolation of patients is not necessary; they can be nursed in an open ward using standard infection control precautions (see Chapter 6 The Principles of Infection Prevention and Control).
* Universal precautions especially when using sharps should be followed at all times.
* The tissues that present the highest risk are the brain, spinal cord, spinal ganglia posterior, eye, dura mater, cranial nerves and cranial ganglia. Special precautions are required for interventions involving these tissues. Table 19.4 categorises tissue infectivity in the transmission of human TSEs.
* Single-use disposable equipment should be used wherever practicable and destroyed by incineration.
* Spillages should be managed as per local Trust guidelines.
* Blood, biopsy and lumbar puncture samples from patients defined in Table 19.3 should only be taken by trained personnel who are aware of the hazards involved.
* Patients undergoing surgical/endoscopic procedures should have a risk assessment of possible prion disease completed at pre-assessment, as detailed in Table 19.4. Any positive responses should trigger further investigations/neurology referral.

Table 19.3 Categorisation of patients at risk

Patients should be categorised as follows, in descending order of risk:

1. Symptomatic patients	1.1 Patients who fulfil the diagnostic criteria for definite, probable or possible CJD or vCJD.
	1.2 Patients with neurological disease of unknown aetiology who do not fit the criteria for possible CJD or vCJD, but where the diagnosis of CJD is being actively considered.
2. Asymptomatic patients at risk from familial forms of CJD linked to genetic mutations	2.1 Individuals who have or have had two or more blood relatives affected by CJD or other prion disease, or a relative known to have a genetic mutation indicative of familial CJD.
	2.2 Individuals who have been shown by specific genetic testing to be at significant risk of developing CJD or other prion disease.
3. Asymptomatic patients potentially at risk from iatrogenic exposure	3.1 Recipients of hormone derived from human pituitary glands e.g. growth hormone, gonadotrophin.
	3.2 Individuals who have received a graft of *dura mater*. (People who underwent neurosurgical procedures or operations for a tumour or cyst of the spine before August 1992 may have received a graft of *dura mater*, and should be treated as at risk, unless evidence can be provided that *dura mater* was not used).
	3.3 Patients who have been contacted as potentially at risk because of exposure to instruments used on, or receipt of, blood, plasma derivatives, organs or tissues donated by a patient who went on to develop CJD or vCJD.

Crown Copyright. Guidance from the Advisory Committee on Dangerous Pathogens and the Spongiform Encephalopathy Committee (Department of Health).
Transmissible spongiform encephalopathy agents: safe working and the prevention of infection. Infection control of CJD and related disorders in the healthcare setting.

SPECIFIC PRECAUTIONS FOR SYMPTOMATIC PATIENTS (DEFINITE, PROBABLE AND POSSIBLE) AND ASYMPTOMATIC PATIENTS POTENTIALLY AT RISK OF CJD

The measures to be taken when performing invasive surgery depend on:

- how likely the patient is to be carrying the infectious agent (risk status); and
- how likely it is that infection could be transmitted by the procedure being carried out.

Table 19.4 Tissue infectivity – CJD/vCJD

High risk tissue	Medium risk (vCJD)	Low risk (CJD/vCJD)
Brain	Tonsil	Peripheral nerve
Spinal cord	Appendix	Skeletal muscle
Dura mater	Spleen	Dental pulp
Cranial nerves	Thymus	Gingival tissue
Cranial ganglia	Other lymphoid tissue	Blood
Posterior eye		Bone marrow
Pituitary gland		CSF
		Placenta
		Urine

Precautionary measures for surgical procedures

Theatre management

For all symptomatic patients (i.e. those who fulfil the criteria for definite, probable or possible CJD or vCJD), the following precautions should be taken:

- Wherever appropriate and possible, the intervention should be performed in an operating theatre.
- Where procedures are performed at the bedside, e.g. a lumbar puncture, care should be taken to ensure the environment may be readily cleaned should a spillage occur. The protective clothing described below should be worn by healthcare personnel performing diagnostic procedures.
- Where possible procedures should be performed at the end of the list, to allow normal cleaning of theatre surfaces before the next session.
- Only the minimum number of healthcare personnel required should be involved.
- The following single-use protective clothing should be worn, and disposed of in line with local policies:

  - liquid repellent operating gown, over a plastic apron
  - gloves
  - mask and goggles, or full-face visor.

- Single-use disposable surgical instruments and equipment should be used where possible, and then destroyed by incineration.

For asymptomatic patients at risk from familial or iatrogenic CJD, the same precautions apply.

Handling of instruments that are not designated as single use

Where single-use instruments are not available, the handling of re-usable instruments depends on a combination of the risk status of the patient, the tissue(s) involved in the procedure, and the type of CJD.

Table 19.5 highlights the actions that should be taken with instruments used on patients with CJD and vCJD.

Table 19.5 Actions to be taken with instruments – CJD other than vCJD and vCJD

CJD other than vCJD

Tissue infectivity	Status of Patient			
	Definite/probable	Possible	At risk	
			Genetic	Iatrogenic
High: • Brain • Spinal cord • Posterior eye	Destroy	Quarantine	Destroy	Destroy
Medium: • Anterior eye • Olfactory epithelium	Destroy	Quarantine	Destroy	Destroy
Low/non detectable	NSP (No special precautions)	NSP	NSP	NSP

vCJD

Tissue infectivity	Status of patient		
	Definite/probable	Possible	At risk
			Iatrogenic
High: • Brain • Spinal cord • Posterior eye	Destroy	Quarantine	Destroy
Medium: • Lymphoid tissue • Anterior eye • Olfactory epithelium	Destroy	Quarantine	Destroy
Low/non detectable	NSP	NSP	NSP

Careful planning is required for the procedure and the management of the equipment to be used.

- All staff directly involved in procedures on patients in the risk groups, or in the subsequent reprocessing or disposal of potentially contaminated items, should be aware of the specific precautions and be adequately trained. These staff should also be made aware of any clinical intervention in sufficient time to allow the necessary preparations for the procedure; this should include notification to the sterile services department (SSD) or reprocessing units, where appropriate. This will allow time to obtain the most suitable instruments and equipment, which may not be those used routinely.
- The number of people incubating vCJD is unknown. The mainstay of reducing risk of transmission via surgical instruments is thorough initial cleaning of instruments after use to remove proteinacious tissue remnants. These otherwise become fixed by initial drying and further fixed by subsequent sterilisation including heat treatment.
- Instruments that have been used on a possible CJD or vCJD patient involving tissues designated as high or medium infectivity must not be used but should be quarantined until the diagnosis is either confirmed or refuted.
- Theatre staff should wear protective clothing and care should be taken to avoid penetrating injuries.
- Single-use instruments should be separated and disposed of by incineration.
- Re-usable instruments should be placed in an impervious rigid plastic container with a close-fitting lid, and the lid sealed with autoclavable tape.
- The container should be labelled with:

    i the hospital number, name and date of birth of the case concerned
    ii the surgical procedure in which the instruments were used
    iii the name of the responsible person (theatre manager).

- The instrument tray should be disposed of by incineration.
- The sealed box should be stored in a suitable designated place in the sterile services department (SSD) until the outcome of any further investigation is known.
- If the patient is confirmed as having CJD, a yellow label must be attached to the outside of the sealed box which must be incinerated without further notice.
- If an alternative diagnosis is confirmed, the instruments may be removed from the box by the responsible person and processed in the normal manner, ensuring instruments are thoroughly clean prior to autoclaving.

Records must be kept of all decisions and the sterile services department must be told of the decision before instruments are sent for routine processing. The records of quarantined instruments should be reviewed at six months and appropriate enquiries made about the diagnosis.

Endoscopy

vCJD infectivity has been detected in lymphoreticular tissues, including tonsils, appendix, lymph nodes and spleen.[647] This raises the theoretical possibility of transfer of abnormal prion protein from the lymphoreticular tissues of a pre-symptomatic patient undergoing certain forms of surgery or invasive procedures, to another patient subsequently receiving treatment with the same instruments or equipment.

In the event of exposure of a flexible endoscope to a possible case of vCJD, it would be necessary to quarantine and perhaps destroy the endoscope.

Sample collecting and labelling

Particular care should be taken with procedures involving the central nervous system. Biopsy and lumbar puncture samples from definite, probable or possible patients should only be taken by trained personnel who are aware of the hazards involved.

- Disposable gloves and eye protection should be worn where splashing may occur.
- Samples should be marked with a 'Danger of Infection' label.
- The laboratory should be given prior warning of the specimen being sent.

Laboratory work

- Particular care should be taken to avoid accidental inoculation or injury when processing samples/specimens. Appropriate protective clothing should be worn. Where possible disposable items should be used and disposed of by incineration.
- The Department of Health suggests blood is unlikely to represent a risk and in laboratories the use of usual control of infection procedures should provide adequate protection for staff, with additional extra care taken to avoid injury. Disposable equipment should be used and subsequently incinerated.
- After laboratory analysis unused CSF should be either autoclaved or immersed in a solution of sodium hypochlorite resulting in 20,000 ppm available chlorine for one hour before final disposal by incineration.
- Instruments of confirmed/known cases of prion disease must be placed in a dedicated sharps bin and labelled 'For incineration'.
- All used instruments and protective clothing should be destroyed by incineration.

After death

- On the death of a patient identified as being in a risk category universal precautions should be applied and the body should be placed in a body bag. The mortician should be notified of diagnosis/suspected diagnosis prior to transfer and a CJD notification form completed by the doctor certifying death.

- Post-mortem examination is recommended to confirm the diagnosis.
- Patients who have died of a suspected prion disease (or any progressive degenerative neurological disease of unknown causation or those who have received pituitary derived hormones, known/assumed to have had human *dura mater* implanted, or with a family history of CJD) should not be considered for organ donation.
- Bodies of patients who have died of CJD must not be used for anatomy/pathology teaching.
- Viewing and superficial contact with the body after death need not be discouraged.

Staff exposed to the prion agent

- The occupational health department should keep a register of any employee who, in the course of their work, may be exposed to the prion agent (in line with COSHH 1999 regulations). In the majority of clinical situations there is no significant risk of exposure. The register will include surgeons, laboratory research staff handling high risk tissue specimens (including CSF) and those who carry out invasive clinical procedures, particularly where there is a risk of exposure to central nervous or eye tissue known to contain the infective agent. Staff should seek advice from occupational health.
- The risks associated with vCJD are still unknown. Current Department of Health recommendations have mainly been targeted at other forms of CJD. If an incident does occur an individual risk assessment should be carried out: the type of prion disease associated with the injury as well as the route of exposure and tissues involved will have a bearing on the suggested line of action. Significant risk of infection by the prion agent is only thought to occur by direct inoculation with central nervous, ocular or lymphoreticular tissues (high risk tissue), for example during ENT surgery. If exposure to this material does occur, the wound should be thoroughly rinsed/washed with detergent. An accident form should be completed.
- Local excision of the inoculated area and secondary prophylaxis treatment may be indicated in some extreme circumstances; advice should be sought from occupational health or the prion unit.

THE REPORTING OF SUSPECTED/CONFIRMED CASES OF CJD IN THE UK

The CJD Surveillance Unit set up in 1990 is still undertaking national surveillance 17 years later. All referrals regarding suspected/definite cases of CJD in the UK are notified to either the CJDSU or the National Prion Unit, and full details of the notification process are available on the CJDSU website.[648]

20 Legionella

INTRODUCTION

In 1976 an outbreak of severe pneumonia, which affected 221 people and killed 34, occurred during a state convention at a hotel in Philadelphia, USA, which was attended by a group of American ex-servicemen at a reunion of the American Legion. Although an airborne disease was suspected given the number of people involved and the nature of the illness, the causative agent went undiscovered for six months, until a fastidious Gram-negative bacillus was identified by two scientists working at the United States Centres for Disease Control and Prevention. The organism responsible for the Philadelphia outbreak was *Legionella pneumophila*, which is now recognised as the cause of 80–90 % of *Legionella* infection in humans. The disease, a relatively rare community acquired pneumonia, is now universally known as Legionnaires' disease, and carries a high morbidity and mortality rate unless diagnosed and treated promptly.[649,650,651]

Legionella is a water-borne pathogen, inhabiting natural aquatic environments and artificial water systems. Since 1976 there have been several notable outbreaks which have occurred in hospitals, hotels and other facilities. The most significant outbreak, which occurred at Stafford General Hospital in 1985[652], is discussed later in this chapter. The largest outbreak of Legionnaires' disease in the world (at the time of writing) was in 2001 in Murcia, Spain. 800 people were diagnosed with pneumonia, of which more than 500 were confirmed as having Legionnaires' disease. Although the actual source was never confirmed, evidence pointed to one or more poorly maintained water cooling towers, which disseminated a contaminated aerosol over the area of the city where the majority of those affected lived.[3,653] The largest outbreak in the UK occurred in 2002 at Barrow-in Furness, Cumbria.[654] 175 people were infected and 7 died because of a poorly maintained air conditioning system at an arts complex run by Barrow-in-Furness Borough Council. The council and a council officer were convicted of health and safety offences at a trial lasting three months, and were eventually acquitted of seven counts of manslaughter. Outbreaks have also occurred in central London; one at the headquarters of the BBC in 1988 affected 79 people and resulted in the deaths of three.[3]

Legionella pneumophila[649] is estimated to cause 1–5 % of all community acquired pneumonias and according to the Health Protection Agency, 300–350 cases of Legionnaires' disease are reported in the UK each year, half of which are associated with travel abroad.[655] A UK survey by the Public Health Laboratory Service (PHLS) found that contamination of domestic hot water systems with *Legionella* bacteria was present in 75 % of business premises, 70 % of hospitals and more than 50 % of hotels.[656]

This chapter discusses the spectrum of illness caused by the *Legionella* bacterium, focussing on Legionnaires' disease and the pathogenesis of infection. As *Legionella* infection is not transmissible between people, there are no specific infection control precautions to be taken for patients with Legionnaires' disease, but the control of *Legionella* within healthcare settings is discussed.

LEARNING OUTCOMES

After reading this chapter the reader will:

- Understand the environmental factors which influence the growth of *Legionella* and how these can be controlled within the healthcare setting
- Be able to describe the clinical features of Legionnaires' disease

THE ORGANISM

Legionella are motile, aerobic Gram-negative bacilli (see Chapter 2 Bacterial and Viral Classification, Structure and Function), and are widely distributed in nature within natural aquatic environments such as rivers and lakes, and man-made aquatic reservoirs such as the ponds in cooling towers of refrigeration plants, in air conditioning systems, domestic hot water systems, air humidifiers, ice-making machines, misting equipment, architectural/decorative fountains, whirlpool spa baths and showers, and respiratory therapy equipment such as nebulisers and oxygen humidifiers.[651,657,658,659] In May 2004, the Medicines and Healthcare Products Regulatory Agency[660] issued an alert warning of the potential risk of transmission of *Legionella* bacteria due to poor drying of re-usable nebulisers after cleaning and recommended that manufacturer's instructions should be followed for cleaning and thorough drying, that no droplets of water remained in the nebuliser before re-use, and that nebulisers which were designated single use items should never be re-used.

Disruption of the domestic water supply, which can result in 'brown' sediment in tap water, recent plumbing work, and residing in a building with an older water system, are environmental risk factors of *Legionella* acquisition, along with community, recreational or travel-related exposures.[650,661,662] Environmental reservoirs for *Legionella* are summarised in Table 20.1.

Legionella often grow in a biofilm with other water organisms, and may be ingested by free-living amoeba, surviving and growing within them as intracellular parasites.[650] They thrive in water temperatures of 20–50 °C, particularly when the

Table 20.1 Environmental risk factors for *Legionella*

Air conditioning systems
Water cooling towers
Domestic water systems – hotels/hospitals/community facilities
Shower heads
Respiratory therapy equipment
Architectural fountains
Ice-making machines
Misting equipment
Whirlpool baths and showers

water is stagnant, but are unable to withstand temperatures of 60 °C or above where they die rapidly, and so the main method of controlling *Legionella* in domestic water systems and in hospitals is to maintain the water temperature below 20 °C and above 60 °C.

There are 45 species of *Legionella* and more than 60 serogroups, of which 18 are opportunistic pathogens causing disease in humans; *Legionella pneumophila* serogroup 1 accounts for most infections in humans.[658] They have exacting growth requirements[659], requiring the use of special media and selective techniques for optimum isolation, and incubation at 35–37 °C in moist air, with the plates 'read' at 3, 5, 7 and 10 days (see Chapter 4 The Microbiology Laboratory). As they stain poorly by Gram-stain, their presence in clinical specimens is best demonstrated by direct or indirect immunofluoresence microscopy.

The organism possesses a number of virulence factors, including pili which promote attachment of the bacteria to macrophages and epithelial cells, flagella which aid motility and promote invasion, and lipopolysaccharide (LPS) which has endotoxic activity.[650]

THE PATHOGENESIS OF INFECTION

Legionellosis is the term used to describe infection caused by *Legionella*, which takes two distinct forms, neither of which are transmissible between humans. Legionnaires' disease is an acute respiratory illness which presents as a rapidly progressive pneumonia. It carries a mortality rate of 5–30 % in healthy individuals, with the higher rate seen in individuals with associated co-morbidities, particularly in situations where the infection is nosocomially acquired.[649,658] Pontiac fever is a milder, febrile, respiratory illness without pneumonia, and often occurs in explosive outbreaks with attack rates of 70–90 %, but the pathogenesis of infection is not fully understood.[650,663] Although *Legionella* are ubiquitous within the environment, they rarely cause disease and certain 'conditions' must be met in order for the process of infection to begin; virulent strains of *Legionella* must be present within an environmental site which supports the survival and multiplication of the organism, and the infectious dose must be disseminated via an infectious aerosol and inhaled by

Table 20.2 Host risk factors for Legionnaires' disease

Smoking
Age > 40 years
Immunocompromised through underlying illness/disease

---

a susceptible individual.[650] Host risk factors for the acquisition of Legionnaires' disease are summarised in Table 20.2.

For a susceptible individual to develop Legionnaires' disease, they need to inhale the bacteria, which then penetrate down to the alveoli. The bacteria are present in water-borne particles suspended in the air as an aerosol. Water droplets evaporate very quickly, although the exact rate depends on the temperature, relative humidity and airflow. A water droplet containing a single *Legionella* bacteria will remain suspended in air for prolonged periods of time and can travel for considerable distances in suitable weather conditions, where it can enter the air conditioning and ventilation systems of buildings.

Following inhalation of an aerosol contaminated with *Legionella*, it enters the lung where it is phagocytosed by the alveolar macrophages. The bacteria replicate within the macrophages, destroying them and then escaping, whereupon they are re-phagocytosed by other macrophages, and this process of re-amplification increases the concentration of bacteria within the lungs. An inflammatory exudate consisting of fibrin, neutrophils, additional macrophages and erythrocytes floods into the area, and the release of cytokines and chemokines from the infected macrophages, along with the virulence factors of the organism, assist the immune system in triggering a severe immune response.[650,663]

INCUBATION PERIOD AND CLINICAL FEATURES

Legionnaires' disease has an incubation period of 2–10 days, and begins with a prodromal illness lasting anything from a few hours to several days. Symptoms are initially non-specific, consisting of a headache (which may be severe), fever with rigors, myalgia and loss of appetite, along with diarrhoea and abdominal pain. Differential diagnoses at this stage may include influenza, a gastrointestinal illness and, given the severity of the headache, subarachnoid haemorrhage.[650] A cough develops after the prodrome, but this is productive in only 50 % of cases, and purulent sputum production is not a clinical feature of Legionnaires' disease.[663] If a chest x-ray is taken within the very early stages of the illness, it may not reveal any clinically significant findings, and the initial clinical picture may be one of a generalised illness with minimal changes, but within a day or so changes will be seen, ranging from patchy infiltrates to multiple areas of consolidation. Some patients may complain of pleuritic chest pain and haemoptysis, and develop pulmonary effusion. Hyponatraemia and abnormal liver function are frequently present and patients with an incubation period of less than five days tend to have a worse prognosis.

Table 20.3 Clinical features of Legionnaires' disease

Prodromal period lasting several days with patients exhibiting:
Headache
Fever and rigors
Abdominal pain
Diarrhoea
Myalgia
Anorexia
Non-productive cough
Chest x-ray taken after the prodromal period will show patchy infiltrates/consolidation
May complain of pleuritic chest pain and haemoptysis
Pleural effusion

The clinical features of Legionnaires' disease are summarised in Table 20.3.

DIAGNOSIS

Diagnosis is difficult because of the non-specific clinical presentation, but Legionnaires' disease should be suspected in those individuals who fail to respond to conventional antibiotic treatment for pneumonia, or where symptoms are so severe that they require admission to an intensive therapy unit. Attempts should be made to establish the patient's travel history, or recreational activities that may have involved the use of whirlpool/spa baths. Detection of *Legionella* antigen in urine is now the gold-standard diagnostic test for serogroup 1 infection and can be performed in minutes by most clinical laboratories. In contrast to the previous tests based on detection of antibody in serum, the test becomes positive shortly after onset of symptoms.

TREATMENT

Patients with Legionnaires' disease are notoriously slow to respond to antibiotic therapy and the treatment of choice remains controversial. Recent evidence suggests that quinolone antibiotics such as levofloxacin are effective, but macrolide agents, including azithromycin and clarithromycin, sometimes in combination with rifampicin, are used.

THE STAFFORD GENERAL HOSPITAL LEGIONNAIRES' DISEASE OUTBREAK[652] – APRIL 1985

The Legionnaires' disease 'incident' at Stafford General Hospital in 1985 in which 22 people died was, like the *Salmonella typhimurium* outbreak at the Stanley Royd

Hospital in Wakefield in 1984 (see Chapter 15 Campylobacter and Salmonella) another spectacularly mismanaged outbreak. Stafford had a population of approximately 57,000 and was served by four hospitals, of which Stafford General, being newly built and opened in 1983, was the flagship. *Legionella* was first isolated from one of the cooling tower ponds in November 1984. The cooling towers had been in service since the hospital opened, without ever being serviced or cleaned, although when *Legionella* was identified, the affected system was drained, cleaned, rechlorinated and then brought back into service. The outbreak that occurred between the 9th and 19th April 1985 was in clinical areas served by that very same cooling tower. Patients attending the outpatients department (OPD) on the ground floor were exposed to an aerosol containing virulent *Legionella pneumophila*; exposure to the organism was brief (less than 25 minutes in one case) and the onset of symptoms was rapid. An increase in admissions to the hospital with severe pneumonia was noted on the 22nd April, and although Legionnaires' disease was on the list of differential diagnoses, it was considered unlikely as there were reports from the community of an outbreak of a severe influenza-like illness. More admissions were seen over the followings days and the severity of the illness became apparent, with some patients requiring intensive care and ventilatory support. At one point 23 out of 24 patients in the admissions ward had been admitted with pneumonia. By the time a meeting of the control of infection committee was organised on the 26th April, 50 patients has been admitted to Stafford General with a severe respiratory infection, 13 were critically ill with 5 on ventilators, and 6 had died. The Communicable Disease Surveillance Centre (CDSC) was contacted and assistance in investigating the outbreak was requested. On the 3rd May, a diagnosis of Legionnaires' disease was made, nearly a week after the first specimens were sent to the laboratory. It was also around this time that the medical staff were first made aware that *Legionella* had been isolated from one of the cooling tower ponds five months previously.

The Committee of Inquiry, set up by the Minister of State for Health (Kenneth Clarke) found that there were several factors relating to the construction of the cooling tower which differed from the usual recommended design, mode of operation (which in this case provided a suitable temperature for the multiplication of *Legionella*), and the condition of its water system, which contributed to the multiplication and dissemination of the organism in sufficient concentration to cause severe infection by the means of an aerosol created in the tower. The aerosol entered the fresh air inlet duct which served maternity (2nd floor), the operating theatres (1st floor) and OPD on the ground floor. The aerosol passed through the air plant on each floor and was subsequently inhaled by patients, visitors and staff in those areas. The resulting infection was particularly severe among vulnerable patients visiting OPD. It was also considered possible that contaminated aerosols may have been carried from the cooling tower down the outside of the building, becoming a source of infection to anyone outside, as well as anyone inside the building and near an open window.

THE PREVENTION AND CONTROL OF LEGIONELLA IN HOSPITALS

The Health Act[22] states that with regard to the prevention of *Legionella* infection: 'Premises should be regularly reviewed for potential sources of infection and a programme should be prepared to minimise any risk. Priority should be given to patient areas, although the exact priority will depend on local circumstances' (page 17).

Water distribution systems in many hospitals are often dated in design and layout given the age of the buildings, and characterised by the presence of long pipe runs (making temperature control difficult) and an over supply of water outlets, some of which may be used infrequently, serving as 'dead-legs'. *Legionella* bacteria have a propensity to colonise these areas, where organic material and waste products from other bacteria form a biofilm (see Chapter 2 Bacterial and Viral Classification Structure and Function) which adheres to the inner surface of the piping, reducing the effectiveness of cleaning and disinfection measures.

The control of *Legionella* in healthcare premises is governed by health technical memorandum (HTM) 04-01[664], which superseded HTM 2040 in 2006. This document combines previous advice on hot and cold water systems with specific *Legionella* advice. The new guidance is also more specific about the value of using additional control systems such as chlorine dioxide and/or silver ion water treatment in addition to water control. There is also an interesting statement that self-draining showers do not work and should be replaced by automatic self-purging showers which run for several minutes a day – potentially an excellent way of preventing ward staff from using ward shower rooms as additional store rooms.

Compliance with *Legionella* control is now a statutory requirement under the following acts and regulations:

- The Health and Safety at Work Act (1974)
- Control of Substances Hazardous to Health (COSHH) Regulations (1988)
- Public Health (Infectious Disease) Regulations (1988)
- Water Supply (Water Quality) Regulations (1989) and Water Supply (Water Quality) Regulations (Amendment) (1991).

A *Legionella* risk assessment, forming the basis of a written operational plan, should identify who has overall accountability for the premises (usually the chief executive) and who is responsible for carrying out the necessary procedures.

The risk assessment should take into account the potential for aerosol formation, water temperature, the means of preventing and controlling the risk, and the likely risk to those who will inhale water droplets.

Basic actions to reduce the risk of *Legionella* outbreaks in healthcare premises include the removal of any redundant pipework, the running of all taps and showers daily (especially those in unoccupied side rooms and rarely used bathrooms), and disconnecting unused showers.

In the event of a suspected outbreak of Legionnaires' disease associated with healthcare premises, an in-depth investigation will be launched to search for the suspected source of the outbreak. Potential sources of *Legionella* infection include domestic hot and cold water distribution systems, showers or spray washing equipment, drainage systems and traps, spas, whirlpool pools or hydrotherapy pools, humidifiers in ventilation systems, cooling coils in air conditioning systems, and fountains and sprinklers.

Exposure to *Legionella* is potentially preventable, outbreaks cause considerable, and justifiable, public concern and those occurring within healthcare environments are particularly worrying given the nature of the vulnerable patient population. Most outbreaks of Legionnaires' disease have been caused by either poor maintenance of air conditioning systems or failure to control water temperature in hot and cold water supplies.

References

1. Gardner A.M.N., Stamp M., Bowgen J.A., Moore B.(1962) The infection control sister: a new member of the control of infection team in general hospitals. *The Lancet* Oct 6, 710–711.
2. Selwyn S. (1991) Hospital infection: the first 2500 years. *Journal of Hospital Infection* **18** (Supplement A), 5–64.
3. Department of Health (2002) *Getting Ahead of the Curve. A Strategy for Combating Infectious Diseases (Including Other Aspects of Health Protection)* A report by the Chief Medical Officer. DoH, London.
4. Ryan K. (2004) Plague and Other Bacterial Zoonotic Diseases. In: Sherris J.C., Ryan K.J., Ray C.G. (eds) *Medical Microbiology: An Introduction to Infectious Diseases.* Fourth Edition. McGraw-Hill, USA, 481–491
5. Corbel M.J., (2002) Yersinia, Pasteurella and Francisella. In: Greenwood D., Slack R.C., Peutherer J.F. (eds) *Medical Microbiology. A Guide to Microbial Infections: Pathogenesis, Immunity, Laboratory Diagnosis and Control.* Sixteenth Edition. Churchill Livingstone, London: 329–336.
6. World Health Organization (1999) *Plague Manual: Epidemiology, Distribution, Surveillance and Control.* Available at: www.who.int/csr/resources/publications/plague/whocdscsredc992a.pdf (accessed 30th May 2007).
7. www.who.int/csr/don/archive/disease/plague/en (accessed 30th May 2007).
8. Lippi D., Conti A.A. (2000) Plague, policy, saints and terrorists: a historical survey. *Journal of Infection* **44** (4), 226–228.
9. Leggiadro R.J. (2000) The threat of biological terrorism: a public health and infection control reality. *Infection Control Hospital Epidemiology* **21**, 53–56.
10. www.dh.gov.uk/en/Policyandguidance/Emergencyplanning/Deliberaterelease/index.htm (accessed 30th May 2007).
11. www.who.int/mediacentre/factsheets/smallpox/en (accessed 30th May 2007).
12. Stewart A.J., Devlin P.M. (2006) The history of the smallpox vaccine. *Journal of Infection* **52** (5), 329–334.
13. www.wikipedia.org/wiki/Smallpox (accessed 30th May 2007).
14. Ray C.G. (2004) Poxviruses. In: Sherris J.C., Ryan K.J., Ray C.G. (eds) *Medical Microbiology: An Introduction to Infectious Diseases.* Fourth Edition. McGraw-Hill, USA, 525–529.
15. www.bt.cdc.gov/agent/smallpox (accessed 30th May 2007).
16. Department of Health (2003) *Guidelines for Smallpox Response and Management in the Post Eradication Era (Smallpox Plan)* DoH, London.
17. Cunningham J.B., Kernohan W.G., Sowney, R. (2005) Bed occupancy and turnover interval as determinant factors in MRSA infections in acute settings in Northern Ireland. *Journal of Hospital Infection* **61** (3), 189–193.

18. Wigglesworth N., Wilcox M.H. (2006) Prospective evaluation of hospital isolation room capacity. *Journal of Hospital Infection* **63** (2), 156–161.
19. Department of Health (2004) *Towards Cleaner Hospitals and Lower Rates of Infection: A Summary of Action*. DoH, London.
20. Department of Health (2000) *The NHS Plan: A Plan for Investment, a Plan for Reform*. DoH, London.
21. Healthcare Commission (2006) *Investigation into Outbreaks of Clostridium Difficile at Stoke Mandeville Hospital, Buckinghamshire Hospitals NHS Trust*. Available at: www.healthcarecommission.org.ik/_db_documents/Stoke_Mandeville.pdf (accessed 30th May 2007).
22. Department of Health (2006) *The Health Act 2006; Code of Practice for the Prevention and Control of Health Care Associated Infections*. DoH, London.
23. Meers P.D., Ayliffe G.A., Emmerson A.M., Leigh D.A., Mayon-White R.T., Mackintosh C.A., Strong J.L. (1981) Report on the national surveillance of infection in hospitals, 1980. *Journal of Hospital Infection* **2** (Supplementary), 1–11.
24. Emmerson A.M., Enstone J.E., Griffin M., Kelsey M.C., Smyth E.M. (1996) The second national prevalence survey of infection in hospitals – overview of results. *Journal of Hospital Infection* **32** (3), 175–190.
25. Department of Health (1995) *Hospital Infection Control: Guidance on the Control of Infection in Hospitals*. HSG (95)10. DoH, London.
26. National Audit Office (2000) *The Management and Control of Hospital Acquired Infection in Acute NHS Trusts in England*. Report by the Comptroller and Auditor General. HC 230 Session 1999–2000. 17 February 2000.
27. Plowman R., Graves N., Griffin M., Roberts J., Swan A.V., Cookson B., Taylor L. (2000) *The Socio-Economic Burden of Hospital Acquired Infection*. Public Health Laboratory Service, London.
28. www.dh.gov.uk/en/Policyandguidance/Organisationpolicy/Financeandplanning/NHS-FinancialReforms/index.htm (accessed 30th May 2007).
29. Department of Health (2006) *Going Further, Faster: Implementing the Saving Lives Delivery Programme. Sustainable Change for Cleaner, Safer Care*. DoH, London.
30. Department of Health (2005) *Saving Lives: A Delivery Programme to Reduce Healthcare Associated Infection, Including MRSA*. DoH, London.
31. www.dh.gov.uk/en/Publicationsandstatistics/Pressreleases/DH_4093533 (accessed 30th May 2007).
32. www.npsa.nhs.uk/health/resources/root_cause_analysis (accessed 30th May 2007).
33. Department of Health (2005) *Action on Health Care Associated Infections in England*. DoH, London.
34. Department of Health (2005) *Standards for Better Health*. DoH, London.
35. Haley R.W., White J.W., Culver D.H., Meade-Morgan W., Emori T.G., Munn V.P., Hooton T.M. (1985) The efficacy of infection surveillance and control programmes in preventing nosocomial infections in US hospitals (SENIC) *American Journal of Epidemiology* **121** (2), 182–205.
36. National Audit Office (2004) *Improving Patient Care by Reducing the Risk of Hospital Acquired Infection: A Progress Report*. Report by the Comptroller and Auditor General. HC 876 Session 2003–2004: 14 July 2004.
37. Burton G.R.W., Engelkirk P.G. (2004) Microbiology: The Science. In: *Microbiology for the Health Sciences*. Lippincott Williams and Wilkins, Philadelphia, USA, 1–4.

38. Barer M.M. (2002) Morphology and the nature of micro-organisms. In: Greenwood D., Slack R.C.B., Peutherer J.F. (eds) *Medical Microbiology. A Guide to Microbial Infections: Pathogenesis, Immunity, Laboratory Diagnosis and Control.* Sixteenth Edition. Churchill Livingstone, London, 9–24.

39. Lindsay D., von Holy A. (2006) Bacterial biofilms within the clinical setting: what healthcare professionals should know. *Journal of Hospital Infection* **65** (4), 313–325.

40. Watnick P., Koiter R. (2000) Biofilm, city of microbes. *Journal of Bacteriology* **182** (10), 2675–2679.

41. Petri W.A., Mann B.J., Huston C.D. (2004) Microbial Adherence. In: Mandell G.L., Bennett J.E., Dolin R.D. (eds) *Mandell's Principles and Practices of Infectious Diseases.* Sixth Edition. Churchill Livingstone, London. PPID Online. www.ppidonline.com (accessed 30th May 2007).

42. Gladwin M., Trattler B. (2004) Cell Structure, Virulence Factors and Toxins. In: *Clinical Microbiology Made Ridiculously Simple.* Edition 3. MedMaster, Inc., Miami, USA, 8–15.

43. Torres B.A., Kominsky S., Perrin G.Q., Hobeika A.C., Johnson H.W. (2001) Superantigens: the Good, the Bad and the Ugly *Experimental Biology and Medicine* **226**, 164–176.

44. Falkow S. (2004) Host-Parasite Relationships. In: Sherris J.C., Ryan K.J., Ray G.C. (eds) M*edical Microbiology: An Introduction to Infectious Diseases* Fourth Edition. McGraw-Hill, London, 149–172.

45. Burton G.W., Engelkirk P.G., (2004) Pathogenesis of Infectious Disease. In: *Microbiology for the Health Sciences.* Lippincott, Williams and Wilkins, Philadelphia, USA, 360–379.

46. Champoux J.J. (2004) Viral Structure. In: Sherris J.C., Ryan K.J., Ray G.C. (eds) *Medical Microbiology: An Introduction to Infectious Diseases.* Fourth Edition. McGraw-Hill, USA, 79–86.

47. www.virustaxonomyonline.com (accessed 30th May 2007).

48. Champoux J.J. (2004) Viral Multiplication. In: Sherris J.C., Ryan K.J., Ray G.C. (eds) *Medical Microbiology: An Introduction to Infectious Diseases* Fourth Edition. McGraw-Hill, USA, 87–104.

49. Peiris J.S.M., Madeley C.R. (2003) Adenoviruses. In: Greenwood D., Slack R.C.B., Peutherer J.F. (eds) *Medical Microbiology. A Guide to Microbial Infections: Pathogenesis, Immunity, Laboratory Diagnosis and Control.* Sixteenth Edition. Churchill Livingstone, London, 392–398.

50. Strohl W.A., Rouse H., Fisher B.D. (2001) Non-Enveloped DNA Viruses. In: Harvey R.A. and Champe P.A. (eds) *Lippincott's Illustrated Reviews. Medical Microbiology.* Lippincott, Williams and Wilkins, Philadelphia, USA, 307–316.

51. Ogilvie M.M. (2004) Herpes Viruses. In: Greenwood D., Slack R.C.B., Peutherer J.F. (eds) *Medical Microbiology. A Guide to Microbial Infections: Pathogenesis, Immunity, Laboratory Diagnosis and Control.* Sixteenth Edition. Churchill Livingstone, London, 399–420.

52. Department of Health (2006) *Immunisation Against Infectious Disease* (Department of Health Green Book) The Stationery Office, London.

53. Burns S.M. (2004) Picornaviruses. In: Greenwood D., Slack R.C.B., Peutherer J.F. (eds) *Medical Microbiology. A Guide to Microbial Infections: Pathogenesis, Immunity, Laboratory Diagnosis and Control.* Sixteenth Edition. Churchill Livingstone, London, 455–467.

54. Peiris J.S.M., Madeley C.R. (2004) Paramyxoviruses. In: Greenwood D., Slack R.C.B., Peutherer J.F. (eds) *Medical Microbiology. A Guide to Microbial Infections: Pathogenesis, Immunity, Laboratory Diagnosis and Control.* Sixteenth Edition. Churchill Livingstone, London, 475–483.
55. www.hpa.org.uk/infections/topics_az/wfhfactsheets/WFHmeasles.htm (accessed 30th May 2007).
56. www/hpa.org.uk/infections/topics_az/vaccination/071102_MMRpreferable.htm (accessed 30th May 2007).
57. www.mmrthefacts.nhs.uk/resources (accessed 30th 2007).
58. Cubitt D. (2004) Caliciviruses. In: Greenwood D., Slack R.C.B., Peutherer J.F. (eds) *Medical Microbiology. A Guide to Microbial Infections: Pathogenesis, Immunity, Laboratory Diagnosis and Control.* Sixteenth Edition. Churchill Livingstone, London, 539–545.
59. Thys J.P., Jacobs F., Bye B. (1994) Microbiological specimen collection in the emergency room. *European Journal of Emergency Medicine* **1** (1), 47–53.
60. Gill V.J., Fedorko D.P., Witebsky F.G. (2004) The Clinician and the Microbiology Laboratory. In: Mandell G.L., Bennett J.E., Dolin R.D. (eds) *Mandell's Principles and Practices of Infectious Diseases.* Sixth Edition. Churchill Livingstone, London. PPID Online. www.ppidonline.com (accessed 30th May 2007).
61. UK Health Departments (1998) *Guidance for Clinical Health Workers: Protection against Infection with Blood Borne Viruses.* Recommendations of the Expert Advisory Group on AIDS and the Advisory Group on Hepatitis. DoH, London.
62. Baxter A., Salter M. (1996) Urinary Catherisation. In: Mallet J., Bailey C. (eds) *The Royal Marsden Hospital Manual of Clinical Nursing Procedures.* Fourth Edition. Blackwell Publishing, London, 590–606.
63. Marwick C.A., Ziglam H.M., Nathwani D. (2006) Your patient has a blood culture positive for *Staphylococcus aureus* – what would you do? *Journal Royal College Physicians Edinburgh* **36**, 350–355.
64. Towner K.J. (2003) Bacterial Genetics. In: Greenwood D., Slack R.C.B., Peutherer J.F. (eds) *Medical Microbiology. A Guide to Microbial Infections: Pathogenesis, Immunity, Laboratory Diagnosis and Control.* Sixteenth Edition. Churchill Livingstone, London, 61–72.
65. Barer M.R. (2003) Bacterial Growth and Physiology. In: Greenwood D., Slack R.C.B., Peutherer J.F. (eds) *Medical Microbiology. A Guide to Microbial Infections: Pathogenesis, Immunity, Laboratory Diagnosis and Control.* Sixteenth Edition. Churchill Livingstone, London, 37–45.
66. Health Protection Agency (2005) National Standard Method – BSOP 54 Inoculation of Culture Media. Available at: www.hpa-standardmethods.org.uk/documents/bsop/pdf/bsop54.pdf (accessed30th May 2007).
67. HPA (2005) National Standard Method – BSOP TP39 Staining Procedures. Available at: www.hpa-standardmethods.org.uk/documents/bsopTP/pdf/bsoptp39.pdf (accessed 30th May 2007).
68. HPA (2005) National Standard Method – BSOP TP10 Coagulase Test. Available at: www.hpa-standardmethods.org.uk/documents/bsopTP/pdf/bsoptp39.pdf (accessed 30th May 2007).
69. HPA (2005) National Standard Method – BSOP 54 Susceptibility Testing. Available at: www.hpa-standardmethods.org.uk/doucuments/bsop/pdf/bsop45.pdf (accessed 30th May 2007).

70. HPA (2005) National Standard Method – BSOP 40 Investigation of Specimens for *Mycobacterium* Species. Available at: www.hpa-standardmethods.org.uk/documents/bsop/pdf/bsop40.pdf (accessed 30th May 2007).

71. HPA (2005) National Standard Method – BSOP ID8 Identification of *Clostridium* Species. Available at: www.hpa-standardmethods.org.uk/documents.bsopid/pdf/bsopid8.pdf (accessed 30th May 2007).

72. HPA (2005) National Standard Method – BSOP 10 Toxin Detection, Isolation, and Identification of *Clostridium Difficile* from Faeces. Available at: www.hpa-standardmethods.org.uk/documents/bsop/pdf/bsop10.pdf (accessed 30th May 2007).

73. Pitt T.L. (2003) Classification and Identification of Micro-Organisms. In: Greenwood D., Slack R.C.B., Peutherer J.F. (eds) *Medical Microbiology. A Guide to Microbial Infections: Pathogenesis, Immunity, Laboratory Diagnosis and Control.* Sixteenth Edition. Churchill Livingstone, London, 25–36.

74. Stewart J (2003) Innate and Acquired Immunity. In: Greenwood D, Slack R.C.B., Peutherer J.F. (eds) *Medical Microbiology. A Guide to Microbial Infections: Pathogenesis, Immunity, Laboratory Diagnosis and Control.* Sixteenth Edition. Churchill Livingstone, London, 121–145.

75. Dieffenbach C.W., Tramont E.D. (2004) Innate (General or Non-specific) Host Defence Mechanisms. In: Mandell G.L., Bennett J.E., Dolin R.D. (eds) *Mandell's Principles and Practices of Infectious Diseases.* Sixth Edition. Churchill Livingstone, London. PPID Online: www.ppidonline.com (accessed 30th May 2007).

76. Ryan K.J. (2004) Normal Microbial Flora. In: Sherris. J.C., Ryan K.J., Ray G.C. (eds) *Medical Microbiology: An Introduction to Infectious Diseases* Fourth Edition. McGraw-Hill, USA, 141–148.

77. Bannister B.A., Begg N.T. Gillespie S.H. (1996) *Infectious Diseases.* Blackwell Science Ltd, London, 1–21.

78. Roitt I., Brostoff J., Male D. (2001) *Immunology.* Sixth Edition. Mosby, London.

79. Staines N., Brostoff J., James K. (1993) *Introducing Immunology.* Second Edition. Mosby, London.

80. Wilson J. (1995) *Infection Control in Clinical Practice.* Bailliere Tindall, London, 77–105.

81. Marchalonis J.J. (2004) Immune Response to Infection. In. Sherris J.C., Ryan K.J., Ray G.C. (eds) *Medical Microbiology: An Introduction to Infectious Diseases.* Fourth Edition. McGraw-Hill, USA, 115–139.

82. Densen P. (2004) Complement. In: Mandell G.L., Bennett J.E., Dolin R.D. (eds) *Mandell's Principles and Practices of Infectious Diseases.* Sixth Edition. Churchill Livingstone, London. PPID Online. www.ppidonline.com (accessed 30th May 2007).

83. www.anaphylaxis.com (accessed 30th May 2007).

84. Simons F.E. (2004) Advances in H_1-antihistamine. *New England Journal Medicine* **351** (21), 2203–2217.

85. www.hse.gov.uk/latex/about.htm (accessed 30th May 2007).

86. Pratt R.J., Pellowe C.M., Wilson J.A., Loveday H.P., Harper P.J., Jones S.R.L.K., McDougall C., Wilcox M.H. (2006) *Epic2: National Evidence-Based Guidelines for Preventing Healthcare – Associated Infections in NHS Hospitals in England.* Available at:www.epic.tvu.ac.uk/Downloads/ (accessed 30th May 2007).

87. Ala'Aldeen D. (2002) Bacterial pathogenicity. In: Greenwood D., Slack R.C.B., Peutherer J.F. (eds) *Medical Microbiology. A Guide to Microbial Infections:*

Pathogenesis, Immunity, Laboratory Diagnosis and Control. Sixteenth Edition. Churchill Livingstone, London, 83–92.

88. O'Connor H. (2002) Decontaminating beds and mattresses. *Nursing Times* **96** (suppl) 46, 2–5.

89. Bannister B.A., Begg N.T., Gillespie S.H. (1996) Bacteraemic Infections. In: *Infectious Diseases.* Blackwell Science, London, 283–300.

90. Slade E., Tamber P.S., Vincent J.L. (2003) The Surviving Sepsis Campaign: Raising Awareness to Reduce Mortality. *Critical Care* **7** (1), 1–2.

91. Offord R. (2002) Causes and features of sepsis. *Hospital Pharmacist* **9** (April), 93–96.

92. Robson W., Newell J. (2005) Assessing, treating and managing patients with sepsis. *Nursing Standard* **19** (50), 56–64.

93. Bone R.C., Balk R.A., Cerra F.B. (1992) American College of Chest Physicians/Society of Critical Care Medical Consensus Conference. Definitions for sepsis and organ failure and guidelines for the use of innovative therapies in sepsis. *Chest* **101** (6), 1644–1655.

94. Vincent J.L. (2002) Sepsis definition. *Lancet Infectious Diseases* **2**, 135.

95. Dellenger R.P., Carlet J.M., Masur H., Gerlach H., Calandra T., Cohen J., Gea-Banachloche J., Keh D., Marshall J.C., Parker M.M. (2004) Surviving Sepsis Campaign guidelines for management of severe sepsis and septic shock. *Critical Care Medicine* **34** (3), 858–873.

96. Ahrens T., Tuggle D. (2004) Surviving sepsis: early recognition and treatment. *Critical Care Nurse* **24** (5) (suppl), 2–13.

97. Garner J.S and the Hospital Infection Control Practices Advisory Committee (1996) Guideline for Isolation Precautions in Hospitals. *Infection Control Hospital Epidemiology* **15** (53), 53–80.

98. Pratt R.J., Pellowe C.M., Loveday H.B., Robinson M., Smith G.W and the Epic Guidelines Development Team (2001) The e*pic* Project: Developing National Evidence-Based Guidelines for Preventing Healthcare Associated Infections. *Journal Hospital Infection* **47** (suppl), S1–S82.

99. Teasley D.G., Gerding D.N., Olson M.M., Peterson L.R., Gebhardt R.L., Schwartz M.J.(1983) Prospective randomised trial of metronidazole versus vancomycin for Clostridium difficile associated diarrhoea and colitis. *The Lancet.* **2** (8358), 1043–1046.

100. Gould D. (1991) Nurses' hands as vectors of hospital-acquired infection: a review. *Journal of Advanced Nursing* **16** (10), 1216–1225.

101. Larson E. (1999) Skin hygiene and infection prevention: more of the same or different approaches? *Clinical Infectious Diseases* **29** (5), 1287–1294.

102. Trampuz A., Widmer A.F. (2004) Hand hygiene: a frequently missed lifesaving opportunity during patient care. *Mayo Clinic Proceedings* **79** (1), 1.109–116.

103. Casewell M., Phillips I. (1977) Hands as a route of transmission of Klebsiella species. *British Medical Journal* **2** (6098), 1315–1317.

104. Reybrouck G. (1982) The role of hands in the spread of nosocomial infections. *Journal Hospital Infection* **4** (2), 103–111.

105. Mackintosh C.A., Hoffman P.N. (1984) An extended model for transfer of microorganisms via the hands: differences between the organism and the effect of alcohol disinfection. *Journal Hygiene* **92**, 45–355.

106. Infection Control Nurses Association (2002) *Guidelines for Hand Hygiene.* ICNA, Bathgate.

107. Garner J.S, Favero M.S. (1985) *Guidelines for handwashing and hospital environmental control*.1st Edition. USA Centres for Infectious Diseases, Atlanta, Georgia.

108. Ehrenkranz N.J., Alfonso B.C. (1991) Failure of bland soap handwash to prevent hand transfer of patient bacteria to urethral catheters. *Infection Control Hospital Epidemiology* **12** (11), 654–662.

109. Hoffman P.N., Cooke P.M., McCarville E., Emmerson A.M. (1985) Micro-organisms isolated from the skin under wedding rings worn by hospital staff. *British Medical Journal* **290** (6463), 206–207.

110. Rotter L.M. (1997) 150 years of hand disinfection: Semmelweis' heritage. *Hyg Med* **22**, 332–339.

111. Taylor L. (1978) An evaluation of handwashing techniques – 1. *Nursing Times* **74** (2), 54–55.

112. Pittet D., Mourouga P., Perneger T.V. (1999) Compliance with hand washing in a teaching hospital; infection control programme. *Annals Internal Medicine* **130** (2), 126–130.

113. Jenner E.A., Fletcher B., Watson P., Jones F.A., Miller L., Scott G.M. (2006) Discrepancy between self-reported and observed hand hygiene behaviour in healthcare professionals. *Journal Hospital Infection* **63** (4), 418–422.

114. Larson E.L., Kretzer E.K. (1995) Compliance with hand washing and barrier precautions. *Journal Hospital Infection* **30** (suppl) 88–106.

115. Pittet D., Boyce J.M. (2001) Hand hygiene and patient care: pursuing the Semmelweis legacy. *Lancet Infectious Diseases* April, 9–20.

116. Boyce J.M., Pettit D., and the Healthcare Infection Control Practices Advisory Committee and the HICPAC/SHEA/APIC/IDSA Hand Hygiene Task Force (2002) Guideline for hand hygiene in healthcare settings: recommendations of the Healthcare Infection Control Practices Advisory Committee and the HICPAC/SHEA/APIC/IDSA Hand Hygiene Task Force. Society for Healthcare Epidemiology of America/Association for Professionals in Infection Control/Infectious Diseases Society of America. *Morbidity Mortality Weekly Review* October 25, **51**, RR–16, 1–45.

117. Bischoff W.E., Reynolds T., Sessler C., Edmond M., Wenzel R.P. (2000) Handwashing compliance by healthcare workers; the impact of introducing an accessible alcohol based hand antiseptic. *Archives Internal Medicine* **160** (7), 1017–1012.

118. Maury E., Alzieu M., Baudel J.L., Haram N. (2000) Availability of an alcohol solution can improve hand disinfection compliance in an intensive care unit. *American Journal Respiratory Medicine* **162** (1), 324–327.

119. Rotter M.L. (1999) Handwashing and hand disinfection. In: Mayhill C.G. (ed) *Hospital Epidemiology and Infection Control*. 2nd Edition. Lippincott Williams and Wilkins, Philadelphia, USA, 1339–1355.

120. www.npsa.nhs.uk/site/media/documents/644_cyh_alert.pdf (accessed 30th May 2007).

121. www.npsa.nhs.uk/display?contentId=3285 (accessed 30th May 2007).

122. www.npsa.nhs/uk/cleanyourhands (accessed 30th May 2007).

123. Department of Health (2004) NPSA cleanyourhands campaign *economic evaluation*. DoH, London.

124. www.supplychain.nhs.uk/portal/page/portal/Hand%20Hygiene/Background (accessed 30th May 2007).

125. Banfield K.R., Kerr K.G. (2005) Could hospital patients' hands constitute a missing link? *Journal Hospital Infection* **61** (3), 183–188.

126. Infection Control Nurses Association (2001) *A Comprehensive Glove Choice*. ICNA, Bathgate.
127. Medical Devices Agency (1996) *Latex Sensitisation in the Health Care Setting (Use of Latex Gloves)*. Medical Devices Agency, London.
128. Dave J., Wilcox M.H., Kellett M. (1999) Glove powder; implications for infection control. *Journal Hospital Infection* **42** (4), 283–285.
129. Johns G. (1999) Avoiding latex allergy. *Nursing Standard* **13** (21), 49–56.
130. Medical Devices Agency (2001) SN 200 (19) – *Safe Use and Disposal of Sharps*. Medical Devices Agency, London.
131. www.opsi.gov.uk/si/si1992/Uksi_19920588_en_1.htm (accessed 30th May 2007).
132. Department of Health (2006) Health Technical Memorandum 0701: *Safe Management of Healthcare Waste*. DoH, London.
133. NHS Executive (1995) HSG (95) 18: *Hospital Laundry Arrangements for Used and Infected Linen*.
134. Barrie D. (1994) How hospital linen and laundry services are provided. *Journal Hospital Infection* **27** (3), 219–235.
135. Babb J.R., Davies J.G., Ayliffe G.A. (1985) Contamination of protective clothing and nurses' uniforms in an isolation ward. *Journal Hospital Infection* **4** (2), 149–157.
136. Wong D., Nye K., Hollis P. (1991) Microbial flora on doctors' white coats. *British Medical Journal* **303** (6817), 1602–1604.
137. Callaghan I. (1998) Bacterial contamination of nurses' uniforms; a study. *Nursing Standard* **13** (1), 37–42.
138. www.rcn.org.uk/resources/mrsa/healthcarestaff/uniforms/infectioncontrol.php (accessed 30th May 2007).
139. www.rcn.org.uk/resources/mrsa/downloads/Wipe_it_out-Guidance_on_uniforms.pdf (accessed 30th May 2007).
140. www.patientexperience.nhsestates.gov.uk/clean_hospitals/ch_content/cleaning_manual/decontamination.asp (accessed 30th May 2007).
141. NHS Estates/Department of Health (2004) *A Matron's Charter: an Action Plan for Cleaner Hospitals*. 19th October. DoH, London.
142. Department of Health (2003) *Winning Ways: Working Together to Reduce Healthcare Associated Infection in England*. DoH, London.
143. www.npsa.nhs.uk/health/resources/peat (accessed 30th May 2007).
144. NHS Estates (2001) *National Standards of Cleanliness for the NHS*. NHS Estates/ DoH, London.
145. www.bics.org.uk (accessed 30th May 2007).
146. www.npsa.nhs.uk/site/media/documents/2140_0429colourcodingsp1D2F4.pdf (accessed 30th May 2007).
147. www.ahcp.co.uk (accessed 30th May 2007).
148. Blythe D., Keenleyside D., Dawson S.T., Galloway A. (1998) Environmental contamination due to MRSA. *Journal Hospital Infection* **38** (1), 67–69.
149. Spach D.H, Silverstein F.E, Stamm W.E. (1993) Transmission of infection by gastrointestinal gastroscopy. *Annals Internal Medicine* **118** (2), 117–128.
150. Medical Devices Agency (2002) *Decontamination of Endoscopes*. MDA DB2002 (05). Medical Devices Agency, London.
151. British Society of Gastroenterology (2003) *BSG Guidelines for the Decontamination of Equipment for Gastrointestinal Endoscopy. The Report of a Working Party of the British Society of Gastroenterology Endoscopy Committee*. BSG, UK.

152. Gould D. (2004) Bacterial infections: antibiotics and decontamination. *Nursing Standard* **18** (40), 38–42.

153. Medical Devices Agency (2000) *Single-Use Medical Devices: Implications and Consequences of Re-Use.* Device Bulletin 2000 (04). Medical Devices Agency, London.

154. MHRA (2006) *Single-Use Medical Devices: Implications and Consequences of Re-Use.* Device Bulletin 2006 (04). MRHA, London.

155. Hospital Infection Society/Infection Control Nurses Association (2006) Third National Prevalence Survey of Healthcare Associated Infections in England. www.his.org.uk (accessed 30th May 2007).

156. Ryan K.J. (2004) Urinary Tract Infections. In: Sherris J.C., Ryan K.J., Ray G.C. (eds) *Medical Microbiology: An Introduction to Infectious Diseases.* Fourth Edition. McGraw-Hill, London, 867–879.

157. Crow R., Mulhall A., Chapman R. (1998) Indwelling catheterisation and related nursing practice. *Journal of Advanced Nursing* **13** (4), 489–495.

158. Saint S., Veenstra D.L., Sullivan S.D., Chenoweth C., Fendrick M. (2000) The potential clinical and economic benefits of silver alloy urinary catheters in preventing urinary tract infection. *Archives Internal Medicine* **160** (9 Sept), 2670–2675.

159. Stamm W.E. (1998) Urinary Tract Infections. In: Bennett J.V., Brachman P.S. (eds) *Hospital Infection.* 4th Edition. Lippincott-Raven, Philadelphia, 477–485.

160. Saint S., Lipsky B. (1999) Preventing Catheter-Related Bacteriuria: Should We? Can We? How? *Archives Internal Medicine* **159** (April), 800–808.

161. Public Health Laboratory Service (1999) *Surveillance of Hospital-Acquired Bacteraemias in English Hospitals 1997–1999.* PHLS, London.

162. Wilson J. (*1995*) Preventing Infection Associated with Urethral Catheters. In: *Infection Control in Clinical Practice.* Bailliere Tindall, London, 215–230.

163. Godfrey H., Evans A. (2000) Management of long-term urethral catheters: minimising complications. *British Journal of Nursing* **9** (2), 74–81.

164. Robinson J. (2001) Urethral catheter selection. *Nursing Standard* **7** (15), 39–42.

165. Neidhardt F.C (2004) Bacterial Processes. In: Sherris J.C., Ryan K.J., Ray G.C. (eds) *Sherris Medical Microbiology: An Introduction to Infectious Diseases.* Fourth Edition. McGraw-Hill, London, 27–51.

166. Simpson L. (2001) In-dwelling urethral catheters. *Nursing Standard* **15** (46), 47–53.

167. Strohl W.A, Rouse H., Fisher D. (2001) Enteric Gram-Negative Rods. In: Harvey R.A. and Champe P.A (eds) *Lippincott's Illustrated Reviews: Medical Microbiology.* Lippincott, Williams and Wilkins, London, 75–190.

168. Sobel J.D., Kaye D. (2004) Urinary Tract Infections. In: Mandell G.L., Bennett J.E., Dolin R.D. (eds) *Mandell's Principles and Practices of Infectious Diseases.* Sixth Edition. Churchill Livingstone, London. PPID Online. www.www.ppidonline.com (accessed 30th May 2007).

169. www.healthcarea2z.org (accessed 30th May 2007).

170. Tambyah P.A., Maki D.G. (2000) The relationship between pyuria and infection in patients with indwelling urinary catheters: a prospective study of 761 patients. *Archives Internal Medicine* **160** (5), 673–677.

171. Morgan M.G., McKenzie H. (1993) Controversies in the laboratory diagnosis of community-acquired urinary tract infection. *European Journal Clinical Microbiology Infectious Disease* **12** (7), 491–504.

172. Health Protection Agency (2005) National Standard Method. *Investigation of Urine.* Available at: www.hpastandardmethods.org.uk/documents/bsop/pdf/bsop41.pdf (accessed 30th May, 2007).

173. Scottish Intercollegiate Guidelines Network (2006) *Management of suspected bacterial urinary tract infection in adults: A national clinical guideline.* SIGN Publication 88. Available at: www.sign.ac.uk/pdf/sign88.pdf. (accessed 30th May, 2007).

174. Makai D., Tambyah P.A. (2001) Engineering out the risk for infection with urinary catheters. *Emerging Infectious Diseases* **7** (2), 342–347.

175. Woodhead S. (2005) Use of lubricant in female urethral catheterisation. *British Journal of Nursing* **14** (9), 1022–1023.

176. Sagripanti J.L. (1992) Metal based formulations with high microbial activity. *Applied Environmental Microbiology* **58** (9), 3157–3162.

177. Lansdown A.B.G. (2002) Silver 1: its antimicrobial properties and mechanisms of action. *Journal of Wound Care* **11** (4), 125–131.

178. Bologna R., Tu L.M., Polansky M., Fraimow H., Gordon D., Whitmore K. (1999) Hydrogel/silver-ion coated urinary catheter reduces nosocomial urinary tract infection rates in intensive care unit patients: a multi-centre study. *Urology* **54** (6), 982–987.

179. Lai K.K., Fontecchio S. (2002) Use of silver-hydrogel urinary catheters on the incidence of catheter-associated urinary tract infections in hospitalised patients. *American Journal Infection Control* **30** (4), 221–225.

180. Gentry H., Cope S. (2005) Using Silver to reduce catheter-associated urinary tract infections. *Nursing Standard* **19** (50), 51–54.

181. Saint S., Elmore J.G., Sullivan S.D., Emmerson S.S., Koepsell T.D. (1998) The efficacy of silver alloy urinary catheters in preventing urinary tract infection: a meta analysis – are we being misled? *American Journal Medicine* **105** (3), 235–241.

182. Davenport K., Keeley F.X. (2005) Evidence for the use of silver-alloy-coated urethral catheters. *Journal of Hospital Infection* **60** (4), 298–303.

183. www.hpa.org.uk/infections/topics_92/rapid_review/pdf/bardex2.pdf (accessed 30th May 2007).

184. Ahearn D.G., Grace D.T., Jennings M.J., Borazjani R.N., Boles K., Rose L.J., Simmons R.B., Ahanotu E. (2000) Effects of hydrogel/silver coatings on in vitro adhesion to catheters of bacteria associated with urinary tract infections. *Current Microbiology* **41** (2), 120–125.

185. Scanlon E. (2005) Wound infection and colonisation. *Nursing Standard* **19** (24), 57–67.

186. Cooper R., Lawrence J. (1996) The prevalence of bacteria and implications for infection control. *Journal of Wound Care* **5** (6), 291–295.

187. American Society of Anaesthiologists (1963) New classification of physical status. *Anaesthesiology* **21**, 111.

188. Garner J. (1984) Guideline for Prevention of Surgical Wound Infections www.cdc.gov/ncidod/hip/Guide/surwound.htm (accessed 30th May 2007).

189. Culver D.H., Horan T.C., Gaynes R.P., Eykyn S.J., Littler W.A., McGowan D.A. (1991) Surgical wound infection rates by wound class, operative procedure and patient risk index. National Nosocomial Surveillance Scheme. *American Journal Medicine* **91** (3), 152–157.

190. Ryan K.J. (2004) Skin and Wound Infections. In: Sherris J., Ryan K.J., Ray G.C. (eds) *Medical Microbiology: An Introduction to Infectious Diseases.* Fourth Edition. McGraw-Hill, London, 867–871.

191. Howarth F.H. (1985) Prevention of airborne infection during surgery. *The Lancet* **1** (8425), 386–388.
192. Dharan S., Pittett D. (2002) Environmental controls in operating theatres. *Journal of Hospital Infection* **51** (2), 79–84.
193. Wilson J. (1995) *Infection Control in Clinical Practice*. Bailliere Tindall, London, 181–201.
194. Cruse P.J.E., Foord R. (1980) The Epidemiology of Wound Infection: A 10-year prospective study of 62,939 surgical wounds. *Surgical Clinics of North America* **60** (1), 27–40.
195. Cruse P.J.E., Foord R. (1973) A five-year prospective study of 23,649 surgical wounds. *Archives Surgery* **107** (2), 206.
196. Tkach J.R., Shannon A.M., Beastrom R. (1979) Pseudofolliculitis due to pre-operative shaving. *AORN Journal* **30** (5), 881–884.
197. McIntyre F.J., McCloy R. (1994) Shaving patients before surgery a dangerous myth? *Annals Royal College of Surgeons of England* **76**, 3–4.
198. Fairclough J., Evans P.D., Eliot T.S.J., Newcomb. RG. (1987) Skin shaving: a cause for concern. *Journal of the Royal College of Surgeons of Edinburgh* **32** (2), 76–78.
199. Scottish Intercollegiate Guidelines Network (2000) *Antibiotic prophylaxis in Surgery*. SIGN Publication Number 45. Available at: www.sign.ac.uk/pdf/sign45.pdf (accessed 30th May 2007).
200. Gould D., Brooker C. (2000) *Applied Microbiology for Nurses*. MacMillan Press Ltd, London, 163–186.
201. Nystrom B., Larson S., Dankert J., Daschner F., Greco D., Gronroos P., Jepson O.B., Lystad A., Meers P.D., Rotter M. (1983) Bacteraemia in surgical patients with intravenous devices: a European multicentre incidence study. *Journal of Hospital Infection* **4** (4), 338–349.
202. Wilkinson R. (1996) Nurses' concerns about IV therapy and devices. *Nursing Standard* **10** (3), 35–37.
203. Turnidge J. (1984) Hazards of peripheral IV lines. *Med J Aust* **141**, 37–40.
204. Infection Control Nurses Association (2001) *Guidelines for Preventing Intravascular Catheter-related Infections*. ICNA, Bathgate.
205. Beekmann S.E., Henderson D.K. (2004) Infections Caused by Percutaneous Devices. In: Mandell G.L., Bennett J.E., Dolin R.D. (eds) *Mandell's Principles and Practices of Infectious Diseases*. Sixth Edition. Churchill Livingstone, London. PPID Online. www.ppidonline.com (accessed 30th May 2007).
206. www.nuigalway.ie/bac/student_info/Infection_With_Indwelling_Devices.html (accesed 30th May, 2007).
207. Dougherty L (1996) Intravenous Management. In: Mallett J., Bailey C. (eds) *The Royal Marsden Hospital Manual of Clinical Nursing Procedures*. Fourth Edition. Blackwell Science, London, 311–337.
208. Royal College of Nursing (2005) *Standards for Infusion Therapy*. RCN, London.
209. www.enturia.co.uk (accessed 30th May 2007).
210. Centres for Disease Control (2002) *Guideline for the Prevention of Healthcare-Associated Pneumonia*. CDC, Atlanta.
211. Chastre J., Fagon J.Y. (2002) Ventilator-associated pneumonia. *American Journal Respiratory Critical Care Medicine* **165** (7), 867–903.
212. Strausbaugh L.J., (2004) Nosocomial Respiratory Tract Infections. In: Mandell G.L., Bennett J.E., Dolin R.D. (eds) *Mandell's Principles and Practices of Infectious*

Diseases. Sixth Edition. Churchill Livingstone, London. PPID Online. www.ppidonline.com (accessed 30th May 2007).

213. American Thoracic Society Ad Hoc Committee of the Scientific Assembly on Microbiology, Tuberculosis and Pulmonary Infections (1995) Hospital-acquired pneumonia in adults; diagnosis, assessment of severity, initial antimicrobial therapy and preventative strategies. *American Journal Respiratory Critical Care Medicine* **153**, 1711–1725.

214. British Society for Antimicrobial Chemotherapy (2005) *Hospital-Acquired Pneumonia.* Consultation Document.

215. Dunn L. (2005) Pneumonia: classification, diagnosis and nursing management. *Nursing Standard* **19** (42), 50–54.

216. Edmondson E.B., Reinarz J.A., Pierce A.K., Sanford J.P. (1996) Nebulization equipment: a potential source of infection in Gram-negative pneumonias. *American Journal of Diseases of Children* **111** (4), 357–360.

217. Hovig B. (1981) Lower respiratory tract infections associated with respiratory therapy and anaesthesia equipment. *Journal of Hospital Infection* **2** (4), 301–315.

218. Wheeler P.W., Lancaster D., Kaiser A.B. (1989) Bronchopulmonary cross-colonization and infection related to mycobacterial contamination of suction valves of bronchoscopes. *Journal Infectious Diseases* **159** (5), 954–958.

219. Gorman L.J., Sanai L., Notman A.W., Grant I.S., Masterton R.G. (1993) Cross-infection in an intensive care unit by *Klebsiella pneumoniae* from ventilator consolidate. *Journal of Hospital Infection* **23** (11), 27–33.

220. Stamm A.M. (1998) Ventilator-associated pneumonia and frequency of circuit changes. *American Journal Infection Control* **26** (1), 71–73.

221. Dodek P., Keenhan S., Cook D., Heyland D., Jaka M., Hand L., Muscedere J., Foster D., Mehta N., Hall R., Brun-Buisson C. (2004) Evidence-Based Clinical Practice Guideline for the Prevention of Ventilator-Associated Pneumonia. *Annals Internal Medicine* **141** (4), 305–313.

222. Kress J.P., Pohlman A.S., O'Connor M.F., Hall J.B. (2000) Daily interruption of sedative infusions in critically ill patients undergoing mechanical ventilation. *New England Journal Medicine* **342** (20), 1471–1477.

223. Machin J (2005) Tracheostomy care and Laryngeal Voice Rehabilitation. In: Mallett J., Bailey C. (eds) *The Royal Marsden Hospital Manual of Clinical Nursing Procedures.* Fourth Edition. Blackwell Science, London, 550–564.

224. Boyce J.M. (1990) Increasing prevalence of methicillin-resistant *Staphylococcus aureus* in the United States. *Journal Infection Control Hospital Epidemiology* **11**(12), 639–642.

225. Talon D. (1999) The role of the hospital environment in the epidemiology of multi-resistant bacteria. *Journal Hospital Infection* **43** (1), 13–17.

226. Government Response to the House of Lords Select Committee on Science and Technology Report (1998) *Resistance to Antibiotics and other Antimicrobial Agents.* The Stationary Office, London.

227. Department of Health (1999) *Resistance to antibiotics and other antimicrobial agents: action for the NHS.* HSC 1999/049. DoH, London.

228. Department of Health (2000) *UK Antimicrobial Resistance Strategy and Action Plan.* DoH, London.

229. Hayden F.G., Belshe R.B., Clover R.D., Hay A.J., Oates M.G. and Soo W. (1989) Emergence and apparent resistance of rimantadine-resistant Influenza A virus in families. *New England Journal Medicine* **321** (25), 1696–1702.

230. Leelapor A., Paulsen I.T., Tennet J.M., Littlejohn T.G., Skurray R.A. (1994) Multi-drug resistance to antiseptics and disinfectants in coagulase-negative Staphylococci. *Journal Medical Microbiology* **40** (3), 214–220.

231. Infection Control Nurses Association (2002) *Antibiotic Resistance: Theory and Practice.* ICNA, Bathgate.

232. Levy S.B. (1998) The challenge of antibiotic resistance. *Scientific American* **278** (3), 46–53.

233. Murray C.J.L., Lopez A.D. (1997) Mortality by cause for eight regions of the world; global burden of disease study. *The Lancet* **349** (9061), 1269–1276.

234. Johnson A.P (1998) Antibiotic-resistance against clinically important Gram-positive bacteria in the UK. *Journal Hospital Infection* **40** (1), 17–26.

235. www.wikipedia.org/wiki/Antibiotics (accessed 30th May 2007).

236. Greenwood D., Ogilvie M.M. (2003) Antimicrobial Agents. In: Greenwood D., Slack R.C.B., Peutherer J.F. (eds) *Medical Microbiology. A Guide to Microbial Infections: Pathogenesis, Immunity, Laboratory Diagnosis and Control.* Sixteenth Edition. Churchill Livingstone, London, 46–60.

237. Greenwood D. (1983) *Antimicrobial Chemotherapy.* Bailliere Tindall, London.

238. Vandenbroucke-Grauls C.M. (1993) The threat of multi-resistant micro-organisms. *European Journal Clinical Microbiology and Infectious Diseases* **12** (suppl 1), 27–301.

239. French G.L., Phillips I. (1997) Resistance. In: O'Grady F., Lambert H.P., Finch H.P. and Greenwood D. (eds) *Antibiotics and Chemotherapy: Anti-infective Agents and Their Use in Therapy.* Churchill Livingstone, London, 23–43.

240. Cohen F.L., Tartsky. D. (1997) Microbial resistance to drug therapy. *American Journal Infection Control* **25** (1), 51–64.

241. Gold H.S, Moellering R.C. (1996) Antimicrobial drug resistance. *New England Journal Medicine* **355** (19), 1443–1445.

242. Livermore D.M., Yuan M. (1996) Antibiotic resistance and production of extended spectrum B-lactamases among Klebsiella species from ICUs in Europe. *Journal Antimicrobial Chemotherapy* **38**, 109–124.

243. Dooley S.W., Villarino M.E., Lawrence M., Salvinas L., Amil S., Rullan J.W. (1992) Nosocomial transmission of multi-drug resistant tuberculosis in a hospital unit for HIV infected patients. *Journal American Medical Association* **267** (7), 2632–2635.

244. Jarvis W.R. (1993) Nosocomial transmission of multi-drug resistant tuberculosis. *American Journal Infection Control* **22** (2), 146–151.

245. Strohl W.A., Rouse H., Fisher BD. (2001) Vaccines and Antibiotics. In: Harvey R.A. and Champe P.A (eds) *Lippincott's Illustrated Reviews. Medical Microbiology.* Lippincott Williams and Wilkins, Philadelphia, 35–50.

246. Ryan K.J. Drew W.L. (2004) Antibacterial and Antiviral Agents. In: Sherris J.C., Ryan K.J., Ray G.C. (eds) *Medical Microbiology: An Introduction to Infectious Diseases.* Fourth Edition. McGraw-Hill, London, 193–213.

247. Gladwin M., Trattler B. (2003) *Clinical Microbiology made ridiculously simple.* Edition 3. MedMaster Inc, Miami, 16–21.

248. Neidhardt F.G. (2004) Bacterial Genetics. In: Sherris J.C., Ryan K.J., Ray G.C. (eds) *Medical Microbiology: An Introduction to Infectious Diseases* Fourth Edition. McGraw-Hill, London, 53–75.

249. Lee V.J., Lomovskaya O. (1998) Efflux mediated resistance to antibiotics in bacteria: challenges and opportunities. *Antibacterial Research* **1**, 39–42.

250. Ryan K.J. (2004) Antimicrobial Resistance. In: Sherris J.C., Ryan K.J., Ray G.C. (eds) *Medical Microbiology: An Introduction to Infectious Diseases* Fourth Edition. McGraw-Hill, London, 193–213.
251. Turnidge J., Christiansen K. (2005) Antibiotic use and resistance – proving the obvious. *The Lancet* **365** (9459), 548–549.
252. Standing Medical Advisory Committee Sub-Group on Antimicrobial Resistance (1998) *The Path of Least Resistance.* DoH, London.
253. Wise R., Hart T., Cars D., Strenulens M., Helmuth R., Huovinen P., Sprenger M. (1998) Antimicrobial Resistance. *British Medical Journal* **317** (7159), 609–610.
254. www.cdc.gov/ncidod/dhqp/ar_acinetobacter.html (accessed 30th May 2007).
255. Association of Medical Microbiologist, British Society for Antimicrobial Chemotherapy, Health Protection Agency, Hospital Infection Society, Infection Control Nurses Association and the Department of Health (2005) *Working Party Guidance on the Control of Multi-Resistant Acinetobacter Outbreaks.* Health Protection Agency, London.
256. www.hpa.org.uk/infections/topics_az/acinetobacter_b/guidance.htm (accessed 19th May 2007).
257. Lucet J.C., Chevret S., Decre D., Vanjak D., Macrez A., Bedos J.P., Wolff M., Regnier B. (1996) Outbreak of multiply-resistant *Enterobacteriaceae* in an Intensive Care Unit: Epidemiology and Risk Factors for Acquisition. *Clinical Infectious Diseases* **22** (3), 403–406.
258. Hobson R.P., Mackenzie F.M., Gould I.M. (1996) An outbreak of multiply-resistant *Klebsiella pneumoniae* in the Grampian region of Scotland. *Journal Hospital Infection* **33** (4), 249–262.
259. www.hpa.org.uk/infections/topics_az/esbl/default.htm (accessed 19th May 2007).
260. Cookson B.D., Macrae M.B., Barrett S.P., Brain D.F.J., Chadwick C., French G.L., Hateley P., Hosein I.K., Wade J.J. (2001) A Report of a Combined Working Party of the HIS/ICNA/BSAC. *Guidelines for the Control of Glycopeptide-Resistant Enterococci in Hospitals.* Hospital Infection Society, London.
261. Moellering R.C. (1992) Emergence of Enterococcus as a significant pathogen. *Clinical Infectious Diseases* **14** (6), 1173–1178.
262. Sigurdardohir B., Vande-Berg J., Hu J., Alamu J., McNutt L.A., Diekeme D.J., Herwaldt L.A. (2006) Descriptive epidemiology and case-control study of patients colonised with vancomycin-resistant Enterococcus and methicillin-resistant Staphylococcus aureus. *Infection Control Hospital Epidemiology* **27** (9), 913–919.
263. Hiramatsu K., Hanaki H., Ino T., Yabuta K., Oguri T., Tenover F.C. (1997) Methicillin-resistant Staphylococcus aureus clinical strain with reduced vancomycin susceptibility. *Journal Antimicrobial Chemotherapy* **40** (1), 135–136.
264. Boyce J.M., Opal S.M., Chow J.W., Zervos M.J., Potter-Bynoe G., Sherman C.B. (1994) Outbreak of multi-drug resistant Enterococcus faecium with transferable vanB class vancomycin-resistant enterococci. *Journal Clinical Microbiology* **32**, 1148–1153.
265. Baden L.R., Thiemke W., Skolnik A., Chambers R., Strymish J., Gold H.S. (2001) Prolonged colonisation with vancomycin-resistant Enterococcus faecium in long-term patients and the significance of 'clearance'. *Clinical Infectious Diseases* **33**, 1654–1660.
266. Sandoe J.A.T., Hall J.M., Collyns T.M., Witherden I.R., Parnell P., Woodrow G. (2002) An outbreak of vancomycin-resistant enterococci associated with major ward refurbishment. *Journal Hospital Infection* **50** (1), 79–80.

267. Patel R. (2003) Clinical impact of vancomycin-resistant enterococci. *Journal Antimicrobial Chemotherapy* **51** (suppl S3) iii13–iii121.

268. Bates J. (1997) Epidemiology of vancomycin-resistant enterococci in the community and the relevance of farm animals to human infection. *Journal Hospital Infection* **37** (2), 89–101.

269. Witte W. (2000) Selective pressure by antibiotic use in livestock. *International Journal Antimicrobial Agents* **16** (suppl), 19–24.

270. Duckworth G.J. (1993) Diagnosis and management of methicillin-resistant Staphylococcus aureus infection. *British Medical Journal* **307** (6911), 1049–1053.

271. Michel M., Gutmann L. (1997) Methicillin-resistant Staphylococcus aureus and vancomycin-resistant enterococci: therapeutic realities and possibilities. *The Lancet* **349** (9069), 1901–1906.

272. Report of a Combined Working Party of the Hospital Infection Society and the British Society for Antimicrobial Chemotherapy (1986) Guidelines for the Control of methicillin-resistant Staphylococcus aureus. *Journal Hospital Infection* **7** (2), 193–201.

273. Working Party Report (1990) Guidelines for the control of epidemic methicillin-resistant Staphylococcus aureus. *Journal Hospital Infection* **16** (4), 351–377.

274. Duckworth G., Cookson G., Humphreys H., Heathcock R. (1998) Revised methicillin-resistant Staphylococcus aureus infection control guidelines for hospitals. Report of a Working Party for the British Society of Antimicrobial Chemotherapy, the Hospital Infection Society and the Infection Control Nurses Association. *Journal Hospital Infection* **39** (4), 253–290.

275. Coia J.E., Duckworth G.J., Edwards D.I., Farrington M., Fry C., Humphreys H., Mallaghan C., Tucker D.R. for the Joint Working Party of the British Society of Antimicrobial Chemotherapy, the Hospital Infection Society and the Infection Control Nurses Association (2006) Guidelines for the control and prevention of meticillin-resistant Staphylococcus aureus (MRSA) in healthcare facilities *Journal Hospital Infection* **63S**, S1–S44. Available at: www.his.org.uk/_db/_documents/MRSA_Guidelines_PDF.pdf (accessed 30th May 2007).

276. Teare E.L., Barrett S.P. (1997) Stop the ritual of tracing colonised patients. *British Medical Journal* **314**, 665–666.

277. Barrett S.P., Mummery R.V., Chattopadhyay B. (1998) Trying to control MRSA causes more problems than it solves. *Journal Hospital Infection* **39** (2), 85–93.

278. Strohl W.A., Rose H., Fisher B.D. (2001) Staphylococci. In: Harvey R.A. and Champe P.A. (eds) *Lippincott's Illustrated Reviews. Medical Microbiology*. Lippincott Williams and Wilkins, Philadelphia, 137–144.

279. Moreillon P., Que Y.A., Glausere M.P. (2004) Staphylococcus aureus (including Staphylococcal Toxic Shock) In: Mandell G.L., Bennett J.E., Dolin R.D. (eds) *Mandell's Principles and Practices of Infectious Diseases*. Sixth Edition. Churchill Livingstone, London. PPID Online. www.ppidonline (accessed 30th May 2007).

280. Humphreys H. (2003) Staphylococcus. In: Greenwood D., Slack R.C.B., Peutherer J.F. (eds) *Medical Microbiology. A Guide to Microbial Infections: Pathogenesis, Immunity, Laboratory Diagnosis and Control*. Sixteenth Edition. Churchill Livingstone, London, 168–173.

281. www.toxicshock.com (accessed 30th May 2007).

282. Newsom S.W.B.(2004) MRSA and its predecessor – a historical overview. Part three: the rise of MRSA and EMRSA. *British Journal Infection Control* **5** (2), 25–28.

283. Aucken H.M., Ganner M., Murchan S., Cookson B.D., Johnson A.P. (2002) A new UK strain of epidemic methicillin-resistant Staphylococcus aureus (EMRSA-17) resistant to multiple antibiotics. *Journal Antimicrobial Chemotherapy* **50** (2), 171–175.

284. Gonzalez B.E., Rueda A.M., Shelburne S.A., Musher D.M., Hamill R.J., Hulten K.G. (2006) Community-acquired strains of methicillin-resistant Staphylococcus aureus as the cause of healthcare-associated infection. *Infection Control Hospital Epidemiology* **27** (10), 1051–1056.

285. Health Protection Agency (2006) Interim guidance on diagnosis and management of PVL-associated Staphylococcal infections in the UK. *CDR Weekly* 27 April, **16** (17).

286. Boubaker K., Diebold P., Blane D.S., Vandenesch F., Praz G., Dupois G., Troillet N. (2004) Panton-Valentine Leukocidin and Staphylococcal skin infections in schoolchildren. Available at: www.cdc.gov/ncidod/EID/vol10no1/03-0144.htm (accessed 30th May 2007).

287. Morgan M. (2005) Editorial. Staphylococcus aureus, Panton-Valentine Leukocidin and necrotising pneumonia. *British Medical Journal* **331** (7520), 793–794.

288. Holmes A., Ganner M., McGuane S., Pitt T.L., Cookson B.D., Kearns A.M. (2005) Staphylococcus aureus isolates carrying Panton-Valentine Leukocidin genes in England and Wales; frequency, characterisation and association with clinical disease. *Journal Clinical Microbiology* **43** (5), 2384–2390.

289. Dennis O., Malaviolle X., Titeca G., Struelens M.J., Garrino M.G., Glupczynski Y., Etienne J. (2004) Emergence of Panton-Valentine Leukocidin positive community-acquired MRSA infections in Belgium. Available at: www.eurosurveillance.org/ew/2004/040610.asp (accessed 19th May 2007).

290. Gould I.M. (2005) The clinical significance of methicillin-resistant Staphylococcus aureus. *Journal Hospital Infection* **61** (4), 7–282.

291. www.hpa.org.uk/infections/topics_az/hai/mrsa_annual_England.xls (accessed 30th May 2007).

292. Grundmann H., Aires-de-Sousa M., Boyce J., Tiemersma E. (2006) Emergence and resurgence of meticillin-resistant Staphylococcus aureus as a public health threat. *The Lancet* **368**, 874–885.

293. Wagenvoort J.H.T. (2000) Dutch measures to control MRSA and the expanding European Union. *Euro Surveillance* **5** (3), 26–28.

294. Department of Health (2006) *Screening for meticillin-resistant Staphylococcus aureus (MRSA) colonisation: a strategy for NHS trusts – a summary of best practice.* DoH, London.

295. Rao G.G., Michalczy K.P., Nayeem N., Walker G., Wigmore L. (2007) Prevention and risk factors for meticillin-resistant Staphylococcus aureus in adult emergency admissions – a case for screening all patients? *Journal Hospital Infection* **66** (1), 15–21.

296. Centres for Disease Control (1997) Staphylococcus aureus with reduced susceptibility to vancomycin. *Morbidity and Mortality Weekly Report* **46**, 765–766.

297. Johnson A.P., Woodford N. (2002) Glycopeptide-resistant Staphylococcus aureus. *Journal Antimicrobial Chemotherapy* **50** (5), 621–623.

298. www.rcn.org.uk/resources/mrsa (accessed 30th May 2007).

299. www.dh.gov.uk/reducingmrsa (accessed 30th May 2007).

300. www.tblaert.org/worldwide/worldwide.php (accessed 30th May 2007).

301. www.who.int/tb/en/index.html (accessed 30th May 2007).

302. Zink A.R., Sola C., Reischi U., Grabner W., Rastogi N., Wolf H., Nerlich A.G (2003) Characterisation of M.tuberculosis complex DNAs from Egyptian mummies by spoli-ogotyping. *Journal Clinical Microbiology* **41** (1), 359–367.

303. www.hpa.org.uk/infections/topics_az/tb/pdf/newsletter_2007_march.pdf (accessed 30th May 2007).

304. Department of Health (2004) *Stopping Tuberculosis in England: An Action Plan from the Chief Medical officer.* DoH, London.

305. World Health Organization (2003) *International Union against Tuberculosis and Lung Disease Global Project on Anti-Tuberculosis Drug Resistance Surveillance.* Report number 3.

306. National Collaborating Centre for Chronic Conditions (2006) *Tuberculosis: clinical diagnosis and management for its prevention and control.* Royal College of Physicians, London.

307. Grange J.M. (2003) Mycobacterium. In: Greenwood D., Slack R.C.B, Peutherer J.F. (eds) *Medical Microbiology. A Guide to Microbial Infections: Pathogenesis, Immunity, Laboratory Diagnosis and Control.* Sixteenth Edition. Churchill Livingstone, London, 200 214.

308. Fitzgerald D., Haas D.W. (2004) *Mycobacterium tuberculosis.* In: Mandell G.L., Bennett J.E., Dolin R.D. (eds) *Mandell's Principles and Practices of Infectious Diseases..* Sixth Edition. Churchill Livingstone, London. PPID Online. www.ppidonline.com (accessed 30th May 2007).

309. Plorde J.J. (2004) Mycobacterium. In: Sherris J.C., Ryan K.J., Ray G.C (eds) *Medical Microbiology: An Introduction to Infectious Diseases.* Fourth Edition. McGraw-Hill, London, 439–456.

310. Strohl W.A., Rouse H., Fisher B.D. (2001) Mycobacteria and Actinomycetes. In: Harvey R.A. and Champe P.A. (eds) *Lippincott's Illustrated Reviews. Medical Microbiology.* Lippincott Williams and Wilkins, Philadelphia, 245–258.

311. British Thoracic Society (2000) Management of opportunistic mycobacterial infection; Joint Tuberculosis Committee Guidelines. *Thorax* **55** (3), 210–218.

312. Gladwin M., Trattler B. (2003) Mycobacterium. In: *Clinical Microbiology made ridiculously simple.* Edition 3. MedMaster Inc, Miami, 102–110.

313. Pratt R.J., Grange J.M., Williams V.G. (2005) *Tuberculosis: A foundation for nursing and healthcare practice.* Hodder Arnold, London, 61–79.

314. Pratt R.J., Grange J.M., Williams V.G. (2005) *Tuberculosis: A foundation for nursing and healthcare practice.* Hodder Arnold, London, 95–108.

315. Granger C. (2005) T-spot: A new test for Tuberculosis infection. *Practice Nursing* **16** (3), 133–136.

316. White V.L.C., Moore-Gillan J. (2000) Resource implications of patients with multi-drug resistant tuberculosis. *Thorax* **55** (11), 962–963.

317. www.searo.who.int/en/Section10/Section2097/Section2106_10680.htm (accessed 30th May 2007).

318. www.who.int/tb/dots/dotsplus/faq/en (accessed 30th May 2007).

319. www.who.int/tb/publications/2006/tb_facts_2006.pdf (accessed 30th May 2007).

320. www.who.int/features/2004/tb_ukraine/en/ (accessed 19th May 2007).

321. www.who.int/tb/xdr/faqs/en/index.html (accessed 30th May 2007).

322. www.cdc.gov/tb/xdrtb/default.htm (accessed 30th May 2007).

323. www.who.int/mediacentre/news/notes/2006/np23/en/index.htm (accessed 30th May 2007).

324. Department of Health (1998) *The Prevention and Control of Tuberculosis in the United Kingdom; UK Guidance on the Prevention and Control of Transmission of HIV-related Tuberculosis and Drug-Resistant, including Multiple-Drug Resistant, Tuberculosis.* The Interdepartmental Working Group on Tuberculosis. DoH, London.

325. Pratt R.J., Curran E.T. (2006) Personal respiratory protection and tuberculosis: national evidence-based guidelines in England and Wales. *British Journal Infection Control* **7** (3) June: 15–17.

326. Humphreys H. (2007) Control and prevention of healthcare-associated tuberculosis; the role of respiratory isolation and personal respiratory protection. *Journal Hospital Infection* **66** (1), 1–5.

327. www.who.int/tb/hiv/faq/en/index/html (accessed 30th May 2007).

328. Daley C.L., Small P.M., Schecter G.F. (1992) An outbreak of tuberculosis with accelerated progression among persons infected with human immunodeficiency virus: An analysis using restriction-fragment-length polymorphisms. *New England Journal Medicine* **326** (4), 231–235.

329. Breathnach A.S., de Ruiter A., Holdsworth G.M., Bateman N.T., O'Sullivan D.G., Rees P.J., Snashall D., Milburn H.J., Peters B.S. (1998) An outbreak of multi-drug resistant tuberculosis in a London teaching hospital. *Journal Hospital Infection* **39** (2), 111–117.

330. www.bbc.co.uk/1/hi/health/564540.stm (accessed 30th May 2007).

331. Pratt R.J., Grange J.M., Williams V.G. (2005) *Tuberculosis: A foundation for nursing and healthcare practice.* Hodder Arnold, London. 149–167.

332. www.who.int/vaccine_research/diseases/tb/vaccine_development/bcg/en (accessed 30th May 2007).

333. www.dh.gov/uk/assetRoot/04/11/49/96/04114996.pdf (accessed 30th May 2007).

334. Meredith S., Watson J.M., Citron K.M., Cockcroft A., Darbyshire J.H. (1996) Are healthcare workers in England and Wales at increased risk of tuberculosis? *British Medical Journal* **313** (7056), 522–525.

335. Department of Health (2007) *Health clearance for tuberculosis, hepatitis B and HIV: New healthcare workers.* DoH, London.

336. www.dh.gov.uk/en/Policyandguidance/Healthandsocialcaretopics/Tuberculosis/index.htm (accessed 30th May 2007).

337. www.stoptb.org/globalplan (accessed 30th May 2007).

338. www.hpa.org.uk/infections/topics_az/tb/menu.htm (accessed 30th May 2007).

339. Hall C., O'Toole E. (1935) Intestinal flora in newborn infants with a description of a new pathogenic anaerobe, Bacillus difficilis. *American Journal Diseases Children* **49**, 390–402.

340. Larson H.E., Parry J.B., Price A.B. (1977) Undescribed toxin in pseudomembranous colitis. *British Medical Journal* **1** (60710), 1246–1248.

341. Wilcox M.H., Cunnliffe J.G., Trundle C., Redpath C. (1996) Financial burden of hospital-acquired Clostridium difficile infection. *Journal Hospital Infection* **34** (1), 23–30.

342. Strohl W.A., Rouse D., Fisher B.D. (2001) Clostridia and other Anaerobic Rods. In: Harvey R.A. and Champe P.A. (eds) *Lippincott's Illustrated Reviews. Medical Microbiology.* Lippincott Williams and Wilkins, Philadelphia, 209–220.

343. Thielman N.M., Wilson K.H. (2004) Antibiotic-associated colitis. In: Mandell G.L., Bennett J.E., Dolin R.D. (eds) *Mandell's Principles and Practices of Infectious Diseases.* Sixth Edition. Churchill Livingstone, London. PPID Online. www.ppidonline.com (accessed 30th May 2007).

344. National Clostridium difficile Standards Group (2003) *Report to the Department of Health.* National Clostridium difficile Standards Group, London.

345. Poutanen S.M., Simor A.E. (2004) Clostridium difficile associated diarrhoea in adults. *Canadian Medical Association Journal* **171** (1), 51–58.

346. Johnson S., Clabots C.R., Linn F.V., Olson M.M., Peterson L.R., Gerding D.N (1990) Nosocomial Clostridium difficile colonisation and disease. *The Lancet* **336** (8707), 97–100.

347. Walker K.J., Gilliland S.S., Vance-Bryan K. (1993) Clostridium difficile colonisation in residents of long-term care facilities: prevention and risk factors. *Journal American Geriatrics Society* **41**, 940–946

348. McFarland L.V (2002) What's lurking under the bed? Persistence and predominance of particular C.difficile strains in a hospital and the potential role of environmental contamination. *Journal Infection Control Hospital Epidemiology* **23** (11), 639–640.

349. Tabaqchali S., Jumaa P. (1995) Fortnightly review: diagnosis and management of Clostridium difficile infection. *British Medical Journal* **310**, 1375–1380.

350. Johnson S., Gerding D.N., Olsen M.M., Weller M.D., Hughes R.A., Clabots C.R. (1990) Prospective controlled study of vinyl glove use to interrupt Clostridium difficile nosocomial transmission. *American Journal Medicine* **88** (2), 137–140.

351. Shim J.K., Johnson M.D., Samore M.D., Bliss D.Z., Gerding D.N. (1998) Primary symptomless colonisation by Clostridium difficile and decreased risk of diarrhoea. *The Lancet* **351** (9103), 633–636.

352. Kyne L., Warny M., Qamar A., Kelly C.P. (2001) Association between antibody response to toxin A and protection against recurring Clostridium difficile diarrhoea. *The Lancet* **357** (9251), 189–193.

353. Wilcox M., Minton J. (2001) Role of antibody response in outcome of antibiotic-associated diarrhoea. *The Lancet* **357** (9251), 158–159.

354. Kyne L., Sougioultzis S., McFarland L.V., Kelly C.P. (2000) Underlying disease-severity as a major risk factor for nosocomial Clostridium difficile diarrhoea. *Infection Control Hospital Epidemiology* **23**, 653–659.

355. Simor A.E., Bradley S.F., Strausbaugh L.J., Crossley K., Nicolle L.E (2002) Clostridium difficile in long-term care facilities for the elderly. *Infection Control Hospital Epidemiology* **23** (11), 697–703.

356. Impallomeni M., Galletly W.P., Wort S.J., Starr J.M., Rogers T.R. (1995) Increased risk of diarrhoea caused by Clostridium difficile in elderly patients receiving cefotaxime. *British Medical Journal* **311** (7016), 1345–1346.

357. Clabots C.R, Johnson S., Olson M.M., Peterson L.R., Gerding D.N (1992) Acquisition of Clostridium difficile by hospitalised patients: evidence for colonised new admissions as a source of infection. *Journal Infectious Disease* **166** (3), 561–567.

358. Brazier J.S. (1998) The diagnosis of Clostridium difficile associated disease. *Journal Antimicrobial Chemotherapy* **41**, Suppl 3, S29–S40.

359. Dial S., Alrasadi K., Manoukian C., Huang A., Menzies D. (2004) Risk of Clostridium difficile diarrhoea among hospital patients prescribed proton pump inhibitors: cohort and case control studies. *Canadian Medical Association Journal* **171** (1), 33–38.

360. Bartlett J.G. (1992) Antibiotic-associated diarrhoea. *Clinical Infectious Diseases* **15** (4), 573–581.

361. Sunenshine R.H., McDonald L.C. (2006) Clostridium difficile associated disease. New challenges from an established pathogen. *Cleveland Clinic Journal of Medicine* **73** (2), 187–197.

362. Kelly C., Pothoulakis C., Lamont J.T. (1994) Clostridium difficile colitis. *New England Journal Medicine* **330** (4), 257–262.
363. Olsen M.M., Shanholtzer C.J., Lee J.T. Jnr., Gerding D.N. (1994) Ten years of prospective Clostridium difficile surveillance and treatment at the Minneapolis VA Medical Centre, 1982–1992. *Infection Control Hospital Epidemiology* **15**, 371–381.
364. Teasley D.G., Gerding D.N., Olson M.M., Peterson L.R., Gebhardt R.L., Schwartz M.J.(1983) Prospective randomised trial of metronidazole versus vancomycin for Clostridium difficile associated diarrhoea and colitis. *The Lancet.* **2** (8358), 1043–1046.
365. Department of Health/Public Health Laboratory Service (1994) *Clostridium Difficile Prevention and Management: A Report by the DoH/PHLS Joint Working Group.* DoH, London.
366. Barbut F., Richard A., Hamadi K., Chomette V., Beurghoffer B., Petit J.C. (2000) Epidemiology of recurrences or re-infections of Clostridium difficile-associated diarrhoea. *Journal Clinical Microbiology* **38**, 2386–2388.
367. Wilcox M.H., Fawley W.N., Settle C.D., Davidson A. (1998) Recurrence of symptoms in Clostridium difficile infection – relapse or re-infection? *Journal Hospital Infection* **38** (2), 93–100.
368. Viscidi R., Laughon BE., Yolken R. (1983) Serum antibody response to toxin A and B of Clostridium difficile. *Journal Infectious Diseases* 148, 93–100.
369. Fekety R., McFarland L.V., Surawicz C.M. (1997) Characteristics of and risk factors for patients enrolled in a prospective randomised double blinded trial. *Clinical Infectious Diseases* **24**, 324–333.
370. Tedesco F.J., Gordon D., Fortson W.C. (1985) Approach to patients with multiple relapses of antibiotic-associated pseudomembranous colitis. *American Journal Gastroenterology* **80**, 867–868.
371. Buggy B.P., Fekety R., Silva J. Jnr. (1987) Therapy of relapsing Clostridium difficile-associated diarrhoea and colitis with the combination of vancomycin and rifampicin. *Journal Clinical Gastroenterology* **9**, 155–159.
372. Leung D.Y., Kelly C.P., Boguniewicz M (1991) Treatment with IV administered gamma-globulin of chronic relapsing colitis induced by Clostridium difficile toxin. *Journal Paediatrics* **118**, 633–637.
373. Salcedo J., Keates S., Pothoulakis C. (2000) IV immunoglobulin therapy for severe Clostridium difficile colitis. *Gut* **41**, 366–370.
374. Kyne L., Warny M., Qamar A. (2000) Asymptomatic carriage of Clostridium difficile and serum levels of IgG antibody against toxin A. *New England Journal Medicine* **342**, 390–397.
375. Surawicz C.M., McFarland L.V., Greenberg R.N., Rubin M., Fekety R., Mulligan M.E. (2000) The search for a better treatment for recurring Clostridium difficile disease; use of high dose vancomycin combined with Saccharomyces boulardii. *Clinical Infectious Diseases* **31**, 1012–1017.
376. D'Souza A.L., Rajkumar C., Cooke J., Bulpitt C.J. (2002) Probiotics in prevention of antibiotic-associated diarrhoea: meta-analysis. *British Medical Journal* **32**, 1361.
377. Lewis S.J., Potts L.F., Barry R.E. (1998) The lack of therapeutic effect of Saccharomyces boulardii in the prevention of antibiotic-related diarrhoea in elderly patients. *Journal of Infection* **36**, 171–174.
378. Starr J. (2005) Clostridium difficile associated diarrhoea: diagnosis and treatment. *British Medical Journal* **331** (7515), 498–501.

379. Loo V.G., Poirier L., Miller M.A., Oughten M., Linman M.D., Michaud S., Bourgault A.M., Nguyen T., Frenette C., Kelly M., Viblen A., Brassard P., Fenn S., Dewar K., Hudson T.J, Horn R., Rene P., Monczak Y., Dascal A. (2003) A predominantly clonal multi-institutional outbreak of Clostridium difficile-associated diarrhoea with high morbidity and mortality. *New England Journal Medicine* **353**, 2442–2449.

380. Brazier J. (2006) Clostridium difficile-associated disease: a case of greater virulence and new risk factors. *Health Protection Matters. The Magazine of the Health Protection Agency* 5 (summer), 20–22.

381. Brierly R. (2005) Clostridium difficile. A new threat to public health? *The Lancet* **5**, 535.

382. Warney M., Pepin J., Fang A. (2005) Toxin produced by an emerging strain of Clostridium difficile associated with outbreaks of severe disease in North America and Europe. *The Lancet* **366**, 1079–1084.

383. Bartlett J.G., Perl T.M. (2005) The new Clostridium difficile. What does it mean? *New England Journal Medicine* **353** (23), 2503–2505.

384. Worsley M.A. (1998) Infection control and prevention of Clostridium difficile infection. *Journal Antimicrobial Chemotherapy* **4**, Suppl C, S59–S66.

385. Cohen S.H., Tang Y.J., Rahman D., Silva J. (2000) Persistence of an endemic (toxigenic) isolate of Clostridium difficile in the environment of a general medical ward. *Clinical Infectious Diseases* **30**, 952–954.

386. Lai K.K., Melvin S., Menard M.J., Kotilainen H.R., Baker S. (1997) Clostridium difficile associated diarrhoea: epidemiology, risk factors and infection control. *New England Journal Medicine* **341**, 1645–1651.

387. Rogers T.R., Petrou M., Lucas C., Chung J.T.N., Barrett AJ., Borreillo S.P. (1981) Spread of Clostridium difficile among patients receiving non-absorbable antibiotics for gut decontamination. *British Medical Journal* **283**, 408–409.

388. Chang V.T., Nelson. K (2000) The role of physical proximity in nosocomial diarrhoea. *Clinical Infectious Diseases* **31**, 717–722.

389. Fawley W.N., Wilcox M. (2001) Molecular typing of endemic Clostridium difficile infection. *Epidemiology and Infection* **126**, 343–350.

390. Wilcox M.H., Fawley W.N., Wigglesworth N., Parnell P., Verity P., Freeman J. (2003) Comparison of the efficacy of detergent versus hypochlorite cleaning on environmental contamination and incidence of Clostridium difficile infection. *Journal Hospital Infection* **54**, 109–114.

391. Lueckerath D., Jones M., Krettek J., Little R., Woodward. J (2005) Reduction of Clostridium difficile infection in a community-based hospital using hypochlorite solution. *American Journal Infection Control* **33** (5), 43–44.

392. Health Protection agency and the Healthcare Commission (2005) *Management, prevention and surveillance of Clostridium difficile: Interim findings from a national survey of NHS Acute Trusts in England.* Health Protection Agency, London.

393. Health Protection Agency (2006) *Clostridium difficile. Findings and recommendations from a review of the epidemiology and a survey of Directors Infection Prevention and Control in England.* Health Protection Agency, London.

394. www.dh.gov.uk/en/Policyandguidance/Healthandsocialcaretopics/Healthcareacquired-generalinformation/DH_4115800 (accessed 30th May 2007).

395. www.hpa.org.uk/infections/topics_az/clostridium_difficile/default.htm (accessed 30th May 2007).

396. www.cdiff-support.co.uk (accessed 30th May 2007).

397. Health Protection Agency Group A Streptococcal Working Group (2004) Interim UK guidelines on management of invasive group A streptococcal disease. *Communicable Disease Public Health* **7** (4), 354–361.
398. Strohl W.A., Rouse D., Fisher B.D (2001) Streptococci. In: Harvey R.A. and Champe P.A. (eds) *Lippincott's Illustrated Reviews. Medical Microbiology.* Lippincott Williams and Wilkins, Philadelphia, 145–156.
399. Ryan K.J (2004) Streptococci and enterococci. In: Sherris J.C., Ryan K.J., Ray G.C. (eds) *Medical Microbiology: An Introduction to Infectious Diseases* Fourth Edition. McGraw-Hill, London, 273–296.
400. Killan J. (2004) Streptococci and enterococci. In: Greenwood D., Slack R.C.B., Peutherer J.F. (eds) *Medical Microbiology. A Guide to Microbial Infections: Pathogenesis, Immunity, Laboratory Diagnosis and Control.* Sixteenth Edition. Churchill Livingstone, London, 174–188.
401. Bisno A.L., Ruoff K.L., (2004) Classification of streptococci. In: Mandell G.L., Bennett J.E., Dolin R.D. (eds) *Mandell's Principles and Practices of Infectious Diseases.* Sixth Edition. Churchill Livingstone, London. PPID Online. www.ppidonline.com (accessed 30th May 2007).
402. Wainwright M. (2005) Childbed fever. *Microbiologist* Sept, 26–29. Available at: www.sfam.org.uk/pdf/features/childbed.pdf (accessed 30th May 2007).
403. Schwartz B., Ussery X.T. (1992) Group A streptococcal outbreaks in nursing homes. *Infection Control Hospital Epidemiology* **13**, 742–747.
404. Harkness G.A., Bentley D.W., Mottley M,. Lee. J (1992) Streptococcus pyogenes outbreak in a long-term care facility. *American Journal Infection Control* **20** (3), 142–148.
405. Dipersio J.R., File T.M., Stevens D.L (1996) Spread of serious disease-producing M3 clones of group A streptococcus among family members and healthcare workers. *Clinical Infectious Diseases* **22** (3), 490–495.
406. Lamagni T.L., Efstratiou A., Vuopio-Varkila J., Jasir A., Schalen C. (2005) The epidemiology of severe Streptococcus pyogenes associated disease in Europe. *Eurosurv* **10** (9), 179–184. Available at: www.eurosurveillance.org/en/v10n09/1009-225.asp (accessed 30th May 2007).
407. Thomson H., Cartwright K. (1995) Streptococcal necrotising fasciitis in Gloucestershire, 1994. *British Journal Surgery* **82** (11), 1444–1445.
408. Neal M.S. (1999) Necrotising fasciitis. *Journal Wound Care* **8** (1), 18–19.
409. Roemmele J., Batdorff D. (2000) *Surviving the flesh-eating bacteria.* Avery, New York.
410. Hasham S., Matteucci P., Stanley P., Hart N. (2005) Necrotising fasciitis. *British Medical Journal* **330**, 830–833.
411. Meleney F.L. (1924) Hemolytic streptococcus gangrene. *Archives of Surgery* 9, 317.
412. Louden I. (1994) Before our time: Necrotising fasciitis, hospital gangrene and phagedema. *The Lancet* **344**, 1416–1419.
413. Brook I., Frazier E.H. (2001) Clinical and microbiological features of Necrotising fasciitis. *Journal Clinical Microbiology* **33** (9), 2382–2387.
414. Holm S.E., Norrby A., Bergholm A.M., Norgreen M. (1992) Aspects of pathogenesis of serious group A streptococcal infections in Sweden, 1989–1998. *Journal Infectious Diseases* **166** (1), 31–37.
415. McHenry C.R., Piotrowski J.J., Teprinic D., Malangoni M.A. (1995) Determinants of mortality for necrotising soft tissue infections. *Annals of Surgery* **221** (5), 558–565.

416. Urschel J.D. (1999) Necrotising soft tissue infections. *Postgraduate Medical Journal* **75**, 645–649.
417. Lille S.T., Sato T.T., Engrac L.H., Foy H., Jurkovich G.J. (1996) Necrotising soft tissue infections: obstacles in diagnosis. *Journal American College Surgeons* **182**, 7–11.
418. Bisno A.L., Stevens D.L. (1996) Streptococcal infections of skin and soft tissues. *New England Journal Medicine* **334** (4), 240–245.
419. Liu S.Y.W., Ng S.S.M., Lee J.F.Y (2006) Multi-limb necrotising fasciitis in a patient with rectal cancer. *World Journal Gastroenterology* **12** (32), 5256–5258.
420. Miller L., Perdreau-Remington F., Reig G., Mehdu S., Perlroth J., Bayer A.S., Tang A.W., Phung T.O., Spellberg B. (2005) Necrotising fasciitis caused by community-associated MRSA in Los Angeles. *New England Journal Medicine* **352** (14), 1445–1453.
421. Elliott D.A., Kufera J.A., Myers R.A.M. (1996) Necrotising soft tissue infections: risk factors for mortality and strategies for management. *Annals of Surgery* **224**, 672–683.
422. Singh G., Sinha S.K., Adhikary S., Babu K.S., Ray P., Khanna S.K. (2002) Necrotising infections of soft tissues – a clinical profile. *European Journal Surgery* **168** (6), 366–377.
423. Stevens D.L. (1996) Invasive Group A Streptococcal disease. *Infectious Agents and Disease* **5** (3), 157–166.
424. Bisno A.L., Cockerill F.R., Bermudez C.T. (2000) The initial patient-physician encounter in Group A Streptococcal necrotising fasciitis. *Clinical Infectious Diseases* **31**, 607–608.
425. Fritzsche S.D. (2003) Soft tissue infection: Necrotising fasciitis. *Plastic Surgical Nursing* Winter, **23**, 155–159.
426. Bain G. (1999) An overview of necrotising fasciitis: primary intention. *Australian Journal Wound Management* **7** (1), 22–25.
427. Childs S. (1999) Necrotising fasciitis: challenging management of a septic wound. *Orthopaedic Nursing* March/April, 11–19.
428. Becker M., Zbaren P., Hermans R., Becker C.D., Marchal F., Kurt A.M., Marre S., Rufenacht D.A., Terrier F. (1997) Necrotising fasciitis of the head and neck: role of CT in diagnosis and management. *Radiology* **202**, 471–476.
429. Ward G.R., Walsh M.S (1991) Necrotising fasciitis: 10 years experience in a district general hospital. *British Journal Surgery* **78** (4), 488–489.
430. Floret D., Stamm D., Cochat P., Delmas P.H., Kohler. W. (1992) Streptococcal Toxic Shock Syndrome in children. *Intensive Care Medicine* **18** (3), 175–176.
431. Baxter F., McChesney J. (2000) Severe Group A Streptococcal Infection and Streptococcal Toxic Shock Syndrome. *Canadian Journal Anaesthesia* **47**, 1129–1140.
432. Green R.J., Dafoe D.C., Raffin T.A (1996) Necrotising fasciitis. *Chest* **110**, 219–227.
433. Edwards J.D. (1993) Management of septic shock. *British Medical Journal* **306**, 1661–1664.
434. Stevens D.L., Tanner M.H., Winship J., Swarts B., Ries K.M., Schlievert P.M., Kaplan. E (1989) Severe Group A Streptococcal infection associated with a toxic shock-like syndrome and scarlet fever toxin A. *New England Journal Medicine* **321** (1), 1–7.
435. Davies H.D., McGeer A., Schwartz B. (1996) Invasive Group A Streptococcal infection in Ontario, Canada. *New England Journal Medicine* **335**, 347–354.
436. www.patient.co.uk/showdoc/450 (accessed 30th May 2007).

437. www.nfsuk.org.uk (accessed 30th May 2007).
438. www.hpa.org.uk/infections/topics_az/streto/pyogenic/GroupA_Strep_FAQ.htm (accessed 30th May 2007).
439. www.who.int/topics/meningitis.htm (accessed 30th May 2007).
440. www.meningitis-trust.org.uk/ (accessed 30th May 2007).
441. Pollard A.J., Begg N. (1999) Meningococcal disease and healthcare workers: the risks to healthcare workers are low. *British Medical Journal* **319** (7218), 1147–1148.
442. Kai J. (1996) What worries parents when their pre-school children are acutely ill and why: a qualitative study. *British Medical Journal* **313** (7063), 983–986.
443. Durland M.L., Calderwood S.B., Webber D.J., Miller S.I., Southwick F.S., Caviness V.S., Swartz M.N (1993) Acute bacterial meningitis in adults. *New England Journal Medicine* **328** (1), 21–28.
444. Heyderman R.S., Lambert H.P., O'Sullivan I., Stuart J.M., Taylor B.L., Wall R.A. on behalf of the British Infection Society (2003) Early management of suspected bacterial meningitis and meningococcal septicaemia in adults. *Journal of Infection* **46** (2), 75–77.
445. Gladwin M., Trattler B. (2003) *Clinical Microbiology Made Ridiculously Simple*. Edition 3. MedMaster Inc., Miami: 49–53.
446. Ryan K.J. (2004) *Neisseria*. In: Sherris J.C., Ryan K.J., Ray G.C (eds) *Medical Microbiology: An Introduction to Infectious Diseases*. Fourth Edition. McGraw-Hill, London, 327–342.
447. Slack R.C.B. (2002) *Neisseria and moraxella*. In: Greenwood D., Slack R.C.B., Peutherer J.F. (eds) *Medical Microbiology. A Guide to Microbial Infections: Pathogenesis, Immunity, Laboratory Diagnosis and Control*. Sixteenth Edition. Churchill Livingstone, London, 242–249.
448. Strohl W.A., Rouse H., Fisher D. (2001) *Neisseriae*. In: Harvey R.A. and Champe P.A. (eds) *Lippincott's Illustrated Reviews. Medical Microbiology*. Lippincott Williams and Wilkins. Philadelphia, 165–174.
449. Apicella M.A. (2004) Neisseria meningitidis. In: Mandell G.L., Bennett J.E., Dolin R.D. (eds) *Mandell's Principles and Practices of Infectious Diseases*. Sixth Edition. Churchill Livingstone, London. PPID Online. www.ppidonline.com (accessed 30th May 2007).
450. World Health Organization (1999) Laboratory methods for the diagnosis of meningitis caused by Neisseria meningitidis, Streptococcus pneumoniae and Haemophilus influenzae. WHO, Geneva.
451. Hart C.A., Thomson A.P.J. (2006) Meningococcal disease and its management in children. *British Medical Journal* **333** (7570), 685–690.
452. www.who.int/mediacentre/factsheets/fs141/en/ (accessed 30th May 2007).
453. Wildersmith A., Barkham T.M., Earnest A., Paton N.I. (2002) Acquisition of W135 meningococcal carriage in Hajj pilgrims and transmission to household contacts: prospective study. *British Medical Journal* **325** (7360), 365–366.
454. www.hpa.org.uk/cdr/archives/2001/cdr1201.pdf (accessed 30th May 2007).
455. www.immunisation.nhs.uk (accessed 24th May 2007).
456. www.meningitis.org (Meningitis Research Foundation) (accessed 30th May 2007).
457. Health Protection Agency (2005) Laboratory reports of invasive meningococcal infections, England and Wales; weeks 50–53/2004. *Communicable Disease Report Weekly* **15** (16).

458. www.hpa.org.uk/infections/topics_az/meningo/data_meni_t03.htm (accessed 30th May 2007).
459. Crowcroft N.S. (1999) What is so good about the new conjugate vaccines? *The Pharmaceutical Journal* **263** (7069), 703–704.
460. National Meningitis Trust (1996) *Meningitis Resource Pack.* National Meningitis Trust, Stroud.
461. De Wals P., Gilquin C., De Mayers S., Bouckaerta A., Noel A., Lechat ME., Lafontaine A. (1983) Longitudinal study of asymptomatic meningococcal carriage in two Belgian populations of school children. *Journal of Infection* **6** (2), 147–156.
462. Goldschneider I., Gotschlich E.C., Artenstein M.S. (1969) Human immunity to the meningococcus II. Development of natural immunity. *Journal Experimental Medicine* **129** (6), 1327–1348.
463. Khan E. (2006) The blood-brain barrier: Its implications in neurological disease and treatment. *British Journal Neuroscience Nursing* **2** (1), 18–25.
464. Bannister B.A., Begg N.T., Gillespie S.H. (1996) *Infectious Diseases.* Blackwell Science, London, 301–330.
465. www.gauchcr.org.uk/bloodbrainmay2005.htm (accessed 30th May 2007).
466. Corless C.E, Guiver M., Borrow R., Edwards-Jones V., Fox A.J., Kazmarski E.B. (2001) Simultaneous detection of Neisseria meningitidis, Haemophilus influenzae and Streptococcus pneumoniae in suspected cases of meningitis and septicaemia using real-time PCR. *Journal Clinical Microbiology* **39** (4), 1553–1538.
467. Health Protection Agency Meningococcus Forum (2006) *Guidance for public health management of meningococcal disease in the UK.* Health Protection Agency, London.
468. DeVoe I.W. (1982) The meningococcus and mechanisms of pathogenicity. *Microbiology Review* **46** (2), 162–190.
469. Abramson J.S., Spika J.S. (1985) Persistence of Neisseria meningitidis in the upper respiratory tract after intravenous therapy for systemic meningococcal disease. *Journal Infectious Diseases* **151** (2), 370–371.
470. Chadwick P.R., Beards G., Brown D., Caul E.O., Cheesborough J., Clarke I., Curry A., O'Brien S., Quigley K., Sellwood J., Westmoreland D. (2000) Report of the Public Health Laboratory Service Viral Gastro-Enteritis Working Group: Management of hospital outbreaks of gastro-enteritis due to small round structured viruses. *Journal Hospital Infection* **45** (1), 1–10.
471. Treanor J.J., Dolin R. (2004) Norovirus and other caliciviruses. In: Mandell G.L., Bennett J.E., Dolin R.D. (eds) *Mandell's Principles and Practices of Infectious Diseases.* Sixth Edition. Churchill Livingstone, London. PPID Online. www.ppidonline.com (accessed 30th May 2007).
472. Ray G.C. (2004) Viruses of diarrhoea. In:. Sherris J.C., Ryan K.J., Ray G.C. (eds) *Medical Microbiology: An Introduction to Infectious Diseases.* Fourth Edition. McGraw-Hill, London, 577–583.
473. www.cdc.gov/ncidod/dvrd/revb/gastro/norovirus-factsheet.htm (accessed 30th May 2007).
474. Vipond I.B., Caul E.O., Lambden P.R., Clarke I.N. (1999) 'Hyperemesis hiemis': new light on an old symptom. *Microbiology Today* **26**, August, 110–111.
475. Bull R.A., Tu E.T., McIver C.J., Rawlinson W.D., White P.A. (2006) Emergence of a new norovirus Genotype II.4 variant associated with global outbreaks of gastroenteritis. *Journal Clinical Microbiology* **44** (2), 327–333.

476. Clarke I.N., Lambden P.R. (2000) Viral gastroenteritis: the human caliciviruses. *CPD Infection* 2, 14–17.
477. www.hpa.org.uk/infections/topics_/norovirus/faq.htm (accessed 30th May 2007).
478. Patterson W., Haswell P., Fryers P.T., Green J. (1997) Outbreak of small round structured virus gastroenteritis arose after kitchen assistant vomited. *Communicable Disease Report* 7 Review 7, 27th June, R101–R103.
479. Caul E.D. (1994) Small round structured viruses – airborne transmission and hospital control. *The Lancet* 343 (8098), 1240–1242.
480. Pether J.V.S., Caul E.O (1983) An outbreak of food-borne gastroenteritis in two hospitals associated with a Norwalk-like virus. *Journal Hygiene (Cambridge)* 91, 343–350.
481. Stevenson P., McCann R., Duthie R., Glew E., Ganguli L. (1994) A hospital outbreak due to Norwalk virus. *Journal Hospital Infection* 26 (4), 261–272.
482. Baker J., Vipond I.B., Bloomfield S.F. (2004) Effects of cleaning and disinfection in reducing the spread of Norovirus contamination via environmental surfaces. *Journal Hospital Infection* 58 (1), 42–49.
483. Cheesbrough J.S., Barkess-Jones L., Brown D.W. (1997) Possible prolonged environmental contamination survival of small round structured viruses. *Journal Hospital Infection* 35 (4), 325–326.
484. Parashur U.D., Dow L., Frankhauser R.L., Humphrey C.D., Miller J., Ando T., Williams K.S., Eddy C.R., Noel J.S., Ingram T., Bresee J.S., Monroe S.S., Glass R.I (1998) An outbreak of viral gastroenteritis associated with consumption of sandwiches: implications for the control of transmission by food handlers. *Epidemiol Inf* 121 (3), 615–621.
485. Goller J.L., Dimitriadis A., Tan A., Kelly H., Marshall J.A. (2004) Long-term features of norovirus gastroenteritis in the elderly. *Journal Hospital Infection* 58 (4), 286–291.
486. Graham D.Y., Jiang X., Tanaka T., Opekun A.R., Madore H.P., Estes M.K. (1994) Norwalk virus infection of volunteers: new insights based on improved assays. *Journal Infectious Diseases* 170 (1), 34–43.
487. Whelan K., Judd P.A., Preedy V.R., Taylor M.A. (2004) Enteral feeding: the effect on faecal output, the faecal microflora and SCFA concentrations. *Proceedings of the Nutrition Society* 63, 105–113.
488. Lewis S.J., Heaton K.W. (1997) Stool form scale as a useful guide to intestinal transit time. *Scandinavian Journal Gastroenterol* 32 (9), 920–924.
489. Green J., Wright P.A., Gallimore C.I., Mitchell O., Morgan-Capner P., Brown D.W.G. (1998) The role of environmental contamination with small round structured viruses in a hospital outbreak investigated by reverse-transcriptase polymerase chain reaction assay. *Journal Hospital Infection* 39 (1), 39–45.
490. Hudson J.B., Sharma M., Petric M. (2007) Inactivation of norovirus by ozone gas in conditions relevant to healthcare. *Journal of Hospital Infection* 66 (1), 40–45.
491. www.who.int/mediacentre/factsheets/fs237/en (accessed 30th May 2007).
492. www.hpa.org.uk/infections/topics_az/noids/food_poisoning.htm (accessed 30th May 2007).
493. A Working Party of the PHLS Salmonella Committee (1995) The prevention of human transmission of gastrointestinal infections, infestations and bacterial infections; A guide for public health physicians and environmental health officers in England and Wales. *CDR Review* 5 (11).

494. Department of Health and Social Security (1984) *The Report of the Committee of Enquiry into an Outbreak of Food Poisoning at Stanley Royd Hospital.* The Stationery Office, London.
495. www.who.int/mediacentr/factsheets/fs255/en (accessed 30th May 2007).
496. www.cdc.gov/ncidod/dbmd/diseaseinfo/campylobacter_g.htm (accessed 30th May 2007).
497. Altekruse S.F., Stern N.J., Fields P.I., Swerdlow D.L. (1999) Campylobacter jejuni – An Emerging Foodborne Pathogen. *Emerging Infectious Diseases* **5** (1). Available at www.cdc.gov/ncidod/eid/vol5no1/altekruse.htm (accessed 30th May 2007).
498. Blaser M.J., Allos B.M. (2004) Campylobacter jejuni and Related Species. In: Mandell G.L., Bennett J.E., Dolin R.D. (eds) *Mandell's Principles and Practices of Infectious Diseases..* Sixth Edition. Churchill Livingstone, London. PPID Online. www.ppidonline.com (accessed 30th May 2007).
499. Ryan K.J. (2004) *Vibrio, Campylobacter* and *Helicobacter.* In: Sherris J.C., Ryan K.J., Ray G.C. (eds) *Medical Microbiology: An Introduction to Infectious Diseases.* Fourth Edition. McGraw-Hill, London, 373–384.
500. Skirrow M.B. (1977) *Campylobacter* enteritis: a 'new' disease. *British Medical Journal* **2** (6078), 9–11.
501. Butzler J.P., Skirrow M.B. (1979) Campylobacter enteritis. *Clinical Gastroenterology* **8**, 737–763.
502. Sudworth S. (2001) Campylobacter: diagnosis, treatment and prevention. www.nursing-times.net/nursingtimes/pages/campylobacterdiagnosistreatmentandprevention. (accessed 24th May 2007).
503. Skirrow M.B. (2002) Campylobacter and helicobacter. In: Greenwood D., Slack R.C.B., Peutherer J.F. (eds) *Medical Microbiology. A Guide to Microbial Infections: Pathogenesis, Immunity, Laboratory Diagnosis and Control.* Sixteenth Edition. Churchill Livingstone, London. 288–295.
504. www.hpa-standardmethods.org.uk/documents/bsop/pdf/bsop30.pdf (accessed 24th May 2007).
505. Skirrow M.B. (1990) Campylobacter. *The Lancet* **336**, 921–923.
506. Campylobacter Sentinel Surveillance Scheme Collaborators (2002) Ciprofloxacin resistance in Campylobacter jejuni: case-case analysis as tool for elucidating risks at home and abroad. *Journal Antimicrobial Chemotherapy* **50** (4), 561–568.
507. Gillespie I.A, O'Brien S.J., Frost J.A., Adak G.K., Horby P., Swan A.V., Painter M.J., Neal K.R and the Campylobacter Surveillance Scheme Collaborators (2002) *A Case-Case Comparison of Campylobacter coli and Campylobacter jejuni infection: A Tool for Generating Hypotheses.* Available at: www.cdc.gov/ncidod/EID/vol8no9/01-0187.htm (accessed 30th May 2007).
508. www.wikipedia.org/salmomellosis (accessed 30th May 2007).
509. Pegues D.A., Ohl M.E., Miller S.I. (2004) Salmonella species, including Salmonella Typhi. In: Mandell G.L., Bennett J.E., Dolin R.D. (eds) *Mandell's Principles and Practices of Infectious Diseases.* Sixth Edition. Churchill Livingstone, London. PPID Online. www.ppidonline.com (accessed 30th May 2007).
510. Chart H. (2004) Salmonella. In: Greenwood D., Slack R.C.B., Peutherer J.F. (eds) *Medical Microbiology. A Guide to Microbial Infections: Pathogenesis, Immunity, Laboratory Diagnosis and Control.* Sixteenth Edition. Churchill Livingstone, London, 250–259.
511. www.foodborneillness.com/salmonella_food_poisoning.htm (accessed 24th May 2007).

512. Ryan K.J. (2004) Enterobacteriaceae. In: Sherris J.C., Ryan K.J., Ray G.C. (eds) *Medical Microbiology: An Introduction to Infectious Diseases* Fourth Edition. McGraw-Hill, London, 343–371.

513. Hansell A.L., Sen S., Sufi F., McCallum A. (1998) An outbreak of Salmonella enteritidis phage type 5a infection in a residential home for elderly people. *Communicable Disease and Public Health* **1** (3), 172–175.

514. www.nutritionandeggs.co.uk (accessed 30th May 2007).

515. www.britegg.co.uk/index.html (accessed 30th May 2007).

516. Health Protection Agency Gastrointestinal Disease Programme (2004) *Controlling the National Outbreaks of Salmonella enteritidis non-Phage Type 4 infection in England and Wales 2002–2004; Report from a multi-agency National Outbreak Team.* Available at: www.hpa.org.uk/cdr/archives/2004/cdr4204.pdf (accessed 30th May 2007).

517. Guard–Petter J., Henzier D.J., Rahman M.M., Carlson RW. (1997) On-farm monitoring of mouse-invasive salmonella enterica serovar enteritidis and a model for its association with the production of contaminated eggs. *Applied Environmental Microbiology* **63** (4), 1588–1593.

518. Bannister B.A., Begg N.T., Gillespie S.H. (1996) *Infectious Diseases.* Blackwell Science, London, 150–182.

519. www.who.int/mediacentre/factsheets/fs139/en/print.html (accessed 24th May 2007).

520. www.who.int/water_sanitation_health/diseases/typhoid/en (accessed 24th May 2007).

521. Ericsson C.D. (2003) Travellers' diarrhoea. *International Journal of Antimicrobial Agents* **21** (2), 116–124.

522. Xavier G. (2006) Management of typhoid and paratyphoid fevers. *Nursing Times* **102** (17), 49–51.

523. World Health Organization (2003) *Background document: The diagnosis, treatment and prevention of typhoid fever.* WHO, Geneva.

524. www.cdc.gov/ncidod/dbmd/diseaseinfo/typhoidfever_g.htm (accessed 24th May 2007).

525. Simmonds P., Peutherer J.F. (2003) Retroviruses. In: Greenwood D., Slack R.C.B., Peutherer J.F. (eds) *Medical Microbiology. A Guide to Microbial Infections: Pathogenesis, Immunity, Laboratory Diagnosis and Control.* Sixteenth Edition. Churchill Livingstone, London, 527–538.

526. Thomas D.L., Ray S.C., Lemon S.M. (2004) Hepatitis C. In: Mandell G.L., Bennett J.E., Dolin R.D. (eds) *Mandell's Principles and Practices of Infectious Diseases.* Sixth Edition. Churchill Livingstone, London. PPID Online. www.ppidonline.com (accessed 30th May 2007).

527. Health Protection Agency (2006) *Eye of the Needle. UK Surveillance of Significant Exposure to Bloodborne Viruses in Healthcare Workers.* HPA, London.

528. UK Health Departments (1998) *Guidance for Clinical Health Care Workers: Protection against Infection with Blood-borne Viruses. Recommendations of the Expert Advisory Group on AIDS and the Advisory Group on Hepatitis.* DoH, London.

529. Durack D.T. (1981) Opportunistic infections and Kaposi's sarcoma in homosexual men. *New England Journal Medicine* **305** (24), 1465–1467.

530. www.cdc.gov/hiv (accessed 30th May 2007).

531. Centres for Disease Control (1982) Update on acquired immune deficiency syndrome – United States. *Morbidity Mortality Weekly Review* 31, 507–514.

532. Pratt R.J. (2003) *HIV and AIDS: A Foundation for Nursing and Healthcare Practice.* Fifth Edition. Hodder Arnold, London, 1–14.

533. Cleghorn F.R., Reitz Jnr M.S., Popvic M., Gallo R.C, (2004) Human Immunodeficiency Virus. In: Mandell G.L., Bennett J.E., Dolin R.D. (eds) *Mandell's Principles and Practices of Infectious Diseases*. Sixth Edition. Churchill Livingstone, London. PPID Online. www.ppidonline.com (accessed 30th May 2007).

534. Champoux J.J., Drew W.L. (2004) Retroviruses, Human Immunodeficiency Virus and Acquired Immune Deficiency Syndrome. In: Sherris J.C., Ryan K.J., Ray G.C. (eds) *Medical Microbiology: An Introduction to Infectious Diseases*. Fourth Edition. McGraw-Hill, London, 601–616.

535. www.cdc.gov/hiv/resources/factsheets/hiv2.htm (accessed 30th May 2007).

536. www.aidsmap.com (accessed 25th May 2007).

537. Pratt R.J (2003) The Clinical Spectrum of HIV disease. In: *HIV and AIDS: A foundation for nursing and healthcare practice*. Fifth Edition. Hodder Arnold, London, 80–122.

538. Strohl W.A., Rouse H., Fisher B.D. (2001) Retroviruses and AIDS. In: Harvey R.A. and Champe P.A. (eds) *Lippincott's Illustrated Reviews. Medical Microbiology*. Lippincott, Williams and Wilkins, Philadelphia, 359–378.

539. Centres for Disease Control (1992) Revised Classification System for HIV infection and Expanded Surveillance Case Definition for AIDS among Adolescents and Adults. *Morbidity Mortality Weekly Review* RR **17**, December 18.

540. British HIV Association (2005) *BHIVA Guidelines for the treatment of HIV-infected adults with antiretroviral therapy*. British HIV Association, London.

541. Pratt R.J (2003) *HIV and AIDS: A Foundation for Nursing and Healthcare Practice*. Fifth Edition. Hodder Arnold, London, 362–379.

542. www.who.int/hiv/drugresistance/en/ (accessed 30th May 2007).

543. World Health Organization Department of Communicable Disease and Response (2002) *Hepatitis B*. WHO, Geneva.

544. www.who.int/mediacentre/factsheets/fs204/en/ (accessed 30th May 2007).

545. Simmonds P., Peutherer J. (2002) Hepadnaviruses. In: Greenwood D., Slack R.C.B., Peutherer J.F. (eds) *Medical Microbiology. A Guide to Microbial Infections: Pathogenesis, Immunity, Laboratory Diagnosis and Control*. Sixteenth Edition. Churchill Livingstone, London, 438–447.

546. Drew W.L. (2004) Hepatitis Viruses. In: Sherris. J.C., Ryan KJ, Ray GC (eds) *Medical Microbiology: An Introduction to Infectious Diseases*. Fourth Edition. McGraw-Hill, London, 541–533.

547. Strohl W.A., Rouse H., Fisher B.D. (2001) Hepatitis B and Hepatitis D (Delta) Viruses. In: Harvey R.A. and Champe P.A. (eds) *Lippincott's Illustrated Reviews. Medical Microbiology*. Lippincott, Williams and Wilkins, Philadelphia, 337–348.

548. Morgan-Capner P., Simmonds P.N. (2004) Togaviruses and Hepaciviruses. In: Greenwood D., Slack R.C.B., Peutherer J.F. (eds) *Medical Microbiology. A Guide to Microbial Infections: Pathogenesis, Immunity, Laboratory Diagnosis and Control*. Sixteenth Edition. Churchill Livingstone, London, 501–512.

549. _www.who.int/vaccine_research/diseases/viral_cancers/en/index2.html (accessed 30th May 2007).

550. National Institute of Clinical Excellence (2006) *Peginterferon alfa and ribavirin for treatment of mild chronic hepatitis C*. NICE, London.

551. Department of Health (2002) *Hepatitis C Strategy for England; Implementing 'Getting Ahead of the Curve' action on blood borne viruses*. DoH, London.

552. Patel K., Muir A.J., McHutchinson J.G. (2006) Diagnosis and treatment of chronic hepatitis C infection. *British Medical Journal* **332** (7548), 1013–1017.

553. Timbury M.C., McCartney A.C., Thakker B., Ward K.N. (2002) *Notes on Medical Microbiology*. Churchill Livingstone, London, 352–364.
554. Anon (1984) Needlestick transmission of HTLV – III from a patient infected in Africa. *The Lancet*. ii: 1376–1377.
555. Department of Health (2004) *HIV Post-Exposure Prophylaxis: Guidance from the UK Chief Medical Officer's Expert Advisory Group on AIDS*. DoH, London.
556. Department of Health (2005) *HIV Infected Healthcare Workers: Guidance on Management and Patient Notification*. DoH, London.
557. Department of Health (2007) *Hepatitis B infected healthcare workers and antiretroviral therapy*. DoH, London.
558. Department of Health (2005) *Hepatitis C infected healthcare workers*. DoH, London.
559. World Health Organization (2003) Chapter 5. SARS. Lessons from a new disease. In: *The World Health Report 2003 – Shaping the Future*. WHO, Geneva.
560. www.who.int/features/2003/07/en (accessed 30th May 2007).
561. World Health Organization (2004) *WHO guidelines for the global surveillance of severe acute respiratory syndrome (SARS) Updated recommendations. October 2004*. WHO, Geneva.
562. www.who.int/topics/sars/en (accessed 30th May 2007).
563. www.hpa.org.uk/infections/topics_az/SARS/menu.htm (accessed 30th May 2007).
564. www.cdc.gov/nicod/sars (accessed 30th May 2007).
565. www.who.int/mediacentre/news/releases/2003/pr56/en/print.html (accessed 30th May 2007).
566. Poon L.L.M., Guan Y., Nicholls J.M., Yuen K.Y., Peiris J.S.M. (2004) The aetiology, origins and diagnosis of severe acute respiratory syndrome. *The Lancet Infectious Diseases* **4** (November) 663–671.
567. World Health Organization (2003) *Severe Acute Respiratory Syndrome (SARS); Status of the outbreak and lessons for the immediate future*. 20th May. World Health Organization Communicable Disease Surveillance and Response. WHO, Geneva.
568. www.who.int/csr/sars/archive/2003_03_12/en/ (accessed 30th May 2007).
569. www.who.int/docstore/wer/pdf/2003/wer7812.pdf (accessed 30th May 2007).
570. www.who.int/whr/2003/chapter5/en/index1.html (accessed 30th May 2007).
571. Ho M.S., Su I.L. (2004) Preparing to prevent severe acute respiratory syndrome and other respiratory infections. *The Lancet Infectious Disease* **4** (November) 684–689.
572. Peiris J.S., Lai S.T., Poon L.L. (2003) Coronavirus as a possible cause of severe acute respiratory syndrome. *The Lancet* **361** (9366), 1319–1325.
573. Ksiazek T.G., Erdman D., Goldsmith C. (2003) A novel coronavirus associated with severe acute respiratory syndrome. *New England Journal Medicine* **348**, 1953–1966. Available at: www.content.nejm.org.cgi/reprint/NEJMoa030781v2.pdf (accessed 30th May 2007).
574. McIntosh K., Anderson L.J. (2004) Coronaviruses, Including Severe Acute Respiratory Syndrome (SARS)-Associated Coronavirus. In: Mandell G.L., Bennett J.E., Dolin R. (eds) *Mandell's Principles and Practices of Infectious Diseases*. Sixth Edition. Churchill Livingstone, London. PPID Online. www.ppidonline.com (accessed 30th May 2007).
575. Yu I.T.S., Wong T.Z., Tam W., Chan A.T., Lee J.H.W., Leung D.YC., Ho T. (2004) Evidence of Airborne Transmission of Severe Acute Respiratory Syndrome Virus. *New England Journal Medicine* **350**, April 22, 1731–1739.

576. Donnelly C.A., Fisher M.C., Fraser C., Ghani A.C., Riley S., Ferguson N.M., Anderson R.M. (2004) Epidemiological and genetic analysis of severe acute respiratory syndrome. *The Lancet Infectious Diseases* **4** (November) 672–683.

577. Lee N., Hui D., Wu A., Chan P., Cameron. P., Joynt G.M. (2003) A major outbreak of severe acute respiratory syndrome in Hong Kong. *New England Journal Medicine* **348**, 1986–1994. Available at: www.nejm.org/cgi/content/abstract/NEJMoa030685v2 (accessed 30th May 2007).

578. Tang K.W., Ho P.L., Ooi G.C., Yee W.K., Wang T., Chan-Yeung M., Lam W.K., Seto W.H., Yam L.Y., Cheung T.M., Wong P.C., Lam B., Ip M.S., Chan J., Yeun K.Y., Lai K.N. (2003) A cluster of cases of Severe Acute Respiratory Syndrome in Hong Kong. *New England Journal Medicine* **348** (20), 1977–1985.

579. Health Protection Agency UK SARS Task Force (2003) *Summary of the UK public health response to Severe Acute Respiratory Syndrome (SARS).* HPA, London.

580. Lipsitch M., Cooper B. (2003) Transmission dynamics and control of severe acute respiratory syndrome. *Science* **300**, 1966–1970.

581. www.wikipedia.org/wiki/SARS (accessed 30th May 2007).

582. Booth C.M., Matukas L.M., Tomlinson G.A., Rachlis R.A., Rose D.B., Dwosh H.A. (2003) Clinical features and short-term outcomes of 144 patients with SARS in the greater Toronto area. *Journal American Medical Association* **289**, 2801–2809.

583. Wong G.W., Hui D.S. (2003) Severe Acute Respiratory Distress Syndrome (SARS); epidemiology, diagnosis and management. *Thorax* **58**, 558–560.

584. www.who.int/cs/sars/postoutbreak/en/print.html (accessed 30th May 2007).

585. Lever F. (2003) SARS: current knowledge and management. *Nursing Times* **99** (18), 26–27.

586. British Infection Society, British Thoracic Society and Health Protection Agency (2004) *Hospital Management of Adults with Severe Acute Respiratory Syndrome (SARS) if SARS Re-emerges.* Available at: www.brit-thoraci.org.uk/c2/iploads/ sars0304.pdf (accessed 30th May 2007).

587. Fowler R.A., Lapinsky S.E., Hallett D. (2003) Critically ill patients with severe acute respiratory distress syndrome. *Journal American Medical Association* **290** (3), 367–373.

588. www.hpa.org.uk/infections/topics_az/SARS/hosp_inf_cont.htm (accessed 30th May).

589. Teleman M.D., Boudville I.C., Hong B.H., Zhu A., Lea Y.S. (2004) Factors associated with transmission of severe acute respiratory syndrome among healthcare workers in Singapore. *Epidemiology and Infection* **132**, 797–803.

590. Christian M.D, Loutfy M., McDonald L.C., Martinez K.F., Ofner M., Wong T., Wallington T., Gold W.L., Mederski B., Green K., Low D.E. on behalf of the SARS Investigation Team (2004) Possible SARS Transmission during Cardio-Pulmonary Resuscitation. *Emerging Infectious Disease* **10** (2). Available at: www.cdc.gov/ncidod/EID/vol10no2/03-0700.htm (accessed 30th May 2007).

591. Wang S.H.X., Li Y.M., Sun B.C., Zhang S.W., Zhao W.H., Wei M.T., Chen K.X., Zhao X.L., Zang Z.L., Krahn M., Cheung A.C., Wang P.P. (2006) The SARS outbreak in a general hospital in Tianjin, China – the cause of the super-spreader. *Epidemiol Infect* **134**, 786–791.

592. Liu J.W., Lu S.N., Chen S.S., Yang K., Lin M.C., Wu C.C., Bloland P.B., Park S.Y., Wong W., Tsao K.C., Lin T.Y., Chen C.L. (2006) Epidemiologic study and containment of a nosocomial outbreak of Severe Acute Respiratory Syndrome in a medical centre in Kaohsiung, Taiwan. *Infection Control Hospital Epidemiology* **27** (5), 466–472.

593. Ofner-Agnostini M., Gravel D., McDonald C., Lem M., Sarwal S., McGeer A., Green K., Vearncombe M., Roth V., Paton S., Loeb M., Simor A. (2006) Cluster of cases of Severe Acute Respiratory Syndrome among Toronto healthcare workers after implementation of infection control precautions: a case series. *Infection Control Hospital Epidemiology* **27** (5), 473–483.

594. Department of Health (2002) *Explaining Pandemic Flu: A Guide from the Chief Medical Officer.* DoH, London.

595. World Health Organization (2005) *Assessing the pandemic threat.* WHO, Geneva.

596. House of Lords Select Committee on Science and Technology (2006)Fourth Report. *Pandemic Influenza.* www.publications.parliment.uk/pa/Id200506/Idselect/Idsctech/88/8805.htm (accessed 30th May 2007).

597. Department of Health (2005) *Pandemic Flu: UK Influenza Pandemic Contingency Plan.* DoH, London.

598. World Health Organization (2005) *WHO Handbook for Journalists: Influenza Pandemic.*

599. www.dh.gov.uk/AdvanceSearchResult/index.htm?searchTerms=Pandemic+Influenza (accessed 30th May 2007).

600. www.hpa.org.uk/infections/topics_az/influenza/pandemic/default.htm (accessed 30th May 2007).

601. www.who.int/csr/disease/avian_influenza/en/index.html (accessed 30th May 2007).

602. Ray G.C (2004) Influenza, Respiratory Syncitial Viruses, Adenovirus, and other Respiratory Viruses. In:. Sherris J.C., Ryan K.J., Ray G.C. (eds) *Medical Microbiology: An Introduction to Infectious Diseases* Fourth Edition. McGraw-Hill, London, 495–524.

603. Sutherland S. (2002) Orthomyoxoviruses: In: Greenwood D., Slack R.C.B., Peutherer J.F (eds) *Medical Microbiology. A Guide to Microbial Infections: Pathogenesis, Immunity, Laboratory Diagnosis and Control.* Sixteenth Edition. Churchill Livingstone, London: 468–474.

604. Treanor J.J. (2004) Influenza Viruses. In: Mandell G.L., Bennett J.E., Dolin R.D. (eds) *Mandell's Principles and Practices of Infectious Diseases.* Sixth Edition. Churchill Livingstone, London. PPID Online. www.ppidonline (accessed 30th May 2007).

605. Strohl W.A, Rouse H., Fisher B.D. (2001) Negative-strand RNA Viruses. In: Harvey R.A. and Champe P.A. (eds) *Lippincott's Illustrated Reviews. Microbiology.* Lippincott, Williams and Wilkins, Philadelphia: 379–396.

606. www.hpa.org.uk/infections/topics_az/influenza/seasona;/flureports0607.htm (accessed 30th May 2007).

607. Kamps B.S, Hoffmann C., Preiser W. (2006) *Influenza Report.* Available at: www.influenzareport.com (accessed 30th May 2007).

608. Department of Health (2006) *The Influenza Immunisation Programme 2006/2007.* DoH, London.

609. www.who.int/csr/disease/avian_influenza/country/cases_table_2007_05_24/en/index (accessed 30th May 2007).

610. www.who.int/csr/don/2005_10_13/en/index.html (accessed 30th May 2007).

611. www.defra.gov.uk/animalh/diseases/notifiable/disease/ai/index.htm (accessed 30th May 2007).

612. Department for Environment, Food and Rural Affairs (2007) *Outbreak of highly pathogenic H5N1 Avian Influenza in Suffolk in January 2007: A Report of the Epidemiological Findings by the National Emergency Epidemiology Group.* DEFRA. 5 April. Available at: www.defra.gov.uk (accessed 30th May 2007).

613. Belshe R.B. (2005) The Origins of Pandemic Influenza – Lessons from the 1918 Virus. *New England Journal Medicine* **353** (21), 2209–2211.
614. Taubenberger J.K., Reid A.H., Lourens R.M., Wang R., Jin G., Fanning T.G (2005) Characterisation of influenza virus polymerase genes. *Nature* **437**, 889–893.
615. www.cdc.gov/flu/about/qa/1918flupandemic.htm (accessed 30th May 2007).
616. www.wikipedia.org/wiki/Spanish_flu (accessed 30th May 2007).
617. www.cytokinestorm.com (accessed 30th May 2007).
618. Health Protection Agency (2005) *Influenza Pandemic Contingency Plan.* HPA, London.
619. World Health Organization (2005) *WHO Global Influenza Preparedness Plan: The Role of WHO and Recommendations for National Measures Before and During Pandemics.* Department of Communicable Disease Surveillance and Response Global Influenza Programme. WHO, Geneva.
620. Department of Health/Health Protection Agency (2005) *Guidance for Pandemic Influenza: Infection Control in Hospitals and Primary Care Settings.* DoH, London.
621. Department of Health (2007) *Pandemic Influenza: Guidance on Preparing Acute Hospitals in England.* (Draft document) DoH, London.
622. Bean B., Moore B.M., Sterner B., Peterson L.R., Gerding D.N., Balfour H.H. Jnr. (1982) Survival of influenza viruses on environmental surfaces. *Journal of Infectious Diseases* **146** (1), 47–51.
623. www.hpa.org.uk/infections/topics_az/SARS/maskFAQs.htm (accessed 30th May 2007).
624. www.dh.gov.uk/PublicationsAndStatistics/PressReleases/PressReleasesNotices (accessed 30th May 2007).
625. Department of Health (2007) *Pre-Pandemic and Pandemic Influenza Vaccines: Summary of the Evidence.* DoH, London.
626. British Infection Society, British Thoracic Society and the Health Protection Agency in collaboration with the Department of Health (2006) *Pandemic Flu: Clinical Management of Patients with an Influenza-like Illness During an Influenza Pandemic. Provisional Guidelines.* British Infection Society, Naphill.
627. Department of Health (2007) *Use of Anti-viral Drugs in an Influenza Pandemic: UK Recommendations and Their Evidence-Base.* DoH, London.
628. www.dh.gov.uk/PandemicFlu/Antivirals/DH_060548 (30th May 2007).
629. Cameron P.A., Schull M., Cooke M. (2006) The impending influenza pandemic: lessons from SARS for hospital practice. *Medical Journal of Australia* **185** (4), 189–190.
630. www.cjd.ed.ac.uk/figures.htm (accessed 30th May 2007).
631. UK CJD Surveillance Unit. www.cjd.ed.ac.uk (accessed 30th May 2007).
632. www.hpa.org.uk/infections/topics_az/cjd/blood_products.htm#one (accessed 30th May 2007).
633. Prusiner S.B (1982) Novel proteinacious infectious particles cause scrapie. *Science* **216**, 136–144.
634. Tyler K.L (2004) Prions and Prion Diseases of the Central Nervous System (Transmissible Neurodegenerative Diseases) In: Mandell G.L., Bennett J.E., Dolin R.D. (eds) *Mandell's Principles and Practices of Infectious Diseases.* Sixth Edition. Churchill Livingstone, London. PPID Online. www.ppidonline.com (accessed 30th May 2007)
635. www.defra.gov.uk/animalh/bse/othertses/index.html (accessed 30th May 2007).
636. www.defra.gov.uk/animalh/bse/general/qa/section1.html (accessed 30th May 2007).

637. Department of Health (2000) *Creutzfeldt-Jakob Disease: Guidance for Healthcare Workers.* DoH, London.
638. Drew W.L (2004) Persistent Viral Infections of the Central Nervous System. In: Sherris J.C., Ryan K.J., Ray G.C. (eds) *Medical Microbiology: An Introduction to Infectious Diseases.* Fourth Edition. McGraw-Hill, USA, 623–628.
639. www.cjdinsight.org (accessed 27th May 2007).
640. Department of Health (2003) *Transmissible Spongiform Encephalopathy Agents: Safe Working and the Prevention of Infection.* Guidance from the Advisory Committee on Dangerous Pathogens and the Spongiform Encephalopathy Committee. Available at: www.advisorybodies.dh.gov.uk/acdp/tseguidance/index.htm (accessed 30th May 2007).
641. Will R.G., Ironside J.W., Zeidler M., Cousens S.N., Estibeiro K., Alperovitch A., Poser S., Pocchiari M., Hoffman A., Smith P.G. (1996) A new variant of Creutzfeldt - Jakob disease in the UK. *The Lancet* **347**, 921–925.
642. www.bseinquiry.gov.uk (accessed 30th May 2007).
643. Department of Health (2005) *Assessing the Risk of Transmission of vCJD Transmission via Surgery: An Interim Review.* Statistics and Operational Research, DoH, London.
644. NHS Estates (2000) *Decontamination Review: the Report on a Survey of Current Decontamination Practices in Healthcare Premises in England.* NHS Estates, London.
645. Engineering and Science Advisory Committee (2006) *The Decontamination of Surgical Instruments with Special Attention to the Removal of Proteins and Inactivation of any Contaminating Human Prions.* Engineering and Science Advisory Committee, London.
646. www.dh.gov.uk/en/Publicationsandstatistics/Pressreleases/DH_4024937 (accessed 30th May 2007).
647. NHS Executive (1999) *Variant Creutzfeldt-Jakob Disease (vCJD), Minimising the Risk of Transmission.* Health Service Circular HSC 1999/178.
648. www.cjd.ed.ac.uk/referralsystem.htm (accessed 27th May 2007).
649. Strohl W.A., Rouse H., Fisher B.D. (2001) Other Gram-negative Rods. In: Harvey R.A. and Champe P.A. (eds) *Lippincott's Illustrated Reviews. Medical Microbiology.* Lippincott, Williams and Wilkins, Philadelphia, 191–208.
650. Edelstein P.H., Cianciotto N.P. (2004) Legionella. In: Mandell G.L., Bennett J.E., Dolin R.D. (eds) *Mandell's Principles and Practices of Infectious Diseases.* Sixth Edition. Churchill Livingstone, London. PPID Online. www.ppidonline.com (accessed 30th May 2007).
651. www.wikipedia.org/wiki/Legionnaires_Disease. (accessed 30th May 2007).
652. *First Report of the Committee of Inquiry into the Outbreak of Legionnaire's Disease in Stafford in April 1985.* The Stationery Office, London.
653. www.hpa.org.uk/infections_az/legionella/gen_info.htm (accessed 30th May 2007).
654. www.hse.gov.uk/legionnaires/barrowreport.pdf (accessed 11 August 2007).
655. http://hpa.org.uk/infections_az/legionella/gen_info (accessed 30th May 2007).
656. Legionella Control Journal. www.Lcj-online.co.uk/legionnaires.php (accessed 30th May 2007).
657. Patterson W.J., Hay J., Seal D.V., McLuckie J.C. (1997) Colonisation of transplant unit water supplies with *Legionella* and protozoa; Precautions required to reduce the risk of legionellosis. *Journal of Hospital Infection* **37**, 7–17.
658. Hood J., Edwards G.F.S. (2003) Legionella. In: Greenwood D., Slack R.C.B., Peutherer J.F. (eds) *Medical Microbiology. A Guide to Microbial Infections: Pathogenesis, Immunity, Laboratory Diagnosis and Control.* Sixteenth Edition. Churchill Livingstone, London, 318–321.

659. Investigation of Specimens for Legionella Species. www.hpa-standardmethods.org/documents/bsop/pdf/bsop47.pdf (accessed 30th May 2007).
660. Medicines and Healthcare Products Regulatory Agency (2004) Medical Devices Alert. MDA/2004/020. 26 May. *Reusable Nebulisers*. www.mhra.gov.uk (accessed 30th May 2007).
661. Bhopal R.S., Fallon R.J., Buist E.C. (1991) Proximity of the home to a cooling-tower and risk of non-outbreak Legionnaires' disease. *British Medical Journal* **302**, 378–383.
662. den Boer J.W., Yzerman E.P., Schellekens J. (2002) A large outbreak of Legionnaires disease at a flower show, the Netherlands 1999. *Emerging Infectious Disease* **8**, 37–43.
663. Ryan K.T (2004) Legionella. In:. Sherris J.C., Ryan KJ, Ray GC (eds) *Medical Microbiology: An Introduction to Infectious Diseases*. Fourth Edition. McGraw-Hill, London, 415–420.
664. Department of Health (2006) *Water Systems. Health Technical Memorandum 04–01. The Control of Legionella, Hygiene, 'Safe' Hot Water, Cold Water and Drinking Water Systems*. DoH, London.

Glossary

Acidosis   Disruption of the acid/base balance (pH) of the body detected by taking an arterial blood sample (pH <7). Can be respiratory (excessive carbon dioxide in the lungs) or metabolic (excess acid in the bloodstream).

Angiodema   Swelling of the deeper layers of the skin, commonly seen as part of an allergic response. Affects the face, and can cause swelling of the eyes and lips, hands and feet. Angiodema affecting the throat is potentially life-threatening.

Antigen   A substance that stimulates the immune system, generating an immune response on behalf of the host.

Anthrax   *Bacillus anthracis*. A disease that predominantly affects grazing animals and which can be transmitted to humans but does not spread through human-to-human transmission. Takes three forms: cutaneous (direct contact with anthrax spores via breaks on the skin), ingestion, or inhalation. Ingestion and inhalation of anthrax spores are associated with high mortality and a deliberate release of anthrax as an aerosol through an act of bio-terrorism could infect large numbers of people with potentially fatal consequences.

Asepsis   The technique used to minimise the risk of contamination.

Biological agent   An infectious disease or its associated toxin that can be deliberately released in an act of bio-terrorism.

Botulism   Food poisoning caused by *Clostridium botulinum* – a Gram-positive anaerobe which is widely distributed in nature. Botulinum toxin is the most poisonous toxin known and therefore it could be used as a biological agent.

Chemoprophylaxis   The use of drugs (antibiotics) to prevent disease; chemoprophylaxis may be given to close contacts of an individual with infectious pulmonary tuberculosis, invasive group A streptococcal disease, or meningococcal disease (**see Prophylaxis**).

Clostridium perfringens   Implicated in food poisoning and wound infections; the commonest cause of gas gangrene.

C-reactive protein (CRP)   An inflammatory marker detected in the blood. Used to check response to treatment.

Crown immunity   Immunity from prosecution for criminal liability.

Disseminated intravascular coagulation   An inappropriate activation of the coagulation pathway which can be fatal. Initially blood starts to coagulate (clot) throughout the body but as clotting factors become depleted, haemorrhaging occurs. It often manifests as large bruises and bleeding at venepuncture sites.

EDTA   (Ethylenediamine tetraacetic acid) Used as an anticoagulant to prevent blood samples from clotting.

Endemic   Occurrence of a disease at a relatively high but constant rate in a population.

Epidemic   Occurrence of new cases of a disease in a population; e.g. an influenza epidemic during the winter months, or a measles epidemic.

Enteric   Refers to the gastro-intestinal tract, i.e. enteric precautions are taken to prevent the spread of infection from intestinal pathogens; stool specimens are examined in the enteric laboratory.

Hypoxia   Depleted levels of oxygen in the blood.

Iatrogenic   Results from medical/healthcare treatment. Another word for nosocomial, or hospital acquired, infection.

Incidence   The number of new cases of an illness/disease in a population at a given time.

Incubation (incubation period)   The time interval between being exposed to an infection and developing symptoms.

Intracranial pressure   Pressure exerted on the brain matter, cerebro-spinal fluid and circulating blood volume, causing damage to the brain itself. Intracranial pressure can be raised as a result of head injury or inflammation/infection of the brain.

Lyses (lysis)   Rupture of the cell membrane resulting in cell death.

Mortality rate   The number of deaths in a population over a period of time. Deaths can be general or due to a specific cause such as infection/disease or following surgery (e.g. mortality rate due to necrotising fasciitis; mortality rate following cardiac surgery).

Myalgia   Muscular pain. Often a feature of influenza.

Neutropenia/neutropenic   Depletion in the number of circulating white blood cells ($< 1,000/mm^3$) which leaves individuals vulnerable to infection. Neutropenic sepsis is a medical emergency.

Notifiable disease   Doctors in England and Wales have a statutory duty to inform the 'Proper Officer' (Consultant, Communicable Disease Control) of suspected/confirmed cases of certain diseases (e.g. food poisoning, bacterial/viral meningitis, viral hepatitis, tuberculosis, measles, mumps). Notification of infectious diseases assists in the detection of outbreaks and epidemics.

Opportunistic   Opportunistic bacteria cause infections in individuals whose immune defence systems are breached. This can be a result of underlying illness/disease, or if the skin is breached (through surgery, the insertion of an invasive device, or through trauma).

Pandemic   A global outbreak of disease.

Pathogen   Capable of causing disease.

Photophobia   Sensitivity to light, causing pain or discomfort.

Prevalence   The total of number of cases of an illness/disease in a population at a given time.

Prodromal illness   Early symptoms of an impending illness.

Prophylaxis   Protection against illness/disease. Antibiotics may be given prophylatically at the time of orthopaedic surgery to reduce the risk of post operative wound infection (see also **Chemoprophylaxis**).

Pruritis   Itching, caused by the release of histamine from mast cells.

Quarantine   Enforced isolation.

Reyes Syndrome   Abnormal collections of body fat which can affect any organ but predominantly affects the liver and the brain. It is almost always associated with recovery from a viral infection. Death can ensue within a couple of days of onset of symptoms, which include vomiting, disorientation and drowsiness.

Rubella   Also known as German measles. Vaccination against rubella is recommended as part of the MMR immunisation programme to protect young adult women from exposure, as rubella contracted during the first eight to ten weeks of pregnancy can cause serious birth defects or fetal death.

Sarcoidosis   A disorder of the immune system that can affect any area of the body but particularly the skin, the eyes and the lungs, with the formation of granulomas. Symptoms can include enlarged lymph nodes, joint pain and blurred vision.

Stevens-Johnson syndrome   An immune-complex-mediated hypersensitivity complex involving the skin and mucous membranes. Mucotaneous lesions develop which slough and blister, and can become ulcerated and necrosed. It often occurs following a viral infection, but can also occur following immunisation (measles, mumps, and hepatitis B) and drugs (penicillins, non-steroidal anti-inflammatory drugs).

Symptomatic   Showing symptoms or signs of a specific disease/injury.

Systemic   Evidence of infection such as high temperature (rigor); hypotension; tachycardia. Patients are said to be systemically unwell.

Surveillance   The routine collection of data on infections for the purposes of preventing and identifying outbreaks and assessing infection rates.

Transient For a short time. Healthcare workers may have transient MRSA carriage, which spontaneously clears when they have time away from the healthcare environment; patients may experience transient bacteraemia on the insertion of an urinary catheter.

Tularaemia A zoonotic infection, endemic in parts of Europe, Asia and North America, which can spread from animals to humans. Caused by *Francisella tularenis* and manifests as an acute, febrile, granulomatous infection. It is highly infectious (requires contact with only 10 organisms to initiate infection) and could potentially be used in bio-terrorism as an airborne agent.

Urticaria An itching, erythematous skin eruption/rash seen during an allergic reaction. Can occur on any part of the skin and may be short-lived or persist for several hours.

Virulent Extremely infectious or malignant. Used to describe a disease caused by a pathogenic organism which commonly overwhelms the immune defences of the host or spreads rapidly among individuals.

Index